Healthcare Analytics

The first COVID-19 case in the United States was reported on January 20, 2020. As the first cases were being reported in the United States, Washington State became a reliable source not just for hospital bed demand based on incidence and community spread but also for modeling the impact of skilled nursing facilities and assisted living facilities on hospital bed demand. Various hospital bed demand modeling efforts began in earnest across the United States in university settings, private consulting and health systems. Nationally, the University of Washington Institute of Health Metrics and Evaluation seemed to gain a footing and was adopted as a source for many states for its ability to predict the epidemiological curve by state, including the peak.

This book therefore addresses a compelling need for documenting what has been learned by the academic and professional healthcare communities in healthcare analytics and disaster preparedness to this point in the pandemic. What is clear, at least from the US perspective, is that the healthcare system was unprepared and uncoordinated from an analytics perspective. Learning from this experience will only better prepare all healthcare systems and leaders for future crisis.

Both prospectively, from a modeling perspective and retrospectively, from a root cause analysis perspective, analytics provide clarity and help explain causation and data relationships. A more structured approach to teaching healthcare analytics to students, using the pandemic and the rich dataset that has been developed, provides a ready-made case study from which to learn and inform disaster planning and preparedness. The pandemic has strained the healthcare and public health systems. Researchers and practitioners must learn from this crisis to better prepare our processes for future pandemics, at minimum. Finally, government officials and policy makers can use this data to decide how best to assist the healthcare and public health systems in crisis.

Healthcare Analytics

Emergency Preparedness for COVID-19

Edited by
Edward M. Rafalski
Ross M. Mullner

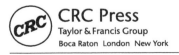

CRC Press
Taylor & Francis Group
Boca Raton London New York

CRC Press is an imprint of the
Taylor & Francis Group, an **informa** business

First edition published 2023
by CRC Press
6000 Broken Sound Parkway NW, Suite 300, Boca Raton, FL
33487-2742

and by CRC Press
4 Park Square, Milton Park, Abingdon, Oxon, OX14 4RN

CRC Press is an imprint of Taylor & Francis Group, LLC

© 2023 selection and editorial matter, Edward M. Rafalski &
Ross M. Mullner; individual chapters, the contributors

ISBN: 978-1-032-06845-9 (hbk)
ISBN: 978-1-032-06846-6 (pbk)
ISBN: 978-1-003-20413-8 (ebk)

DOI: 10.1201/9781003204138

Typeset in Sabon
by SPi Technologies India Pvt Ltd (Straive)

Special thanks to: Asif Alauddin, Bob Costello, Ashish Jain, Zak Hanano, Muyuan Li, Michael Mana, Deborah Pergolizzi, Jeffrey Thiel and Alan Weiss for their insightful observations regarding pandemic data analytics.

Contents

Foreword   xi
Contributors   xiii

Introduction   1
EDWARD M. RAFALSKI

SECTION I
Epidemiology and analytics   **7**

1 What is an epidemic, a pandemic?   9
JONATHAN A. MCCULLERS

2 A brief history of pandemics   17
JONATHAN A. MCCULLERS

3 The healthcare continuum   25
EDWARD M. RAFALSKI

4 The fog of war and data   35
EDWARD M. RAFALSKI AND ROBERT MARKSTHALER

5 Sources of data/modeling   43
EDWARD M. RAFALSKI AND ROBERT MARKSTHALER

6 Quantifying and responding to COVID's financial
   and operational impact   61
MARK GRUBE AND ROB FROMBERG

SECTION 2
State case studies   71

7 Measuring and addressing healthcare employee well-being
   in an Alabama health system during COVID-19   73
   KATHERINE A. MEESE, ALEJANDRA COLON-LOPEZ, ASHLEIGH M. ALLGOOD
   AND DAVIS A. ROGERS

8 Colorado state case study   89
   ADOM NETSANET, SERA SEMPSON AND WILLIAM CHOE

9 Case study: A Florida COVID-19 dashboard   107
   ZACHARY PRUITT AND JASON L. SALEMI

10 State case study: Illinois   143
    HELEN MARGELLOS-ANAST, FERNANDO DE MAIO, C. SCOTT SMITH,
    PAMELA ROESCH, EMILY LAFLAMME AND EVE SHAPIRO

11 Tennessee case study   161
    CORI COHEN GRANT, DAVID SCHWARTZ AND ARASH SHABAN-NEJADO

12 Regional modeling   177
    MADELEINE MCDOWELL, MEGHAN ROBB AND JIM JACOBSOHN

SECTION 3
Topics   193

13 Healthcare analytics: The effects of the pandemic on
    behavioral health   195
    KASEY KNOPP AND NAAKESH (NICK) DEWAN

14 Digital transformation in healthcare: How COVID-19
    was an agent for rapid change   219
    BALA HOTA AND OMAR LATEEF

15 Telehealth   235
    RICHARD FINE

16 The COVID-19 pandemic and development of drugs
    and vaccinations   243
    PRADEEP S. B. PODILA

17 Value of health information exchanges to support
public health reporting 263
PRADEEP S. B. PODILA

Conclusion 279
EDWARD M. RAFALSKI AND ROSS M. MULLNER

Epilogue 281
EDWARD M. RAFALSKI

Index 285

Foreword

Contemporary management is all about getting the proper arrangement and alignment of your organization's internalities and the externalities that you face at any given moment. Internalities are, of course, the business conditions that are generally under your control, while externalities are the conditions that are generally beyond your control.

At times you find that internalities are ascendant, and at other times externalities are ascendant. The healthcare CEO must constantly tinker with and adjust his or her organization's operating style and strategy: Be more aggressive when internalities are ascendant, and show more care when externalities have the upper hand.

Today, the external business conditions have never been more formidable. Consider just a few elements of the unpredictable environment:

• The unknown post-COVID care and economic environment
• Unprecedented business technological changes
• Rapidly evolving consumer demand
• The demands of the social justice movement
• The fast developing business demands of climate change
• A divisive political/business environment
• An American culture that is increasingly difficult to both interpret and navigate

In the thoughtful, practical book *Healthcare Analytics: Emergency Preparedness for COVID-19*, Edward Rafalski and his co-authors do a great service to an industry that is struggling to quantify the effects of roiling externalities. The chapters in this book present a detailed examination of how to assess COVID-19 and other external forces, measure their effects on hospital and health system performance, and translate that understanding into strategy for the uncertain post-COVID-19 period.

The stubbornly persistent effects of the COVID-19 pandemic remind us that the organizational goal today for hospitals and health systems is not to find the way back to a pre-COVID comfort zone, but rather to negotiate and navigate toward being the best performing healthcare organization possible within a fast-changing and uncertain post-COVID business environment. As this book reminds us, when developing strategy in such an environment, a basis of solid and sophisticated analytics is more important than ever.

Kenneth Kaufman,
Managing Director and Chair,
Kaufman Hall

Contributors

Ashleigh M. Allgood
The University of Alabama at Birmingham
Birmingham, Alabama

William Choe
South Denver Cardiology Associates
Littleton, Colorado

Alejandra Colon-Lopez
The University of Alabama at Birmingham
Birmingham, Alabama

Fernando De Maio
American Medical Association
DePaul University
Chicago, Illinois

Naakesh (Nick) Dewan
GuideWell-Florida Blue
Jacksonville, Florida

Richard Fine
Zocdoc
New York, New York

Robert Fromberg
Kaufman Hall, Chief Communications Officer
Chicago, Illinois

Cori Cohen Grant
University of Tennessee Health Science Centner
Memphis, Tennessee

Mark Grube
JMP Ventures
Delray Beach, Florida

Bala Hota
Tendo Systems
Chicago, Illinois

Jim Jacobsohn
SG2
Chicago, Illinois

Kasey Knopp
University of Maryland School of Medicine
Baltimore, Maryland

Emily Laflamme
American Medical Association
Chicago, Illinois

Omar Lateef
Rush University Medical Center
Chicago, Illinois

Helen Margellos-Anast
Sinai Urban Health Institute
Chicago, Illinois

Robert Marksthaler
Epic Systems
Verona, Wisconsin

Jonathan A. McCullers
Department of Pediatrics, College
Medicine
University of Tennessee Health
Science Centner
Memphis, Tennessee

Madeleine McDowell
Sg2/Vizient
Carbondale, Colorado

Katherine A. Meese
The University of Alabama at
Birmingham
Birmingham, Alabama

Ross M. Mullner
University of Illinois School of
Public Health (retired)
Chicago, Illinois

Adom Netsanet
University of Colorado School of
Medicine
Denver, Colorado

Pradeep S. B. Podila
Clinical Research Assistant
Methodist Le Bonheur Healthcare
Memphis, Tennessee

Zachary Pruitt
College of Public Health University
of South Florida
Tampa, Florida

Edward M. Rafalski
University of Illinois School of
Public Health
Chicago, Illinois
and
University of South Florida College
of Public Health
Tampa, Florida

Meghan Robb
Vizient
Annapolis, Maryland

Pamela Roesch
Sinai Urban Health Institute
Chicago, Illinois

Davis A. Rogers
The University of Alabama at
Birmingham
Birmingham, Alabama

Jason L. Salemi
College of Public Health University
of South Florida
Tampa, Florida

David Schwartz
University of Tennessee Health
Science Centner
Memphis, Tennessee

Sera Sempson
University of Colorado School of
Medicine
Denver, Colorado

Arash Shaban-Nejado
University of Tennessee Health
Science Centner
Memphis, Tennessee

Eve Shapiro
West Side United
Chicago, Illinois

C. Scott Smith
DePaul University
Chicago, Illinois

Introduction

Edward M. Rafalski

University of Illinois School of Public Health
Chicago, IL, USA
University of South Florida College of Public Health
Tampa, FL, USA

CONTENTS

What would Alexis de Tocqueville have observed? 2
What did we learn from the last flu pandemic in 1918, or not? 2
    Section 1: Epidemiology and analytics 3
    Section 2: State case studies 4
    Section 3: Topics 4
References 6

As we are writing this book the pandemic is still with us. We have learned, and continue to learn, from the experience but the story is not yet over and there will be significantly more to learn. COVID-19, the disease caused by the severe acute respiratory syndrome coronavirus 2 (SARS-CoV-2), has placed a severe strain on the United States (U.S.) healthcare system. It has been observed to have done the same in other countries around the world that preceded the pandemic arriving in the United States. With the discovery of SARS-CoV-2, there are now seven types of coronaviruses known to infect humans, four of which regularly circulate among humans and mostly cause mild to moderate upper respiratory tract infections or common colds. The remaining three jumped from animal hosts to humans, resulting in more serious disease.

The outbreak of COVID-19 was officially announced as a pandemic by the World Health Organization (WHO) on March 11, 2020. The first case was reported by the Chinese Center for Disease Control and Prevention on December 8, 2019, and then quickly spread throughout the Wuhan City and Hubei Province.[1] There is some current research taking place that may show that the virus was spreading in the general population earlier than initially reported as the variant observed in Wuhan was not the ordinal strain.

DOI: 10.1201/9781003204138-1

1

WHAT WOULD ALEXIS DE TOCQUEVILLE HAVE OBSERVED?

When Alexis de Tocqueville visited the United Sates in 1831 he observed, among many other things, the delicate balance between federal and state approaches to legal and policy issues. While observing the strengths of township government in New England he made the broader case that local government is particularly strong in the United States. He further argued that Americans corrected their laws and saved the country by adopting a federal system with clearly defined responsibilities for the state and national government.[2] Had he jumped into a time machine and travelled to 2020 he may have noted that the contrasting strengths and weaknesses observed in the past were still playing out in the present, namely that the federal, state and township responses to the pandemic were a complex quilt of different textures, materials and styles not all of which were aligned in an organized fashion. One may observe, as did de Tocqueville, that this may be both a strength and a weakness of our Republic. Data and analytics have provided lessons to be learned regarding our response to one of the greatest public health challenges in recent memory. How may we apply these lessons for future public health disasters?

WHAT DID WE LEARN FROM THE LAST FLU PANDEMIC IN 1918, OR NOT?

The last world-wide pandemic occurred in 1918 and hit the shores of the United States with a fury not unlike COVID-19, the disease caused by the severe acute respiratory syndrome coronavirus 2 (SARS-CoV-2) which has again placed a severe strain on the U.S. public health and healthcare systems.[3] There is a marked difference between the two systems. The distinction is that the public health system is funded and managed largely by government at the local, state and federal levels whereas the healthcare system is largely privately managed and partially funded by government through the Medicare and Medicaid programs. In the former, insurance coverage is provided to the disabled and those over the age of 65 by the Federal government. In the latter, insurance coverage is provided to the poor largely by the states. Neither program existed in the last pandemic as both came into existence in 1965 as a legislative effort made by the Great Society during President Lyndon Johnson's administration. Public health agencies, as we know them today, were much smaller in both scope and funding at the turn of the last century. In 1918 public health represented less than 5% of the Federal budget and in the recent decade it represents approximately 8% of GDP. In 1918, the healthcare system represented 3% of GDP and currently it is estimated to represent approximately 18% of the GDP heading into the pandemic. Clearly, the United States has added significant resources to the nation's public health and health systems in the last 100 years. It is estimated that approximately 292,000 people or .27% of the population died from the pandemic between 1918 and 1920 in four waves. To date, 639,000 people have died of COVID-19 to date or.19% of the population has died to date from the COVID-19 pandemic in four waves. If we were to calculate a very crude return on investment (ROI), the United States spent approximately $118 per life lost in 1918 dollars (roughly $3,074 in 2020 dollars) and $8,631 per life lost to date in 2020. While the United States has invested heavily in the healthcare industrial complex, our investment in analytics has largely been driven by the private sector. In the chapters that follow, we highlight some observations on analytics that have resulted because of the pandemic and the need to thoughtfully react to a crisis in preparation for future healthcare disasters. We have organized the material into three primary sections: 1) epidemiology and analytics, 2) case studies and 3) topics.

Section 1: Epidemiology and analytics

We begin by discussing the difference between epidemics and pandemics and provide some context for the current pandemic when observed in the context of the history. We then shift to an overview on the healthcare continuum, its structure and general level of preparedness and evolution during the pandemic. There is a distinction between the public health and healthcare systems in the United States. However, there is an even broader level of distinction in the latter beginning with screening and testing through, primary care, urgent care, emergency care, hospital acute care, field hospitals, transition hotel to home, post-acute care, hospital at home, home health, the physician house call, palliative care and hospice care. Some portions of the continuum existed prior to the pandemic (i.e. emergency room (ER)/emergency department (ED), others had been out of use and re-instituted anew (i.e. field hospital) and yet others were created (i.e. triage chat bots). The pandemic created new levels of analytics across the continuum and created a deeper understanding of the interconnectedness of the care of health ecosystem.

Sources of data for modeling are reviewed. Early in the pandemic, little was known about how the incidence of disease would place demands on health system resources. This chapter will explore the art of assumptions, leveraging data as it becomes available and the analytics of early warning signs in addition to modeling approaches. We evolve the dialogue to discuss modeling techniques. Various modeling resources became available as the pandemic progressed and datasets became richer. This chapter will catalog various modeling approaches that became publicly available and how they were used to predict demand for health system resources. A variety of techniques and approaches were developed, and this body of work has arguably advanced the art and science of modeling and predictive analytics in healthcare.

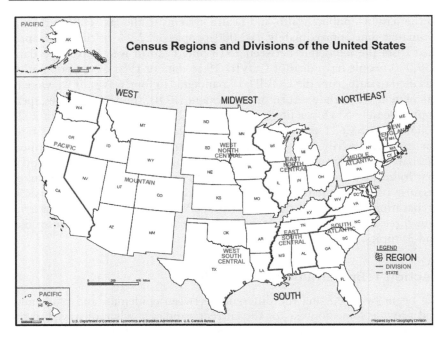

Figure I.I Census regions and divisions of the United States.

Section 2: State case studies

Federalist vs antifederalist analytics and what we have learned from the United States? This series of chapters will review state responses to the pandemic, provide the local flavor & richness of data analytics and summarize how health systems were affected. Each contributing author brings to bear their professional experience and area of subject matter expertise to the discussion. For example, those that are in academia discuss the value of analytics from the research and teaching point of view. Others discuss healthcare disparity and the impact of the pandemic on discrete populations and their access to health services. Health system executives and physicians provide a perspective on how the pandemic strained hospital resources and affected care. We present case studies from states around the Union to provide some level of context of how regional responses led to lessons learned from each part of the country. Attempting to provide a sample from each CDC Census region, we review lessons from Alabama, California, Colorado, Illinois, Florida, New York, Tennessee and Texas (see Figure I.1).

Section 3: Topics

We shift to discuss the effects of the pandemic on behavioral health. The poor mental and behavioral health of the population have been sequelae of the pandemic and are not well understood. There are many more sequelae, such as clinical comorbidities, and more longitudinal data is needed to understand these changes in patient acuity. In the case of behavioral health, how has physical distancing affected the childhood development of children who were required to stay at home and learn online? We make the distinction between social distancing and physical distancing. Unfortunately, our public health leaders used the former when speaking without perhaps noting the behavioral health effects of socially distancing. Did they really mean we should not provide moral support to our senior neighbors or virtual support to our families at the time of death? There are some early indicators of the effects of the pandemic on behavioral health and those are shared in this chapter.

We discuss the evolution of technology and the digital landscape. The digitization of healthcare has provided an opportunity to discuss how technology can be used to analyze and manage through a pandemic. We cover the opportunity technology presents to prepare society for the next public health crisis in the context of innovation. Necessity is the mother of invention and the pandemic created an opportunity to stand up new solutions and bolster others.[4] This chapter will highlight areas of innovation, how cycle time was reduced and the data it created for analytics.

We discuss the development of drugs and vaccines shedding light on the importance of computational modeling toward the development of drugs and vaccines, as well as highlight a general overview of the different categories related to the development of vaccine candidates, their challenges and the progress made to date. We follow this conversation with an overview of health information exchanges. The HHS Office of the National Coordinator for Health Information Technology (ONC) is the principal federal entity charged with coordination of health IT efforts and work on the strategic efforts to propel the adoption of health information technology (HIT) and promotion of nationwide health information exchange to improve healthcare. The creation of ONC back in 2004 has popularized the terms "Health Information Exchange (HIE or HIX) and Regional Health Information Organization (RHIO)." The goal of a HIE is to provide the medical staff with access to a patient's clinical data and enable the cooperation between the care providers across organizations from both healthcare and non-healthcare domains. In addition to that, the utilization of Master Patient Index (MPI) to accurately resolve the identity of individuals by filling in the missing details and their ability to protect the privacy and security of Personal Health Information (PHI) places the HIEs in a unique position to develop a more realistic picture of health outcomes in the community. In addition to their role in population health management, HIEs also play a crucial role within the overall healthcare ecosystem. The COVID-19 pandemic has stressed the importance of timely, accurate and complete reporting to enable quick response to outbreaks that threaten the health of the public. The Health and Human Services (HHS) requires labs to report patients' sex, race and ethnicity with COVID-19 tests in order to combat disparities. This is where HIEs can help in empowering the public health infrastructure by (a) filling in the missing data on key demographic identifiers, (b) attaching the lab results and (c) merging pre-existing data to enrich the information and for elevating the real burden by means of data visualizations at the community level. This chapter sheds light on the importance of HIEs, issues with interoperability and how they can aid with public health reporting during the pandemics.

Finally, we conclude with some final observations in the midst of the fourth wave of the pandemic in the United States and provide an epilogue with any new information coming to light. Healthcare analytics have evolved in the last 2 years and sharing observations will advance administrative knowledge in preparation for the next pandemic/health disaster in the United States.

REFERENCES

1 Wu, Z. and McGoogan, J.M. 2020. Characteristics of and Important Lessons from the Coronavirus Disease 2019 (COVID-19) Outbreak in China. JAMA. Downloaded from: https://jamanetwork.com on 3/16/2020.
2 De Tocqueville, A. 1835 and 1840. De La Democratie en Amerique, Volumes 1 and 2. Translated by Reeve, H. New York. George Dearborn & Co.
3 Barry, J. 2005. The great influenza: the story of the deadliest pandemic in history. New York. Penguin Books.
4 Wycherley, William. 1671. Love in a Wood. London.

Section 1

Epidemiology and analytics

Chapter 1

What is an epidemic, a pandemic?

Jonathan A. McCullers

University of Tennessee Health Science Center
Memphis, TN, USA

CONTENTS

Definition(s) of epidemics and pandemics..9
Why do pandemics occur?...11
Perspective for the healthcare system..14
References 15

DEFINITION(S) OF EPIDEMICS AND PANDEMICS

On March 11, 2020, the World Health Organization (WHO) declared the novel coronavirus outbreak (COVID-19) a global pandemic. The WHO describes a pandemic on its website as "the worldwide spread of a new disease" [1]. The first known usage of the term pandemic appears to have been in the mid-17th century [2], a relatively recent development compared to the history of the term epidemic, which dates to at least 5th century BCE [3]. Epidemic derives from the Greek *epi* meaning "on" and *demos* meaning "the people" or "place of the people," interpreted later as "country." Hippocrates first gave epidemic its disease connotation around 400 BCE in his seven-volume work titled *Epidemics*, which described various diseases and used the term epidemic to mean outbreaks that had spread over a large part of a country. The later introduction of pandemic then substituted the prefix *pan*, meaning "all," describing pandemics as disease outbreaks that spanned all known countries. Pandemic and epidemic were used interchangeably in many texts and dictionaries throughout the 17th through 19th centuries, until the striking global emergence of the influenza pandemics of 1889 and 1918 solidified the usage of pandemic for worldwide disease outbreaks.

Despite its seeming simplicity, the WHO definition "the worldwide spread of a new disease" has its controversies. First, does a pandemic need to be worldwide? Many authors in the scientific and popular press use pandemic in the sense of a very large epidemic, one that covers much of a country, or multiple countries or regions, but is not truly worldwide. Reports of historical pandemics such as the bubonic plague are limited to the author's context; the disease may have spread across the "known" world, but much of the world was unknown at that time. Attempts have been made to codify types of pandemic, e.g., "trans-regional," "inter-regional," and "global" [2] to add precision, but no nomenclature is widely accepted. In the declaration of COVID-19 as a pandemic, the WHO used the term "pandemic" alone, but many of the reports on this event added the (potentially redundant) modifier "global" describing it as a global pandemic.

Second, must the disease be new to be described as a pandemic? The recent confirmation by DNA sequencing of materials from victims of the Plague of Justinian (541–543 ACE) demonstrates that *Yersinia pestis* was the cause of this ancient pandemic [4], adding to its toll as the agent of the Black Death (14th century) and the Third Plague (ca. 1855–1960). Each outbreak began in a different century and spread across the known world, but all were caused by the same pathogen. The strains causing the Black Death and the Third Plague are near identical by DNA sequencing, so the most recent pandemic from the Plague is not even from a new strain of *Y. pestis*, just a new incursion in time. Similarly, influenza viruses cause periodic pandemics without being a new virus entirely; typically one of the surface proteins changes by swapping its encoding gene segment with an animal strain, but many other parts of the virus are identical to circulating strains [5]. These viruses can thus be characterized as a new strain, but not a new virus, or a new disease.

Finally, must a pandemic be an infectious disease, or can any disease be characterized as a pandemic? Since the time of Hippocrates, the terms epidemic and pandemic have typically referred to widespread outbreaks of infectious agents. However, the lay press and practitioners in certain fields such as public health increasingly refer to the ubiquitous nature of certain chronic diseases (e.g., diabetes) or lifestyle choices, such as obesity or smoking, as pandemics. [2] The WHO and the Centers for Disease Control and Prevention (CDC) both refer to the worldwide (at least in westernized countries) increase in obesity as an epidemic, but not a pandemic, perhaps adding additional confusion. In the scientific literature, a pandemic is usually described as being contagious and spreading between persons, such that the term's usage is confined to infectious agents.

Much of our current worldview on pandemics is due to the devastation wrought by the 1918 influenza pandemic and the current parallels of that worldwide disaster to the COVID-19 pandemic. The overwhelming nature of the 1918 pandemic led to a discussion of the differences between pandemic and epidemic influenza. The most compelling framework came from Dr. Edwin D. Kilbourne following the swine influenza outbreak at Fort Dix, New Jersey, which caused great fear of a repeat of 1918 but never attained global or even significant regional spread. His answer to this question of "What is a pandemic?" framed the general criteria scientists who study influenza and other viruses have used to distinguish pandemic strains from epidemic strains since that time. According to Kilbourne, a pandemic strain

Table 1.1 The Kilbourne framework for defining a pandemic

Disease	Novel?	Worldwide spread?	Deadly?	Pandemic?
Seasonal Influenza	No	Yes	Yes	**No**
Common human coronaviruses	No	Yes	No	**No**
1918 H1N1 Influenza	Yes	Yes	Yes	**Yes**
2009 H1N1 Influenza	Yes	Yes	No	**No**
2003 SARS	Yes	No	Yes	**No**
2019 COVID-19	Yes	Yes	Yes	**Yes**

must be antigenically novel, cause severe illness, and spread easily through the susceptible population. [5] Antigenic novelty for influenza viruses has typically meant the spread of a virus with an antigenically distinct hemagglutinin (HA) protein, the surface glycoprotein that is most targeted by the human immune system. Antigenically distinct in this context means it would not be recognized by the immune systems of most people of the world. There has been significant concern that the H5N1 strains infecting humans in Asia and Europe over the last two decades could develop into pandemic viruses, since they meet two of these three criteria, lacking only ease of transmission to qualify (Table 1.1).

The WHO caused great consternation in 2009 when an antigenically novel H1N1 strain began to circulate globally. This new strain spread easily from person to person, had an HA protein descended from the 1918 strain to which few globally had immunity, but did not cause severe disease. In the decade prior the WHO had developed a pandemic warning system that relied on the novelty of the agent and its proven spread across multiple regions, but at the time of the 2009 outbreak it did not take severity into account [6]. Earlier versions of the WHO phases of a potential pandemic included language about "enormous numbers of deaths and illness," but this language had been removed by the time of the declaration. The result was WHO declaring a pandemic that did not meet Kilbourne's criteria (Table 1.1). This declaration led to aggressive activation of pandemic plans by numerous countries with measures that differed from their responses to annual epidemics, engendering significant public confusion and concern. The fallout from this controversy has been an erosion in trust for public health agencies, which has undergirded a number of problems with the ongoing COVID-19 response.

WHY DO PANDEMICS OCCUR?

Ultimately, pandemics are the end result of human activity. The needs of a burgeoning population now approaching 8 billion, together with technological advances that enable massive changes to how humanity works, lives,

Table 1.2 Contributions of global changes in climate and environment to human epidemics and pandemics

Global change	Relevant environmental impact	Disease impact
Increased CO_2	Increased density and longevity of foliage	Greater range in latitudes and altitude of disease vectors such as mosquitoes, ticks, rodents
Increased temperature	Fewer frosts, more extreme weather events such as floods	Increased range, better overnight and over-winter survival, and faster cycle times of disease vectors; more frequent contamination of water sources during flooding
Deforestation	Overlap of human and disease vector ranges/ habitats, decreased bio-diversity	Increased contact and disease transmission to both humans and domesticated animals; proliferation of disease vectors with a decrease in predation
Urbanization	Increased density and poorer sanitation	Higher rate of disease transmission at same vector density; more water-borne disease outbreaks, more vector breeding sites
Technological advances	Increased worldwide trade and travel	Geographic dispersion and homogenization of vectors; more rapid spread of infectious diseases worldwide

and plays, have resulted in disruption of pathogen and vector ecosystems and increasing contact with humans. Global climate change, the alteration of pathogen and vector habitats by human activity, and changes to civilization itself have all contributed to this new paradigm in which the risk of pandemics is as great or greater than it has ever been (Table 1.2). Regardless of the precise method of ingress of severe acute respiratory syndrome coronavirus 2 (SARS-CoV-2), the cause of COVID-19, into humans, environmental and societal changes that brought humans into closer proximity to bats are the underlying cause.

Climate change in the modern era is the result of increased release of carbon dioxide (CO_2) into the atmosphere from human activities such as large-scale industry, travel, and agriculture. Multiple mass-extinction events occurred in prior eras due to disruption of the worldwide carbon cycle by climate change. These were from non-human events, however, such as massive meteorite strikes or increased activity by mega-volcanoes [7]. Climate change today increases the risk of disease in several ways. A rise in global CO_2 emissions allows greater growth of foliage, increased longevity for a greater mass of foliage, and an expanded range in latitude and altitude, resulting in increased sites for breeding of disease-causing vectors such as mosquitoes, ticks, and mice and rats. The rising average global temperatures that accompany higher atmospheric CO_2 levels lead to decreased stability of weather patterns due to the injection of more energy into these systems. The result is decreased extreme cold events, which would typically have suppressed or killed pathogens and vectors, and increased warm events, which allow more generations of pathogens and vectors to occur before any die off. The net effect plays out on a local and regional level with increased density and geographic range of the agents that cause epidemics and pandemics and the vectors that might shepherd them to humans [8]. Associated extreme weather events (e.g., Hurricane Katrina) may also lead to flooding, disruptions and contamination of water supplies, and increased exposure to pathogens such as mosquito-vectored diseases or *Vibrio cholerae*, the agent of cholera.

The population of the world has been growing explosively for much of the last four centuries. It would take around 700 years to double the population a mere 1500 years ago, e.g., from 250 million in the year 837 to 500 million in 1534, but doubling times were as short as 37 years from 1950 to 1987. [9] Although population growth has been slowing since 1962, there are nearly eight-fold more people on the planet now than in the year 1800. This has led to massive deforestation to make room both for living spaces for humans and for the agriculture to support them [8]. The impact of deforestation can be seen in two ways. First, encroachment by humans and domesticated farm animals into the native habitats of potential disease vectors presents more opportunities for exposure to zoonotic illnesses. An example is the Nipah virus epidemic in Southeast Asia – Nipah first emerged in 1998 in pig farmers in Malaysia, causing devastating outbreaks of viral encephalitis. The disease was transmitted to them from fruit bats who had lived in forests that were cleared for farms and orchards, and now had an overlapping range with humans and more frequent contact [10]. Because bats are the source of many zoonotic pathogens with significant risk for pandemic spread, including SARS-CoV-2, the cause of COVID-19, continued deforestation is a worldwide concern. A linked issue is the decreased biodiversity that is coupled to elimination of natural habitats; if the predators responsible for controlling disease vectors such as mosquitoes, mice, or rats are displaced or extinct, diseases can proliferate along with their vectors.

The changing face of civilization as the human population has increased from about 1 billion in 1800 to nearly 8 billion today has altered our interactions with pathogen vectors in numerous other ways. In 1800 only 3% of the world's population lived in cities, compared to 56% now. In 1950 there were only two mega-cities (urban areas with more than 10 million inhabitants), compared to 34 today. Increased urbanization and density as humanity have clustered in cities have several negative impacts on the spread of epidemic and pandemic diseases. Sanitation becomes more difficult, aiding proliferation of vectors and increasing exposure to deadly diseases, and a pathogen such as SARS-CoV-2 can infect many more hosts much more rapidly at the same relative level of infectivity than in non-urban settings. In addition, urbanization has increasingly led to the industrialization of the poultry industry – consumption of chicken meat has increased six-fold in the last century, and chickens and other domestic fowl are now the leading source of human protein worldwide. Zoonotic pathogens such as avian influenza have ever-increasing opportunities to "cross-over" into humans both due to the large-scale nature of poultry factories and due to increased contact of humans with poultry as utilization rises.

Increased air travel and the accompanying increases in worldwide trade allow rapid transit of not only people and goods, but vectors and diseases as well. Trade has increased more than forty-fold in the last century alone, and passenger air travel has increased five-fold in the last 40 years. This has led not only to the obvious problem of expanding geography of pathogens and their vectors to new geographies as they hitch-hike on planes, trains, and boats but also to homogenization of vector populations and resultant decreased barriers for disease spread. Numerous mosquito-borne diseases such as Chikungunya fever, West Nile virus, and Zika virus disease have spread worldwide over the last several decades not only because infected humans transported the causative agents during travel allowing introduction into mosquitoes in a new geography but also because the particular mosquito species that can host these viruses had also spread across a wider geography through increased opportunities for travel and ever-increasing connectivity. Indigenous mosquito species that may not have been able to serve as hosts for these viruses have been, in many cases, competed out or now co-exist with the relevant vectors.

PERSPECTIVE FOR THE HEALTHCARE SYSTEM

In the aftermath of the COVID-19 pandemic, it is now abundantly clear that pandemics are not a relic of the past that can be easily handled with technological advances in medicine and healthcare delivery. Indeed, technology and outgrowths of technology like global warming are likely accelerating the pace and scope of pandemics and making it more urgent that hospitals and healthcare systems be well prepared. The precise definition of a pandemic is one of academic interest that is perhaps not of urgent importance to the healthcare sector, but this designation does drive government-level responses. When the WHO or CDC declares an outbreak to be the next pandemic, it will trigger a different and more aggressive level of response than is expected during routine seasonal epidemics, as has been seen during the COVID-19 experience. Hospitals and healthcare systems should be aware of State and Federal disaster plans for upcoming pandemics and should have their own disaster plans that specifically include pandemic planning. Pandemic planning needs cover a gamut of areas within a hospital, including facility planning, staffing, policies and procedures, government relations, and supply chain concerns (particularly for PPE). It will not be a full century before the next pandemic as severe as the 1918 influenza or COVID-19 strikes, and hospitals and healthcare systems need to be better prepared the next time.

REFERENCES

[1] World Health Organization (WHO) Pandemic Definition. 7 May 2022. [Online]. Available: https://www.who.int/csr/disease/swineflu/frequently_asked_questions/pandemic/en/

[2] D. M. Morens, G. K. Folkers and A. S. Fauci, "What is a pandemic?," *J Infect Dis*, vol. 200, pp. 1018–1021, 2009.

[3] P. M. Martin and E. Martin-Granel, "2500-year evolution of the term epidemic," *Emerg Inf Dis*, vol. 12, no. 6, pp. 976–980, 2006.

[4] D. M. Wagner, J. Klunk, M. Harbeck and et al., "Yesrsinia pestis and the Plague of Justinian 541-542 AD: a genomic analysis," *Lancet Infect Dis*, vol. 14, pp. 319–326, 2014.

[5] J. A. McCullers, "Preparing for the next influenza pandemic," *Ped Infect Dis J*, vol. 27, pp. S57–S59, 2008.

[6] P. Doshi, "The elusive definition of pandemic influenza," *Bull World Health Org*, vol. 89, pp. 532–538, 2011.

[7] P. Brannen, *The ends of the world: volcanic apocalypses, lethal oceans, and our quest to understand Earth's past mass extinctions*, New York City: Ecco Press, 2017.

[8] R. W. Sutherst, "Global climate change and human vulnerability to vector-borne diseases," *Clin Microbiol Rev*, vol. 17, no. 1, pp. 136–173, 2004.

[9] M. Roser, H. Ritchie and E. Ortiz-Ospina, "World population growth," Online, https://ourworldindata.org/world-population-growth, 2013.

[10] V. S. Pillai, G. Krishna and M. V. Vettil, "Nipah virus: past outbreaks and future containment," *Viruses*, vol. 12, no. 465, pp. 1–15, 2020.

Chapter 2

A brief history of pandemics

Jonathan A. McCullers
University of Tennessee Health Science Center
Memphis, TN, USA

CONTENT

References 23

Pre-history likely claims many pandemics that have not survived into the written record. Diseases such as smallpox, measles, and typhoid fever achieved worldwide spread millennia ago and have re-emerged many times, so have likely caused pandemics lost to human knowledge. As one example, the mummy of the Pharaoh Ramesses V (ca. 1196–1145 BCE) clearly shows evidence of smallpox lesions [1], speaking to the antiquity of that disease. Thus, dating the first pandemic, well before the word was in use and in acknowledgment of how fraught with difficulties defining the word is (c.f. Chapter 1), seems an exercise in futility. Nevertheless, most historians point to the "Plague of Athens" as the first recorded pandemic [2].

The Peloponnesian War, a 27-year-long conflict between the ancient Greek civilizations of Athens and Sparta, broke out in 431 BCE. The 4-year-long Plague of Athens erupted in 430 BCE and was estimated by the Athenian general Thucydides to have killed one-quarter of the population occupying Athens during the war, including the city-state's leader, Pericles. The death of Pericles and loss of the war is generally considered by historians to mark the end of the "Golden Age" of Ancient Greece [2]. Thucydides suffered from the plague himself and wrote down careful observations in his *History of the Peloponnesian War* that have been used by modern scholars in attempts to ascribe a pathogen to the plague, paleobiological remains being absent. Thucydides described the disease as having a sudden onset, accompanied by a high fever, sore throat, and a red rash that descended from the head down the body. Later disease signs including cough, vomiting, copious diarrhea, small blisters and sores, and sleeplessness followed, before recovery or death around day eight or nine of the illness.

Possible causes of this first pandemic have been debated, including anthrax, the bubonic plague, typhoid fever, epidemic typhus, smallpox, or measles. No one disease fits the descriptions of Thucydides precisely, leaving doubt as to the real cause and laying open the question of whether there were multiple causes [1]. As Sparta was carrying out an assault by land and laying siege to the city, citizens who would normally have lived in the countryside outside the walls were now forced to shelter inside for multiple years in very poor living conditions. It is conceivable that contaminated and overburdened sanitation systems led to one or more waterborne outbreaks, while, simultaneously, the crowding encouraged spread of both gastrointestinal and respiratory diseases. At least one disease must have predominated at some point, however, as the outbreak spread out of the city and across the Mediterranean and into North Africa in three distinct waves, thus encompassing most of the known world and earning the distinction of being a pandemic as defined in Chapter 1 [2].

There are several obvious parallels between the Plague of Athens and the COVID-19 pandemic. The environment clearly played a role in both pandemics – disease spread was aided by close, indoor conditions, while improving sanitation and ventilation has been shown to slow the spread of COVID-19. Doctors were among the first to die in Athens as they tended the sick, leaving others as caretakers who also became ill more readily than the general population [1, 3]. During COVID-19, healthcare workers were among the groups at highest risk for contracting the disease, and inter-familial spread was common, particularly in crowded living situations linked to poverty and multi-generational housing [4]. Despair during the Plague of Athens led citizens to abandon social mores, disobeying orders intended to protect the public health in a "lawless extravaganza," as Thucydides described it [3]. This finds parallels today in those who opposed masking during the pandemic on political grounds, in the "COVID-deniers," and the "anti-vaxxers" who follow opinion rather than science and reject public health directives as infringing on personal autonomy.

Many further epidemics and pandemics have occurred in the two and a half millennia since the Plague of Athens. These can be broadly classified by mode of transmission, which is useful when considering infection control measures in the context of government policy or in healthcare delivery settings. Common modes of transmission for significant (region-, country-, or world-wide) spread of infections include vector-borne, airborne, and oral ingestion from a common source (Table 2.1). Other modes of transmission, such as direct person-to-person contract and fomite spread, may account for local or (rarely) regional spread, but do not lend themselves to pandemic spread. Ebola is an example of a disease which is spread directly person-to-person; it is acquired by contact with infected bodily fluids from an ill individual. Because persons who are contagious with Ebola exhibit significant signs of infection including hemorrhage from mucus membranes, outbreaks can be limited through education, community engagement, and standard infection control measures. The 2014–2016 Ebola outbreak in West Africa encompassed Guinea, Sierra Leone, and Liberia and was the largest in scope to this point. Fomite spread of organisms is a concern in hospitals, where spread from an infected person to another patient via the intermediary of contaminated objects can occur for many viral and bacterial organisms, but this is a limited mode of transmission.

Prior to our understanding of the germ theory of disease, diseases such as the plague were thought to be caused by "miasmas" or pockets of unclean air, and the role of insect and rodent vectors was unappreciated. The Justinian Plague, named after the Byzantine Emperor Justinian I, began in Southeast Asia, spread to Constantinople, capital of the Byzantine Empire and the major trading port linking Asia and Europe, and spread in waves throughout Europe, North Africa, and the Middle East in 8–12 year intervals from 541 to 750 CE [5]. The plague is caused by a bacterium, *Yersinia pestis*, which is carried by fleas and lice. These vectors live on rodents including black rats but can pass the disease on to humans when the rats are in close proximity. The grain ships traveling to Constantinople were a rich environment for these rats and brought the plague with them.

Three forms of the plague are recognized – the bubonic plague, characterized by buboes or infected and swollen lymph nodes, septicemic plague, often occurring if the bubonic plague was untreated with the infected person progressing to sepsis, and pneumonic plague, which can be transmitted by respiratory droplets person-to-person (Table 2.1) and caused rapid and almost certain mortality. Overall, mortality during the Justinian Plague was estimated at between 15 and 40%. Two subsequent plague pandemics occurred; the Black Death spread out of Asia and through Europe from 1347 to 1351 and is thought to have killed as much as one-third of all Europeans living at the time. It recurred in Europe five times between 1351 and 1400. The Third Plague also originated in China in 1855 and spread worldwide. The last major outbreak of the plague was in Cuba and Puerto Rico in 1912, but it remains endemic today in Africa and the Americas. Most cases in the United States are confined to the "four corners" states of the Southwest, where *Y. pestis* is endemic in rats and prairie dogs. From molecular typing we know that the Black Death and the Third Plague were caused by the same strain of *Y. pestis* that is extant today; the Justinian Plague was caused by a strain that is now extinct.

History's second most deadly pandemic after the Black Death was caused by an avian influenza virus that emerged in 1918 and spread around the globe, carried initially on troop ships engaged in World War I [6]. Influenza viruses also caused the pandemics of 1889, 1957, 1968, 2009, and likely others in history prior to the discovery of viruses. Influenza is spread by respiratory droplets (Table 2.1), but depending on the host and environmental conditions, it can also spread via aerosol or fomites. Smallpox, caused by the variola virus, is spread in a similar manner and has been causing epidemics since prehistoric times. In modern history, smallpox caused many regional epidemics at the level of a city or country. One example was the introduction into the island nation of Japan in 735; smallpox spread rapidly and is estimated to have killed up to one-third of the population [7]. Recurrences

Table 2.1 Significant pandemics and epidemics

Agent	Disease	Transmission	Years	Extent	Pan-/Epi-demic	Notes
Vector-Borne Transmission						
Yersinia pestis	Bubonic Plague	Fleas and lice	541–750	Known World	Pandemic	Named the Justinian Plague after the Byzantium Emperor Justinian I
			1347–1667			European spread during 1337–1351 known as the Black Death
			1855–present			"Third" Plague is now endemic; last major outbreak was in Cuba and Puerto Rico in 1912
Yellow Fever virus	Yellow Fever	Mosquitos	1793–1905	Americas	Epidemic	Major outbreaks in US cities on the East Coast and Mississippi valley, as well as in Cuba and Panama during US military incursions
Zika virus	Zika virus disease	Mosquitos	2013–present	Worldwide in tropical climes	Pandemic	Mild infections unless exposed congenitally
Chikungunya virus	Chikungunya	Mosquitos	2014–present	Worldwide in tropical climes	Pandemic	From the Makonde language meaning "that which bends up"; rarely fatal
Airborne person-to-person transmission						
Variola major	Smallpox	Droplet, direct contact, and fomite spread	Prehistory	Worldwide	Pandemic	Multiple major epidemics throughout known history (e.g., Japan in 735)
			1520–?	South and Central America	Epidemic	Introduced into the Americas by the Spanish - killed half the population of Mexico in the first year
Yersinia pestis	Pneumonic plague	Respiratory droplets	Intermittent	Known World and Worldwide	Pandemic	Pneumonic plague was a more deadly form of transmission that occurred alongside the more common vector-borne illnesses

Mycobacterium tuberculosis	Tuberculosis	Respiratory droplets	Prehistoric	Worldwide	Pandemic	Endemic throughout recorded history
Influenza A virus	Influenza	Respiratory droplets	1889, 1918, 1857, 1968, 2009	Worldwide	Pandemic and Epidemic	Causes seasonal epidemics with periodic zoonotic incursions leading to pandemics. Controversy over whether 2009 H1N1 was a pandemic. May have been responsible for multiple other pandemics prior to 1889.

Ingestion from a common source

Vibrio cholerae	Cholera	Waterborne	1817–1824 and multiple recurrences	Worldwide	Pandemic and Epidemic	Seven major pandemics from 1817–1961; significant epidemics continue to occur almost annually
Salmonella typhi	Typhoid Fever	Waterborne	Multiple	Regional to countrywide	Epidemics	May have been responsible for the Plague of Athens and for wiping out the Jamestown colony; significant epidemics continue to occur almost annually

were common until 1206, occurring 5–32 years apart. Smallpox was also the centerpiece of what is known in history as the "Columbian Exchange" where the ships of Spanish explorers including Columbus carried syphilis from Central America back to Europe in 1494 and seeded smallpox and other diseases in Mexico in 1520 [8]. Syphilis spread rapidly through Europe following invasions during the Italian Wars, killing an estimated 50,000 persons [1]. Smallpox is thought to have killed half the population of Mexico City in the first year after introduction, and it may have wiped out as much as 95% of the indigenous populations of South and Central America in subsequent decades.

The third major mode of transmission, oral ingestion from a common source, is best exemplified by the cholera pandemics of the 19th century (Table 2.1). Cholera, a disease characterized by acute watery diarrhea, is caused by the bacterium Vibrio cholerae. It had been endemic for centuries in the Ganges basin of India, but first spread globally beginning in 1817 through Asia, and thence into India, Russia, Europe, and the Americas. Six subsequent pandemics occurred over the next 130 years, and it continues to cause epidemics worldwide affecting millions annually [9]. The third cholera pandemic is best known for the observations of the epidemiologist John Snow in England, who demonstrated the waterborne nature of the illness by removing the pump handle on a well in one district, and comparing disease there to other city districts. The current strain causing epidemics, known as the "El Tor biotype," first arose in "quarantine stations" in El Tor, Egypt where travelers back from Mecca after attending the Hajj were kept in squalid conditions for weeks or months prior to being allowed into European countries [9].

Many other pandemics have afflicted the world throughout history, and doubtless many more will emerge from animal reservoirs and cause significant morbidity, mortality, and societal disruption. Understanding the past is a vital key to preparing for the future, as our recent experience with COVID-19 has demonstrated. There are numerous examples from past pandemics that could have informed many of the so-called controversies that arose in 2020 had world and local leaders been better educated. The uneven and sometimes defiant response to authority has been a staple of pandemics since the Plague of Athens and was amply documented in the 1918 influenza pandemic; public resistance by a minority of citizens to public health measures such as business closures, mask mandates, and vaccination should have been anticipated. The heavy burden on frontline healthcare workers and the resulting stress and burnout have been well appreciated throughout history. The roles of over-crowding, poor ventilation, and close living spaces linked to poverty have likewise been seen as important factors in the ease of spread and severity of pandemics for millennia. Finally, the impact on the economy and on disease spread of school closures, limitations on businesses, banning of mass gatherings, and mask mandates have all been studied during previous pandemics and epidemics, and the utility of these measures should not be controversial [6]. Health systems likewise should use this knowledge from past history and lived experience from the COVID-19 pandemic to revise and update disaster and pandemic plans.

REFERENCES

[1] B. A. Cunha, "The cause of the plague of Athens: plague, typhoid, typhus, smallpox, or measles?," *Infect Dis Clin N Amer*, vol. 18, pp. 29–43, 2004.

[2] D. M. Morens, P. Daszak, H. Markel and J. K. Taubenberger, "Pandemic COVID-19 joins history's pandemic legion," *mBio*, vol. 11, no. 3, pp. 1–9, 2020.

[3] J. J. Fins, "Pandemics, protocols, and the Plague of Athens: Insights from Thucydides," *Hastings Cent Rep*, vol. 50, no. 3, pp. 50–53, 2020.

[4] N. Truong and A. O. Asare, "Assessing the effect of socio-economic features of low-income communities and COVID-19 related cases: An empirical study of New York City," *Glob Publ Health*, vol. 16, no. 1, pp. 1–16, 2021.

[5] D. M. Wagner, J. Klunk and M. Harbeck, "Yersinia pestis and the Plague of Justinian 541–543 AD: A genomic analysis," *Lancet Infect Dis*, vol. 14, pp. 319–326, 2014.

[6] J. M. Barry, *The Great Influenza: The Story of the Deadliest Pandemic in History*, New York: Viking, 2004.

[7] A. Suzuki, "Smallpox and the epidemiologic heritage of modern Japan: Towards a total history," *Med Hist*, vol. 55, no. 3, pp. 313–318, 2011.

[8] N. Nunn and N. Qian, "The columbian exchange: A history of disease, food, and ideas," *J Econ Perspect*, vol. 24, no. 2, pp. 163–188, 2010.

[9] J. D. Clemons, G. B. Nair, T. Ahmed, F. Qadri and J. Holmgren, "Cholera," *Lancet*, vol. 390, pp. 1539–1549, 2017.

Chapter 3

The healthcare continuum

Edward M. Rafalski
University of Illinois School of Public Health
Chicago, IL, USA
University of South Florida College of Public Health
Tampa, FL, USA

CONTENTS

Introduction 25
Public health 27
Healthcare systems.. 27
The evolution of the healthcare continuum 28
    Screening and testing 28
    Primary care 29
    Urgent and emergent care 29
    Hospital acute care and the re-establishment of the field hospital ... 30
    Post-acute care... 30
    Transition hotel to home, Hospital at Home®, home health
        and the physician house call... 31
    Palliative care and hospice care... 32
Conclusion.. 32
References 33

INTRODUCTION

The last world-wide pandemic, The Great Influenza, occurred in 1918 and hit the shores of the United States with a fury not unlike COVID-19, the disease caused by the severe acute respiratory syndrome coronavirus 2 (SARS-CoV-2) which has again placed a severe strain on the United States (U.S.) public health and healthcare systems.[1] Both systems are distinct and, for the most part, uncoordinated in the United States. The public health system is funded and managed largely by government at the local, state and federal levels whereas the healthcare system is largely privately managed and partially funded by government through the Medicare and Medicaid programs, the insurance programs for primarily the elderly and poor, respectively. In the former, insurance coverage is provided to the disabled and those over the age of 65 by the Federal government. In the latter, insurance coverage

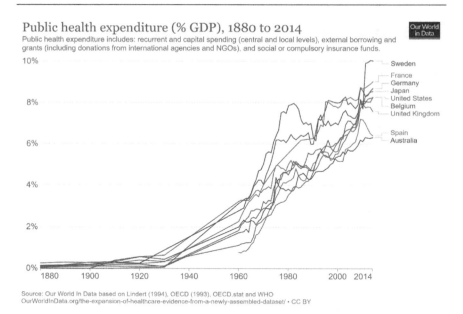

Figure 3.1 Public health expenditure.

is provided to the poor largely by the states. Neither program existed in in the last pandemic as both came into being in 1965 during President Lyndon Johnson administration's Great Society legislative effort.

Public health agencies, as we know them today, were much smaller in both scope and funding at the turn of the last century. For example, in 1920 public health expenditures as a percentage of GDP were .40% and 8.28% in 2014 (see Figure 3.1).[2] In contrast, overall healthcare system spending was 3.03% at the end of the 1920s and grew to 8.98% of total GDP by the mid-2010s (see Figure 3.2).[3] Recent estimates are that the United States has spent 18% of its GDP on overall healthcare, inclusive of public health and health system expenditures, at the beginning of this decade heading into the pandemic.[4]

Once the pandemic has subsided/ended and more data becomes available, it will be a worthwhile exercise to update funding of efforts to fight the pandemic and isolate which portions of the overall U.S. healthcare enterprise used resources to combat COVID-19. One question left to be answered will be, was the U.S. effective and efficient in our mixed use of public and private resources or could they have been used more effectively and efficiently? Further, comparisons of the U.S. approach vs those of other developed nations around the world will further provide insights for public health policy formulation in preparation of future pandemics and healthcare disasters.

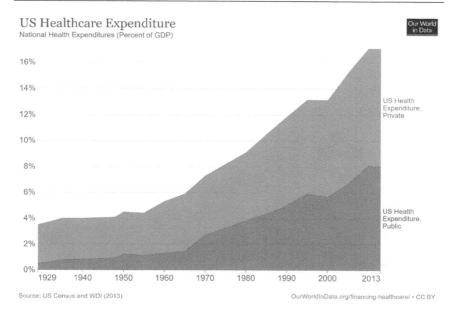

US Healthcare Expenditure
National Health Expenditures (Percent of GDP)

Figure 3.2 U.S. healthcare expenditure.

PUBLIC HEALTH

As noted above, there is a distinction between the public health and health-care systems in the United States. It is fair to say that the U.S. public health infrastructure was unprepared to deal with the scale of this healthcare crisis. For example, testing sites were stood up by private industry in many markets across the U.S. as the public heath infrastructure to do so was lacking. Arguably, testing is a public health function, not a private health system function, yet, private industry was asked to lead in this effort as evidenced by the fact that most testing sites are privately managed.[5] In the case of public health agencies reflective of the level of lack of preparation, it has been noted that a significant percentage of leaders of public health departments have turned over as a result of lack of resources, stress, public pressure, etc.[6]

HEALTHCARE SYSTEMS

In the case of healthcare systems, organizations were also largely unprepared for what was to come in March of 2020 and since the inception of the pandemic. Certain portions of the healthcare continuum were arguably more hardened for crisis, such as those in critical care. Other portions of the continuum were less hardened, such as those in primary care and specifically telehealth. Some portions of the continuum existed prior to the pandemic

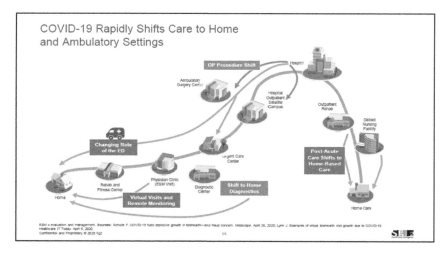

Figure 3.3 Healthcare continuum.

such as the emergency room (ER)/emergency department (ED), others had been out of use and re-instituted anew such as the field hospital, and still others were created such triage chat bots (an automated form of self-triage based on clinical criteria and algorithms). In all cases, care shifted closer to the home as a result of the pandemic and quickened the pace of a process that was underway prior to the pandemic with a projected shift of 15% by the end of the decade (see Figure 3.3). The pandemic created new levels of analytics across the continuum and created a deeper understanding of the interconnectedness of the care of health ecosystem.

THE EVOLUTION OF THE HEALTHCARE CONTINUUM

Screening and testing

Screening is used as a primary public health prevention technique focused on avoiding disease altogether, generally by preventing disease development.[7] National screening guidelines have been developed for a variety of disease states such as breast cancer, hypertension and diabetes drawing on the expertise of such groups as the United States Preventative Services Task Force (USPSTF).[8] In the case of COVID-19, testing, a form of screening for the disease and a prevention measure used in the Swiss cheese defense model, standardization of process and requirements evolved during the pandemic. The Swiss cheese model of accident causation was updated to address the need for defense against respiratory infection prevention, such as SARS-CoV-2, the virus that causes COVID-19.[9] Specific and sensitive testing and tracing is a critical component of the model. Other components include physical distancing, masking, hand hygiene/cough etiquette,

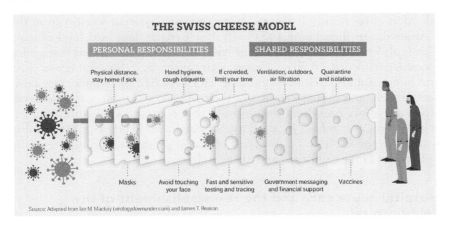

Figure 3.4 Swiss cheese (public health) model.

avoiding touching your face, limiting crowds, ventilation/air filtration, government messaging/financial support, quarantine/isolation and vaccines (see Figure 3.4). Private organizations, mostly healthcare systems, took it upon themselves to develop an approach to testing in the broader community. Access was provided to established patients and new patients alike, at a cost born not by public health but by private institutions. This was done for the public good and acted as the first line of defense and gathering of early knowledge of the extent of community spread of the virus.

Primary care

Primary care evolved in the pandemic. Telehealth, healthcare provided using video, audio and diagnostic technology, was available prior to the pandemic but not widely adopted by providers and consumers. It is estimated that between 5% and 15% of all primary care encounters were being delivered prior to the pandemic. At the height of the first wave when the United States was in shutdown, there were instances where telehealth was representing upward of 80% of all clinical visits. While not sustained nationally as shutdown measures were eased, the industry has settled back to slightly higher than pre-pandemic levels estimated at approximately 22%, but this varies by system, region and specialty. For example, behavioral health utilization has maintained higher than average utilization as high as 68% nationally. It is projected that the industry will reach a tipping point where 40%–50% of all visits will be delivered using telehealth technology.[10]

Urgent and emergent care

Urgent care (UC), care provided in a clinical setting other than an emergency room, has been one of the areas that has struggled with maintaining volumes during the pandemic, arguably given the evolution and wider adoption of telehealth. Patients can now access physician services from the convenience of their home and in effect, self-triage their next level of care. This is also true of emergent care provided in the hospital-based emergency room/department (ER/ED). Urgent care providers, hospital-based ERs and non-hospital-based free-stranding ERs have had to rethink their business models and perhaps right-size their operations given softer demand. However, it has been long documented that consumers over-utilize emergency rooms as a default location for ongoing care.[11] Perhaps a silver lining within the pandemic is a right-sizing of access points delivering care at the right place, at the right time and at the right cost.

Hospital acute care and the re-establishment of the field hospital

Hospital-based acute care has been transformed. Infection control and clinical treatment methods have evolved during the pandemic. It is both the simplest steps – handwashing – and the most sophisticated of mechanisms – clinical excellence guidance – that contribute to good medical care. Throughout the pandemic health systems reminded healthcare personnel of basic infection control measures while simultaneously working to assimilate public health data and research to learn best practices and to plan for optimal patient care. Clinical techniques evolved to treat patients including lying patients prone to prevent the onset of pneumonia. The field hospital, the first of which was created at the battle of Shiloh in the U.S. Civil War, was employed to create additional capacity during the worst peaks of the pandemic.[12] In New York the field hospital constructed in Central Park was the first time a field hospital was stood up since the Civil War.[13]

Post-acute care

Post-acute care includes: assisted living, skilled nursing, long-term care and most recently super skilled nursing facilities (Super-SNFs) a new designation created by certain states to accommodate the most skilled post-acute care for COVID-19 patients.[14] Assisted living is housing for the elderly or disabled that provides nursing care, housekeeping and prepared meals as needed. Skilled care is nursing and therapy care that can only be safely and effectively performed by, or under the supervision of, professionals or technical personnel. It is healthcare given when skilled nursing or skilled therapy to treat, manage, and observe the condition, and evaluation of care is needed. Long-term care involves a variety of services designed to meet a person's health or personal care needs during a short or long period of time. These services help people live as independently and safely as possible when they can no longer perform everyday activities on their own. Long-term care is provided in different places by different caregivers, depending on a person's needs. Most long-term care is provided at home by unpaid family members and friends. It can also be given in a facility such as a nursing home or in the community, for example, in an adult day care center.[15]

The coordination between hospitals and the post-acute portions of the continuum proved challenging, particularly early in the pandemic as COVID-19 spread through this population of elderly patients.[16] Arguably, this segment of the healthcare continuum was overwhelmed and unprepared. Opportunities for improved communication, a review of infection control practices and a centralized process for tracking and testing the target population were identified.[17] Telemonitoring was deployed to assist in monitoring patients in this environment and projects such as The Project for Extension of Community Healthcare Outcomes (ECHO) were employed as a best practice.[18]

The super skilled nursing facility (Super-SNF) was created as a result of the pandemic and the need to create a higher level of infection prevention, care and safety for COVID-19 patients. These facilities were designated centers for congregating patients and were put in place temporarily early in the pandemic to deal with surges in hospital admissions and discharges among the elderly. As vaccination rates improved in this population, the need for these units subsided.

Transition hotel to home, Hospital at Home®, home health and the physician house call

As bed capacity was constrained, new locations for care to decompress the hospital setting were created. Transition hotel to home was an offering whereby traditional hotel space was leased and staffed by clinical personal to observe patients in transition to home. The clinical acuity of these patients was between that required for observation in a hospital setting and that provided by home care health nursing in the home.

Hospital at Home®, first named by Johns Hopkins Medicine, was already a concept in place prior to the pandemic, but largely in the early stages of adoption across the United States. It is an innovative care model for adoption by healthcare organizations that provides hospital-level care in a patient's home as a full substitute for acute hospital care. The program has been implemented at numerous sites around the United States by Veterans Administration (VA) hospitals, health systems, home care providers and managed care programs as a tool to cost-effectively treat acutely ill older adults, while improving patient safety, quality and satisfaction. The pandemic afforded an opportunity for health systems around the country to establish their own nascent programs enabling the discharge of stable COVID-19 patients to home with the ability to monitor remotely with telehealth and provide at home health visits with clinical personnel thereby freeing up beds for more acutely ill patients.

Home healthcare, a service delivered primarily by licensed home health registered nurses (RNs), is an offering where the patient must require skilled qualifying services, the care needed must be intermittent (part time) and the care must be a medical necessity (must be under the supervision of a physician). Home healthcare is a wide range of healthcare services that can be given in your home for an illness or injury. Home healthcare is usually less expensive, more convenient, and just as effective as care one receives in a hospital or skilled nursing facility (SNF).[19] This mature offering has been part of the healthcare continuum in the United States since 1909 when the first home health insurance policy was offered by Metropolitan Life. Home health services supported both the transition hotel to home and Hospital at Home® during the pandemic.

For as long as physicians have been practicing the art and science of medicine they have visited the home of the patient to provide care. House calls used to make up 40% of U.S. doctors' visits in the 1940s before going into decline in the 1960s. By 1980, house calls accounted for only 0.6% of encounters. The financial pressures for gaining efficiency following the creation of the Medicare and Medicaid programs arguably led to the decline of visits to the home in addition to other developments such as the growth of biomedical knowledge and technology, a growing medical care system and liability concerns.[20] While the same pressures existed during the pandemic, the home visit may still have a place in the healthcare continuum given the risk of acquiring disease by congregating in clinic waiting rooms. Companies such as Dispatch Health were created pre-pandemic and provided yet another safe access point for patients.[21]

Palliative care and hospice care

At the end of the healthcare continuum we find palliative and hospice care. Palliative care is specialized medical care that focuses on providing patients relief from pain and other symptoms of a serious illness, no matter the diagnosis or stage of disease. Palliative care teams aim to improve the quality of life for both patients and their families. This form of care is offered alongside curative or other treatments you may be receiving. Like palliative care, hospice provides comprehensive comfort care as well as support for the family, but, in hospice, attempts to cure the person's illness are stopped. Hospice is provided for a person with a terminal illness whose doctor believes he or she has six months or less to live if the illness runs its natural course.[22] In the experience of some health systems, the nature of end of life care for COVID-19 patients was such that hospice care was not an option given the rapid nature of the progression of the disease and the highly critical acuity.

CONCLUSION

Some aspects of healthcare continuum, such as primary, urgent, emergency, acute, skilled and home care, were well established prior to the pandemic and were essential in serving as the last line of defense and care in the pandemic. Other aspects, such as the field hospital and physician home visit were old concepts that found a useful place of service. Yet other aspects, such as telehealth and Hospital at Home®, were in existence but still not widely adopted. It may be that we have reached the tipping point at which these services become ubiquitous in the wake of the pandemic, although in this case it was a very big thing that made a difference.[23]

REFERENCES

1 Barr, J.M. 2005. The Great Influenza: The epic story of the deadliest pandemic in history. New York, Penguin Books.
2 https://ourworldindata.org/grapher/public-health-expenditure-share-gdp-owid. Accessed August 30, 2021.
3 https://ourworldindata.org/grapher/public-health-expenditure-share-gdp-owid. Accessed August 30, 2021.
4 https://www.statista.com/statistics/184968/us-health-expenditure-as-percent-of-gdp-since-1960/. Accessed August 30, 2022.
5 https://www.hhs.gov/coronavirus/community-based-testing-sites/index.html#fl. Accessed August 30, 2021.
6 Axe Files Podcast.
7 Mayzell, G. 2016. Population health: An implementation guide to improve outcomes and lower costs. Boca Raton, FL, CRC Press.
8 https://www.uspreventiveservicestaskforce.org/uspstf/. Accessed August 30, 2021.
9 https://www.infectioncontroltoday.com/view/wiss-cheese-model-how-infection-prevention-really-works Accessed August 30. Accessed August 30, 2021.
10 https://www.sg2.com/media-center/press-releases/vizient-analysis-telehealth-data-visits-trend-above-prepandemic-levels/. Accessed August 30, 2021.
11 Ho V. et al. 2017. Comparing utilization and costs of care in freestanding emergency department, hospital emergency departments, and urgent care centers. *Annals of Emergency Medicine*. Vol. 70(6): pp. 846–857.
12 Fahey J.H. Bernard. 2006. John Dowling Irwin and the development of the field hospital at Shiloh. *Mil Med*. May; Vol. 171(5): pp. 345–351. doi: 10.7205/milmed.171.5.345. PMID: 16761879.
13 Cunningham, O.E. 2007. Shiloh and the western campaign of 1862. New York: Savas Beatie.
14 https://www.nia.nih.gov/health/what-long-term-care. Accessed August 30, 2021.
15 https://www.nia.nih.gov/health/what-long-term-care. Accessed August 30, 2021.
16 Lavery, A. et al. 2020. Characteristics of hospitalized COVID-19 patients discharges and experiencing same-hospital readmission. Morbidity and mortality weekly report. Vol. 69(45): pp. 1695–1699.
17 Kim, G. et al. 2020. A health system response to COVID-19 in long-term care and post-acute care: a three-phase approach. *Journal of the American Geriatrics Society*. Vol. 68(6): pp. 1155–1161.
18 Gleason, L.J. et al. 2020. Using telemonitoring to share best practices on COVID-19 in post-acute and long- term care facilities. *Journal of the American Geriatrics Society*. Vol. 68(11): pp. E58–E60.

19 https://www.medicare.gov/what-medicare-covers/whats-home-health-care. Accessed August 30, 2021.
20 Leff, B. and Burton, J.R. 2001. The future history of home care and physician house calls in the United States. *Journal of Gerontology*. Vol. 56A(10), pp. M603–M608.
21 https://www.dispatchhealth.com/. Accessed August 30, 2021.
22 https://www.nia.nih.gov/health/what-are-palliative-care-and-hospice-care. Accessed August 30, 2021.
23 Gladwell, M. 2002. The tipping point: How little things can make a big difference. Boston. Little, Brown and Company.

Chapter 4

The fog of war and data

Edward M. Rafalski
University of Illinois School of Public Health
Chicago, IL, USA
University of South Florida College of Public Health
Tampa, FL, USA

Robert Marksthaler
Epic Systems
Verona, WI, USA

CONTENT

References 40

A phrase now much used to describe the complexity of military conflicts, the fog of war is often attributed to Carl Philipp Gottfried Clausewitz, a Prussian general and military theorist, but is in fact a paraphrase of what he said: "War is the realm of uncertainty; three quarters of the factors on which action in war is based are wrapped in a fog of greater or lesser uncertainty."[1] The Fog of War was also the title of Errol Morris's 2004 award-winning documentary about Robert S. McNamara, US Secretary of State during the Vietnam War. In that conflict, data on casualties and deaths were significantly understated during the war. This lack of clarity led to assumptions about where the United States stood in the conflict which then led to policy decisions that may have been incorrect in retrospect. The fog of data created by the COVID-19 pandemic, which some have referred to as a war, has had arguably similar policy results.

COVID-19, the disease caused by the severe acute respiratory syndrome coronavirus 2 (SARS-CoV-2), has placed a severe strain on the United States (U.S.) healthcare system. It has been observed to have done the same in other countries around the world that preceded the pandemic arriving in the United States. With the discovery of SARS-CoV-2, there are now seven types of coronaviruses known to infect humans, four of which regularly circulate among humans and mostly cause mild to moderate upper respiratory tract infections or common colds. The remaining three jumped from animal hosts to humans, resulting in more serious disease.

DOI: 10.1201/9781003204138-6

The outbreak of COVID-19 was officially announced as a pandemic by the World Health Organization (WHO) on March 11, 2020. The first case was reported by the Chinese Center for Disease Control and Prevention on December 8, 2019, and then quickly spread throughout the Wuhan City and Hubei Province.[2] There is some current research taking place that may show that the virus was spreading in the general population earlier than initially reported as the Wuhan strain was not the ordinal strain. In the early research on what is now a pandemic, key findings were shared that were adopted by various modeling teams around the country in the U.S. Key findings included: the distribution or spectrum of disease from mild (81%; 36,160 cases) to severe (14%; 6,198 cases) to critical (5%; 2,087 cases), and a case fatality rate (CFR) of 2.3%, among other findings. Some have viewed the data from China as suspect, but for those modeling what may happen in the United States prior to its arrival on our shores, it was the best information available at the time.

The clinical opinion by many was that a significant portion of critical COVID-19 patients would develop pneumonia which would lead to intensive care unit (ICU) bed utilization, isolation room (rooms with negative air flow pressure) utilization and ventilator (vent) utilization.[3,4] Applying this logic, the United States already had data from various sources that could be used to begin modeling inpatient bed demand. Central to bed demand modeling was the creation of length of stay (LOS) modeling assumptions for COVID-19 patients with pneumonia. Length of stay is a hospital operating statistic reflecting the number of days between admission and discharge in which a patient occupies a bed. These patients would place a strain on existing ICU, isolation bed and vent capacity. For example, three quarters of inpatients hospitalized for pneumonia (74.2%) do not have an ICU stay. Pneumonia inpatient hospitalizations resulting in acute care (short-term care received in a hospital, typically on a medical/surgical unit) instead of an ICU stay have an average length of stay (ALOS) of 4.2 days. If the inpatient hospitalization included time in the ICU, the average LOS increased to 7.2 days.[5]

As the pandemic spread to other parts of the world, most importantly the European continent, the data set for modeling became richer, varied and more easily accessible. Organizations, such as Statista, began making raw COVID-19 data including incidence rates, readily available.[6] Italy was arguably the first, most significantly affected of the European countries and well suited because of the timing for modeling an aggressive scenario in the United States. One early finding comparing the Italian and Chinese experience was that the CFR was identical at 2.3%. Additionally, case fatalities in Italy appeared to be in the elderly group of age 60 and above, and comorbidities appeared to be important contributors in deaths in both countries.[7] Furthermore, surge planning recommendations were becoming available from Italy including increasing ICU surge capacity and implementing measures of containment. In the Italian experience, the proportion of ICU admissions represented 12% of total positive cases and 16% of all hospitalized patients compared to China where only 5% of patients who tested positive for COVID-19 required an ICU admission.

Three planning principles were introduced. First, linear and exponential models should be created to forecast demand for ICU beds. Second, laboratory capacity to test for SARS-CoV-2 should be increased immediately. Third, in parallel to the surge ICU capacity response, a large dedicated COVID-19 facility (or units) should be converted more quickly.[8] Additional operational suggestions were made including: creating cohort ICUs for COVID-19 patients; organizing triage areas where patients could receive mechanical ventilation if necessary; establishing local protocols for triage of patient with respiratory symptoms to test them rapidly; ensuring that adequate personal protective equipment (PPE) for health personnel is available; reporting every positive or suspected critically ill COVID-19 patient to a regional coordinating center; and to quickly make available ICU beds and personnel; nonurgent procedures should be cancelled. Standard public health measures of quarantine were introduced to attempt to contain and mitigate spread of the disease. Many of these early Italian principles were adopted throughout the United States.

The first COVID-19 case in the United States was reported on January 20, 2020.[9] As subsequent cases were being reported in the United States, Washington State became a reliable source not just for hospital bed demand based on incidence and community spread but also for modeling the impact of skilled nursing facilities (SNFs) and assisted living facilities (ALFs) on hospital bed demand.[10,11] Various hospital bed demand modeling efforts began in earnest across the United States in university settings, private consulting and health systems. Nationally, the University of Washington Institute of Health Metrics and Evaluation (IHME) seemed to gain a footing and was adopted as a source in many states for its ability to predict the epidemiological curve(s) by state, including the peak(s) of each wave.

Once the first peak of the first pandemic wave passed in certain locales, and state restrictions on stay-at-home orders loosened, focus shifted to post-first peak, first-wave pandemic modeling and planning assumptions. At least one group suggested the use of scenario planning to anticipate four different unique pandemic behaviors: (1) quick recovery, (2) long slog, (3) secondary surge and (4) seasonal surge.[12] The consensus view by many, including the Centers for Disease Control and Prevention (CDC) and the (WHO was that a quick recovery was unlikely, thereby reducing the probability of the first scenario. For the remaining three, new assumptions were required for each approach. For example, how many waves should we expect after the first? Would the second, third and fourth peaks/waves be more, or less, severe than the first? How long would the pandemic last?

There is emerging consensus that we will see multiple peaks and perhaps waves in this pandemic over multiple years and that surveillance for SARS-CoV-2 should be maintained since a resurgence in contagion could be possible as late as 2024.[13] Complicating matters is a resurgence in the Northern Hemisphere during the seasonal flu season, with other virus strains thereby compounding the demand for critical care inpatient hospital beds. Further, seasonal variation in SARS-Co-V-2 transmission could differ between geographic regions. The Ro, a measure of the mean number of infections from

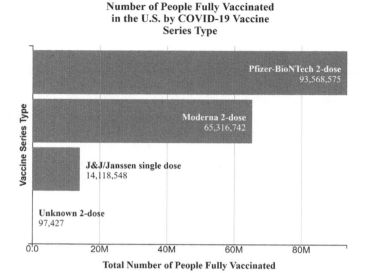

Figure 4.1 People vaccinated by type.

one case, for influenza in New York declines in the summer by approximately 40%, while in Florida the decline is closer to 20%. Current strains could further mutate as has been experienced with the UK B.1.1.7, South African V501, V2 clade, and Brazilian B 1.1.28.

The vaccination rates for the Pfizer, Moderna and Johnson & Johnson vaccines have differed by region, thereby creating variability in herd immunity in the general population (see Figures 4.1, 4.2, 4.3).[14]

Last is the effect of increasing social distancing policies put in place heading into the first wave and subsequent waves/peaks of the pandemic to "flatten the curve," which is a reference to the SIR (number of susceptible, infectious and recovered/diseased/immune individuals) epidemiological curve and the adjustments made to the policy since the development of vaccines. Under all scenarios, according to one study, there was a resurgence of infection when the simulated social distancing measures were lifted.[15]

Creating further confusion when making assumptions in predictive modeling has been the variability of public health policies by state, county and township in the United States. Unlike other countries in the world, such as New Zealand, where country-wide lockdown polices were employed to flatten the curve in multiple waves/peaks, the United States employed the technique only once. As a result, states, counties and townships were left to their own devices to implement curve flattening polices. In any given metropolitan statistical area (MSA), a modeler may encounter four different county policies and a variety of township policies, many of which may not be aligned with policy at the state level. For example, if there is no consistent policy for mandating the wearing of masks or vaccination in schools, the

Total Doses Administered Reported to the CDC by State/Territory and for Select Federal Entities per 100,000 of the Total Population

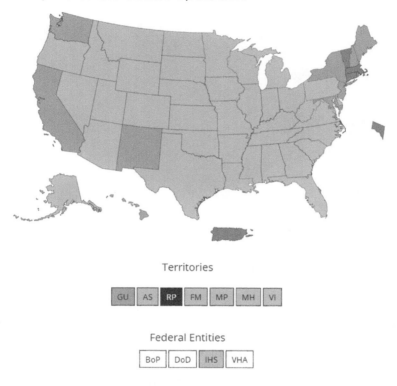

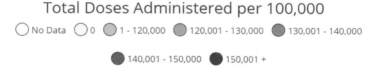

Figure 4.2 Doses by state.

ability to predict the effects of each becomes a fool's errand. How is one to make an assumption regarding incidence when there is no consistency? As a result, anticipating the end of a wave/peak for surge capacity planning has been hampered and made less effective calling into question the benefit of a patchwork of solutions as opposed to a more coordinated approach with consistent policy formulation and guidance.

Percentage of residents age 12+ that are fully vaccinated by county and state

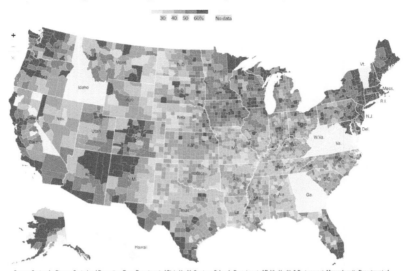

Source: Centers for Disease Control and Prevention, Texas Department of State Health Services, Colorado Department of Public Health & Environment, Massachusetts Department of Public Health, U.S. Census Bureau | Note: No C.D.C. data available for Hawaii, Texas and some counties. Four other states were excluded because more than a quarter of data is missing. Data from Texas and Colorado excludes shots given by most federal agencies.

Figure 4.3 Fully vaccinated population.

REFERENCES

1 Knowles, E.M. 2005. The Oxford Dictionary of Phrase and Fable. Oxford University Press. DOI: 10.1093/acref/9780198609810.001.0001.
2 Wu, Z. and McGoogan, J.M. 2020. Characteristics of and Important Lessons from the Coronavirus Disease 2019 (COVID-19) Outbreak in China. *JAMA*. Downloaded from: https://jamanetwork.com on 3/16/2020.
3 Li, Q. Guan, X. Wu, P. et al. 2020. Early Transmission Dynamics in Wuhan, China, of Novel Coronavirus-infected Pneumonia. *New England Journal of Medicine*. 382: 1199–207.
4 Gaythrope, K., Imai, N. Cuomo-Dannenburg, G. et al. Symptom Progression of COVID-19. Imperial College London. 3/11/2020. https://www.imperial.ac.uk/media/imperial-college/medicine/sph/ide/gida-fellowships/Imperial-College-COVID19-symptom-progression-11-03-2020.pdf.
5 Williams, S., Gousen, S. and DeFrances, C. 2018. National Hospital Care Survey Demonstration Projects: Pneumonia Inpatient Hospitalizations and Emergency Department Visits. U.S. Department of Health and Human Services, Centers for Disease Control and Prevention, National Center for Health Statistics. Number 116.
6 https://www.statista.com/
7 Porcheddu, R. et al. 2020. Similarity in Case Fatality Rates (CFR) of COVID-19/SARS-COV-2 in Italy and China. *The Journal of Infection in Developing Countries*. 14(2): 125–128.

8 Graselli, G., Pesenti, A. and Cecconi, M. 2020. Critical Care Utilization for the COVID-19 Outbreak in Lombardy, Italy. Early Experience and Forecast During an Emergency Response. JAMA.

9 Holshue, M.L., DeBolt, C. Lindquist, S. et al. 2020. First Case of 2019 Novel Coronavirus in the United States. *New England Journal of Medicine*. 382: 929–936.

10 McMichael, T. et al. COVID-19 in a Long-Term Care Facility—King County, Washington, February 27–March 9, 2020. *Morbidity and Mortality Weekly Report*. Vol. 69, No. 12. March 27, 2020.

11 Kimball, A. et al. Asymptomatic and Presymptomatic SARS-CoV-2 Infections in Residents of a Long-Term Care Skilled Nursing Facility – King County, Washington, March 2020. *Morbidity and Mortality Weekly Report*. Vol, 69, No. 13. April 3, 2020.

12 Grube, M. and Patel, C. Hospital Post-COVID Demand Modeling. Kaufman Hall. April 2020.

13 Kissler, S. et al. Projecting the Transmission Dynamics of SARS-CoV-2 through the Post-pandemic Period. *Science*. 10.1126/science.abb5793. 2020.

14 https://covid.cdc.gov/covid-data-tracker/#vaccinations_vacc-total-admin-rate-total

15 Kissler, S. et al. Projecting the Transmission Dynamics of SARS-CoV-2 through the Post-pandemic Period. *Science*. 10.1126/science.abb5793. 2020.

Chapter 5

Sources of data/modeling

Edward M. Rafalski

University of Illinois School of Public Health
Chicago, IL, USA
University of South Florida College of Public Health
Tampa, FL, USA

Robert Marksthaler

Epic Systems
Verona, WI, USA

CONTENTS

Introduction 43
Constants and assumptions 45
Early public data modeling – SIR 47
Health system experiential modeling 52
Publicly available models 54
    Proprietary models 55
    Institutional proprietary models 55
Conclusion 56
References 57

INTRODUCTION

Various modeling resources became available as the COVID-19 pandemic progressed and datasets became richer. This chapter catalogs the various modeling approaches that became publicly available and how they were used to predict demand for health system resources in the United States (US). Applying a cursory meta-analysis, we review and summarize multiple modeling approaches. In addition to publicly available models, propriety modeling was created by a variety of consultancies and a variety of techniques and approaches were developed by healthcare systems. This body of work has arguably advanced the art and science of modeling and predictive analytics in healthcare, which should be hardwired for the future. Concepts such as deciding when to shift from a population-based model to a health system-experiential model, determining when isolation beds would no longer be necessary and applying shifting variables to modeling were all found to be critical to model accuracy and predictive value for healthcare administrators. National, regional, state, and local experiences varied through the early days of the pandemic (and continue to do so) and determining when to apply local knowledge over other sources of information was an elusive concept because no one source of truth was validated by a central authority.

The value of modeling to healthcare administrators addressed a multitude of needs including surveillance, market observations, trends in patient care, and prediction. The need for surveillance was most acute in the very early days of the pandemic in the United States when the first cases of COVID-19 appeared in skilled nursing facilities (SNFs) and hot spots began to appear in these congregate living facilities occupied primarily by the elderly, many of whom had chronic conditions and were at higher risk for contracting the virus. Understanding where these hot spots in the community were located allowed for anticipated hospital admission planning and preparation.[1] Further, where possible, hospitals could plan to load balance admission activity across a community to prevent any one facility from being overwhelmed. Surveillance data points included nurse triage, laboratory testing, consumer mobility, digital search, SNF infection rates, school-based infection rates, employee infection rates, international incidence rates by region and by season, i.e. Northern vs Southern Hemisphere comparing seasonal flu to COVID-19 rates.

Market data, including share of COVID-19 patients, was central to understanding impact on financial performance. In the United States there are 6,090 hospitals of which 5,141 are community hospitals. Community hospitals are defined as all nonfederal, short-term general, and other special hospitals. Other special hospitals include obstetrics and gynecology; eye, ear, nose, and throat; long-term acute-care; rehabilitation; orthopedic; and other individually described specialty services. Community hospitals include academic medical centers or other teaching hospitals if they are nonfederal short-term hospitals. Excluded are hospitals not accessible by the general public, such as prison hospitals or college infirmaries. We have a mixture of nongovernmental private not-for-profit community hospitals (2,946), investor-owned private (for-profit) hospitals (1,233) and state and local government community hospitals (962), federal government hospitals, such as the Veterans Administration (VA) hospitals (208), non-federal psychiatric hospitals (625), and other hospitals (116). Other hospitals include non-federal long-term care hospitals and hospital units within an institution such as a prison hospital or school infirmary. Long-term care hospitals may be defined by different methods; here they include other hospitals with an average length of stay (LOS) of 30 or more days. 1,805 hospitals are in rural communities, 3,336 are located in urban communities, and 3,453 hospitals are part of a larger system.[2]

Each model of hospital operational structure has its nuances, but the way in which each were managed throughout the pandemic arguably varied with different areas of focus and performance. One example is the use of observation beds versus inpatient beds. In the first instance, patients are placed in observation if it is clinically deemed that they will not stay in the hospital for an extended period, usually seventy-two (72) hours. The contracted payment rates for this level of care are markedly lower than that for an inpatient admission. The proportion of patients admitted under observation versus those admitted as inpatients varied greatly by market and provider, in some cases ranging from as little as 1% to as much as 35%. The suspension of elective surgery also varied widely, though not always the same way in each wave.

There has been some discussion regarding whether we have experienced one continuous wave with peaks and valleys or multiple waves.[3] For purposes of this discussion, we will refer to the pandemic as having multiple waves. In the case of the United States, there have been four distinct waves to date (see Figure 5.1). The first wave peaked on or about April 11, 2020, the second, on or about July 23, 2020, the third on or about January 9, 2021 (which ended with a very small surge at the of seasonal flu season on or about April 15, 2021), and the fourth which has not yet peaked as of August 26, 2021.[4] In the first wave of the pandemic in 2020, certain states mandated suspension of elective surgeries to create capacity for critically ill patients and intensive care beds, in a way influencing the effect seen above. The financial impact on the hospital industry was significant and resulted in the federal government providing relief funding to mitigate the financial strain. In the subsequent waves/peaks certain healthcare organizations voluntarily suspended elective procedures to create capacity, depending on the severity of the wave/peak in their geographic area. These decisions also had financial implications, but because they were not mandated, certain systems may have disproportionately benefited from others suspending services that they were willing to provide thereby gaining market share and experiencing financial gains.

Trends in patient care provided insights for clinical staff and administrators to better manage daily needs, especially in the context of demand for protective personal equipment (PPE) such as masks, respirators, shields, gowns, gloves, pharmaceuticals, etc. Being able to anticipate surges in volume and ensure that enough supplies were on hand was critical to patient care and staff safety. The value of predictive modeling was invaluable especially in the area of bed management and staffing, most acutely in nursing and support staff. For example, the demand for traveling nurses grew significantly over time and the ability to predict future surges to secure adequate staff in advance of a wave was critical, especially since healthcare providers were all in a competition to secure temporary staffing. One organization may have had enough beds, but those beds would be useless if there were not sufficient staff to care for patients.

CONSTANTS AND ASSUMPTIONS

Early in the pandemic and prior to it reaching the United States, modeling techniques focused on public health, population-based modeling. The first wave of general-population interest stemmed from limited access to

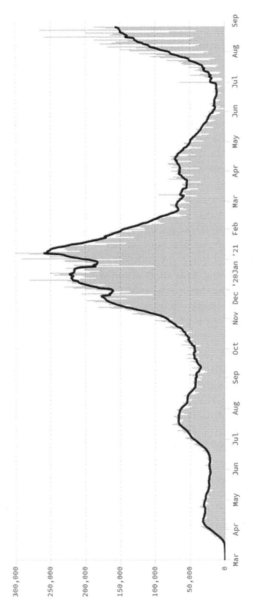

Figure 5.1 US COVID-19 cases.

real-time local data, coupled with a heavy reliance upon third-party data, particularly from overseas. This in turn caused case prediction using the SIR model (susceptible, infected, recovered) and peer-reviewed acute care literature sources to result in less accurate and wide-ranging forecasts based on the variety of assumptions employed. Various modeling teams employed techniques to predict the trajectory of the pandemic over the broadest levels of geography – i.e., the national and state levels – with the exception of the University of Chicago model which honed in on the local community level (see Table 5.1). For the most part, these early models focused on community incidence of disease, from which hospital demand could be derived by employing additional assumptions. Some were collaborative efforts, such as the COVID Act Now team which included Georgetown University, Stanford Medicine, and Harvard Global Health Institute, and some came from standalone institutions such as the University of Washington's institute for Health Metrics and Evaluation (IHME) and Johns Hopkins University & Medicine. As the pandemic progressed and local data became more readily available, particularly at the local hospital level, modeling techniques evolved to include local datasets with actual COVID-19 admissions, as opposed to expected admissions based on incidence rates. As such, the models that resulted from this new-found data targeted hospital capacity rather than the population at large, converging on a smaller and more consistent set of parameters. The models became much more accurate in their predictive capabilities, in particular reflecting tight fit for medical/surgical (Med/Surg) hospital census and intensive care unit (ICU) hospital census (see Figures 5.2 and 5.3).

EARLY PUBLIC DATA MODELING – SIR

An SIR model is an epidemiological model that computes the theoretical number of people infected with a contagious illness in a closed population over time. As explained earlier, the name of this class of models derives from the fact that they involve coupled equations relating the number of susceptible people $S(t)$, number of people infected $I(t)$, and number of people who have recovered $R(t)$. One of the simplest SIR models is the Kermack-McKendrick model, originally developed in the wake of numerous plague and cholera epidemics in London.[5] As local COVID data became available, incidence, which is a measure of the proportion of new cases per time period, became a useful variable to predict hospital admission using proportion assumptions. For example, based on acuity, a certain proportion of new cases would require admission and the exact opposite proportion would not. Additionally, as testing became more readily available and accessible, positive testing and the infection rates in the general population also became useful variables against which to project trends. This was especially useful for health systems that were operating their own testing sites. Prevalence, which is reflective of the proportion of persons who have a condition at or

Table 5.1 Public health population-based model sample

Variables	IHME[a]	COVIDActNow[b]	Penn Chime[c]	UChicago[d]	Johns Hopkins[e]	SG2	Chartis	Health Systems
Regional Population (by age)				×		×	×	×
Hospital Types				×				×
Hospital Market Share (%)			×					
Currently Hospitalized COVID-19 Patients			×					
Epidemic doubling time (every x days)							×	
R(t) infection rate		×				×	×	×
Ro (mean number of infections from first case)		×				×	×	×
SIR			×					×
LOS (Med/Surg & ICU)							×	×
Incidence rate (new cases per 100,000)	×	×			×			
Infection rate	×	×						
Positive testing rate	×	×			×			
Prevalence					×			
% population vaccinated (first dose and second dose)	×	×						
Hospitalizations/Admissions/Rates		×	×			×		×
Deaths (cumulative; daily; excess)	×	×			×	×	×	
Mask use	×							
Physical (social) distancing	×					×		
Vulnerability/risk level		×						
Susceptible, infected and recovered patients			×					

	a	b	c	d	e
Cluster detection					
Supplies (PPE)			x		
Treatments (Pharmaceutical)		x			
Licensed beds					x
Staffed beds (Med/Surg & ICU)	x		x		x
Staff-able beds					x
Swing beds					x
Triage beds					
Observation beds					
Ventilators			x	x	x
Average Daily Census (ADC)		x	x		x
Bed occupancy rate (Med/Surg & ICU)			x	x	x

a University of Washington. Institute for Health Metrics and Evaluation. http://www.healthdata.org/

b COVIDActNow. U.S. COVID Risk & Vaccine Tracker. https://covidactnow.org/?s=2223149

c Penn University of Pennsylvania. Penn Medicine Predictive Healthcare. The COVID-19 Hospital Impact Model for Epidemics. https://penn-chime.phl.io/

d The University of Chicago. The Center for Spatial Data Science. https://spatial.uchicago.edu/content/us-covid-19-atlas

e Johns Hopkins University & Medicine. Coronavirus Resource Center. https://coronavirus.jhu.edu/map.html

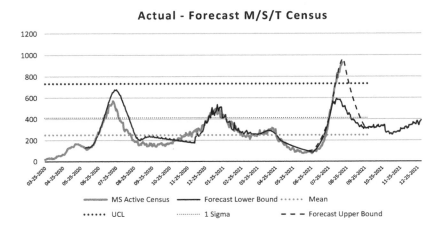

Figure 5.2 Actual – forecast M/S/T census.

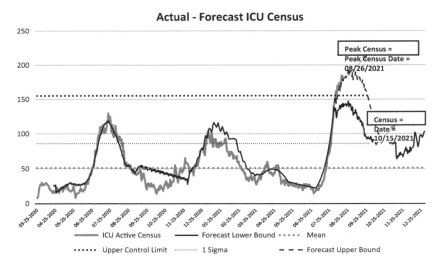

Figure 5.3 Actual – forecast ICU census.

during a particular time period, was less useful in modeling because it was not sensitive enough to predict surges in new cases which were the primary concern of hospital modeling teams.

$R(t)$ infection rate, also known as $R(t)$ or "R-effective," was a crucial element of the SIR formula because it estimates how quickly COVID-19 was spreading at a given moment. For example, an $R(t)$ of 3 indicates that one infected person will most likely infect three other people, and those three people will each go on to infect three more people. The $R(t)$ could be influenced by modifying community behavior (whether there were large gatherings or inter-community travel) and non-pharmaceutical intervention (NPI) practices (whether people wore masks and maintained physical distancing). Depending on the policy directives at the local, state, and federal levels, the $R(t)$ assumption can be adjusted to reflect those policies. In the early days of the pandemic, prior to vaccine development, the flexibility of $R(t)$ became important given that policies varied widely by region, down to the local township level. As an example, masking within schools where local school boards made the policy decision, at times in conflict with city and state mandates, could reduce $R(t)$ for that school district relative to the rest of its region. Conflicts over school policies also highlight the variability of NPI effectiveness across age groups, which along with the wide range of times that any particular intervention can be effective, makes modeling the NPI-related aspect of $R(t)$ a challenge.[6]

R_0 (a measure of the mean number of infections from 1 case), R-naught (R_0), represents the natural ability of a virus to spread in an unprotected population where no special precautions are being taken. $R(t)$, in contrast, takes into account public health measures or the development of a vaccine. This makes $R(t)$, the actual or "effective rate" of the virus under current conditions, a more accurate reflection of the number of people that a single infected person is expected to infect in a specific area at a specific time. It is also more relevant than R_0 in directing public policy and informing private behavior, given that these actions can demonstrably affect the outcome. The value of $R(t)$ can change over time, depending on such factors as how many people are staying home or wearing masks. The COVID Act Now team used $R(t)$, or infection rate, because it represented more closely what was happening at a given moment and was calculated based on actual case data.[7,8]

Epidemic doubling time, the rate in days at which the size of an infected population doubles, proved to be another valuable predictive metric as it led to the identification of hot spots that needed to be monitored more closely. This was of particular use when modeling the spread of the virus in the SNF population which was disproportionately leading to hospital admissions in the first wave/peak.[9]

Various mathematical modeling techniques were used in addition to the SIR model. The exponential model has been widely successful in capturing the increase in COVID-19 cases during the phases that developed most rapidly and thus were the most difficult to mitigate. Based on a similar principle as doubling time, the exponential model takes a simple form and essentially captures the effect of repeated doubling over time (1, 2, 4, 8, …). In this modeling, predicted values of the exponential were determined by linear regression conducted on log (numbers of cases). Another was the Polynomial (2nd-order) model. A 2nd-order polynomial ($y \sim x2 + x$) captures quadratic growth and is the expected outcome when the growth rate changes and when that rate of change is constant. The rate of increase in this model is initially faster than that of the exponential model. From this model were obtained predicted values using numerical optimization of parameters and curve fitting. Logistic modeling was also used. When exponential growth slows and tapers-off, the growth curve often becomes logistic, that is, "S" shaped. The rate of increase in this model is initially exponential but slows as an upper limit is approached. Predicted values could be obtained from this model using numerical optimization of parameters and curve fitting.

The SEIR-SD model is an epidemiological model that attempts to predict the changes in numbers of people who are susceptible to COVID-19 infection, who have been exposed to COVID-19, who have been infected and are symptomatic, and who have recovered. The SEIR model uses the total population size of your chosen location (source: US Census 2010–2019), the date of the first COVID-19 case in your chosen location, the average incubation period of COVID-19 (default = 5 days), average infectious period (default 7 days), and an initial reproductive number (default = 4). The 'SD' in the model pertains to the inclusion of social distancing as a measurable factor. The model assumes that social distancing naturally becomes more prevalent as the percent of the population infected with COVID-19 increases. The model also assumes, as we saw in real life during the first wave, that testing for COVID-19 was initially low but increased during the weeks following the first reported cases in the United States. Coefficients of Determination (also known as r-square values) were also used in modeling. These pertain to the relationship of observed values to predicted values, and so reveal the percent of variation in the observed values explained by those predicted by the model.

As vaccines became available later in the pandemic (with the Pfizer-BioNTech vaccine receiving emergency approval December 11 and the Moderna vaccine one week later), the percent of the vaccinated population could be used to reduce the probability of hospital admissions using proportions of population given the rate of breakthrough cases was statically insignificant. Applying the proportions of population receiving the first dose and the second dose of vaccine provided further refinement of projections.

HEALTH SYSTEM EXPERIENTIAL MODELING

As local datasets became available leveraging the electronic medical record (EMR), health systems could now further refine modeling using actual experience. Market share is one example of a variable that could be used to reflect the proportion of cases being admitted by facility. Traditionally, market share is calculated by dividing local facility inpatient admissions by the total inpatient admissions to all facilities in a geography. It could be further refined to reflect observation status admissions as a proportion of inpatient admissions which reflect a higher acuity and typically have longer lengths of stay i.e. >72 hours.

Hospital inpatient admission rates were used considering that a wide range of 6% to as many as 56% of positive cases would be admitted overall.[10,11,12,13] Age-adjusted admission activity had to be considered, particularly for those aged greater than 65 years, which was viewed as the most at-risk sub-population along with those with chronic comorbidities. Early assumptions considered the possibility that 67% of cases would be potentially admitted to Med/Surg. Survival rates and expiration rates were also applied to inform Med/Surg discharge rates and capacity.[14,15,16] ICU admission rates were used considering the possibility that a range of 5% to as many as 33% of cases would be admitted to ICU. Survival rates and expiration rates could also be applied to inform ICU discharge rates/capacity. Assumptions included ICU mortality rates that considered a range of 17% to as high as 49%.

COVID-19 LOS, a measure reflecting the number of days from admission to discharge, was a critical measure in predicting observation and inpatient hospital census, the number of patients in a bed at midnight (or at other times during the day). A function of admissions, discharges, patient days, location days, discharge days, and census, all are hospital statistics concepts that were first standardized by Florence Nightingale.[17] Further refining LOS, modeling the movement of a patient between levels of care was critical in predicting hospital census. Med/Surg LOS is a function of survivability and mortality and includes the average number of days that a patient requires a med/surg bed who will survive will need to be hospitalized and the average number of days that a patient requiring a med/surg bed who will expire will need to be hospitalized. During the early days of the pandemic, prior to the evolution of clinical treatment of COVID-19, such as lying patient prone to prevent the onset of pneumonia, the data ranged from 10 to 14 days. ICU LOS is a function of the average number of days that a patient who will be admitted to the ICU and survive and will spend in an ICU bed which includes survivability and mortality. LOS can be measured for two separate cohorts of patients: the average number of days that a patient who is likely to survive will require an ICU bed when hospitalized and the average number of days that a patient who is likely to expire will require an ICU bed when hospitalized. The data ranged from 1 to 56 days early in the pandemic.[18,19]

Additional LOS measures included ventilator days, reflecting the length of time a patient was on a ventilator, which were approximately 9 days. Further, early assumptions were that 3% of infected patients would require ventilators, which helped to inform the supply chain needs for ventilators which were in high demand. Finally, isolation room LOS was also a further refinement of hospital census projections given that not all critical care beds had negative air flow capability providing an additional level of protection for staff caring for COVID-19 patients.

For a more advanced approach to LOS, models could also factor in multiple possible pathways during the stays of the patient population. Along with Med/Surg/floor-only and ICU-only stays, several models account for a selection of stays with patient transfers included, such as: floor-to-ICU, ICU-to-floor, floor-to-ICU-to-floor, floor-to-ventilated ICU, and ventilated ICU-to-floor.[20] These intricacies allowed for a more realistic picture of the flow of patients between multiple wards, which then gave model users a more accurate understanding of the changes in resources needed to address the current wave appropriately. This level of detail would not have been possible without the state, city, and community-based data that made calculating average LOS across different pathways a more manageable task.

On top of patient pathways, a hospital system's capacity could also be measured by the types of beds available for patients. These included licensed beds, the number of beds for which a facility it licensed by a state to operate; staffed beds, the number of beds that are acknowledged to be staffed for utilization by a state; staff-able beds, the number of beds a facility can theoretically safely staff at maximum critical care capacity (this is a function of the skill mix of caregivers trained to operate at the highest level of care needed); swing beds, staff-able beds that can be converted to observation of inpatient beds such a post-surgical recovery beds; triage beds, beds used to determine the level of patient acuity before placement such as emergency room beds that could be scaled up in triage tents, i.e. field hospitals; observation beds, beds that are not licensed inpatient beds but are so for observational use, i.e. up to 72 hours; and overflow beds, any other beds that could be used for care such as a gurney in a hallway. Each category of bed type was used in modeling to determine need at every level of care and to determine the maximum capacity a hospital could muster before ethical triage criteria were employed (deciding who gets a bed and lives and who does not).

Modeling outputs included, most importantly, average daily census (ADC) which reflected the number of patients in any type of bed which subsequently drove staffing needs. ADC also drove supply chain demand modeling which included personal protective equipment (PPE) such as masks by type, gowns, shields, and gloves. Finally, other supply chain modeling included the demand for ventilators, oxygen, pharmaceuticals, and vaccines.

PUBLICLY AVAILABLE MODELS

Many modeling teams around the country worked to develop publicly available models. Many universities, particularly those with schools of public health, provided various alternatives for modeling including Penn, Cornell, Columbia, Johns Hopkins, The University of Chicago, and The University of South Florida. Collaborative groups were also formed most notably, The University of Washington's ESRI COVID, Institute for Health Metrics and Evaluation (IHME). No two models were identical, but each gave health system modeling team's reference points against which to test their own models and assumptions. At a certain level, these university driven models provided some solace that no one really knew where the pandemic was heading and when it would end.

Proprietary models

Proprietary modeling also took place with a variety of consultancies, each providing their own interpretation of the art and science of predictive modeling. Foremost among these included The Chartis Group, Rush and SG2, among others such as Kaufman Hall, E&Y Parthenon, and McKinsey & Company.

The Chartis Group is a comprehensive advisory and analytics services firm dedicated to the healthcare industry. Early in the pandemic the consultancy created a predictive model to assist healthcare administrators with anticipating bed need for COVID patients, including isolation rooms. SG2, a Vizient company which focuses on healthcare performance improvement, also developed modeling capabilities for their members which could be used to exclusively predict demand or as a reference for local modeling efforts. Rush and The Center for Quality, Safety & Value Analytics created a model that forecasted cases, hospital census and PPE needs including surgical gloves, vinyl and nitrile examination gloves exam vinyl, masks face procedure anti fog, mask procedure fluid resistant, gown isolation x-large yellow, mask surgical anti fog w/film, shield face full anti fog w/film, shield face full anti fog, and respirator particulate filter regular.[21]

Institutional proprietary models

Institutional health system models such as these were built by healthcare systems across the United States. In some instances, these models were shared among system leaders to, at minimum, create some sense of validity and reliability of directional accuracy of prediction. Arguably, the entire industry became smarter and more skilled in predictive analytics as a result of this work. Efforts were collaborative in nature and drew from a variety of disciplines including strategic planning, marketing, clinical, finance, performance improvement, information systems, and operations. The establishment of cross-functional modeling teams enabled cross-pollination of techniques, ideas, and approaches (see Figure 5.4).[22] Perhaps most valuable was the ability to test assumptions from a variety of perspectives, with no one approach being necessarily the correct one.

The process of forming a modeling team required suspending one's ego and inviting members that brought subject matter expertise of their own to the math table. This created an environment of intellection tension that led to better work product.[23] Teams needed to be cross-functional to leverage insight from every perspective. The process of data acquisition and processing was essential in building successful models. Perhaps most important was leveraging the EMR and supporting electronic data warehousing (EDW)

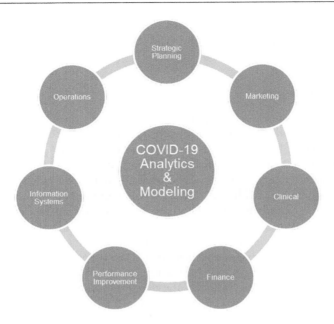

Figure 5.4 Cross-functional modeling team design.

techniques.[24] The cadence of meetings needed to be weekly at minimum to inform leadership, particularly hospital incident command system (HICS) teams which were meeting daily during surge periods. HICS is an incident management system based on principles of the Incident Command System (ICS), which assists hospitals and healthcare organizations in improving their emergency management planning, response, and recovery capabilities for unplanned and planned events. HICS is consistent with ICS and the National Incident Management System (NIMS) principles.[25]

Finally, employing the triple aim, focusing on continuous improvement and iterative learning across the dimensions of service, outcome, and cost afforded modeling teams the ability to look through the lens of each dimension and consider the implications of the model on each. Namely, was the organization positioning itself to provide the highest possible clinical care with the best outcomes, at a level of service commensurate with consumer expectations and at a cost that the organization could absorb? This approach allowed the team to focus on the most important goals of the work – saving lives.

CONCLUSION

The first lesson learned from this meta-analysis is that model accuracy greatly improved with actual local data. Reliance on other states' and countries' data, while useful in the stage of modeling when having some data was better than having no data, proved unstable; localized data enabled expanded analysis, particularly in allowing NPIs to be analyzable as a parameter. Predictive analytics enabled a new perspective of data-driven decision making, data acquisition, and analysis that requires dedicated cross-functional teams and starting simple. Manually collecting data and iterating versions over time ultimately led to more accurate modeling.

The healthcare industry could have arguably benefited from a more coordinated collaborative modeling effort, gaining efficiency insights and applying new techniques. Where collaboration has occurred, particularly within institutions, we have seen better modeling techniques stemming from the ability to share and adapt ideas among a larger group. Creating super-collaboratives among academic, private, and institutional teams could have added to the collective wisdom of the industry. Conducting a more formal meta-analysis of all models created during the pandemic will most assuredly address that opportunity.

At the same time that model builders learn from each other, they can also learn from current epidemiological research to identify and incorporate parameters outside of those discussed in this analysis. As much as focusing on the direct scope of the hospital system allowed for more accurate modeling, additional factors, some already used during the initial wave of modeling, can be helpful in describing the population being modeled. Characteristics like socioeconomic status, race, profession, and the presence of certain comorbidities have been shown to adversely affect a person's susceptibility and risk of death to COVID-19.[26,27] Even environmental factors such as temperature and humidity have altered the rate of spread.[28] With time, these factors can be acknowledged and incorporated into the frameworks of the most successful models, allowing demographic and meteorological information to tailor predictions to the situation and needs of individual communities.

Finally, once the pandemic ends, sharing of best practices in predictive analytics should begin in earnest to prepare for the next health system disaster, pandemic or otherwise.[29] The industry will only get better through sharing of knowledge and hardening the analytics skills of future generations of healthcare professionals. Much like we prepare hospital facilities for hurricanes through a hurricane hardening processes of the physical plant and infrastructure, so must we harden the analytics intellect of healthcare leaders.

REFERENCES

1 Cutts, T., Rafalski, E., Grant. C. and Marinescu, R. February, 2014. Utilization of hot spotting to identify community needs and coordinate care for high-cost patients in Memphis, TN. *Journal of Geographic Information System (JGIS)*, 6(1), 23–29.

2 American Hospital Association. https://www.aha.org/statistics/fast-facts-us-hospitals.
3 Cacciapaglia, G. et al. 2021. Multiwave pandemic explained: how to tame the next wave of diseases. *Scientific Reports*, 11(6638), 2. https://doi.org/10.1038/s41598-021-85875-2
4 https://covidactnow.org/?s=22231149. Accessed August 31, 2021.
5 Brauer, F. 2005. The Kermack-McKendrick epidemic model revisited. *Mathematical Biosciences*. 198: 2.
6 Kunst, Andrea Luviano, Yadira Peralta, Marissa Reitsma, Jose Manuel Cardona Arias Andrews, Liz Chin, Anneke Claypool, Hugo Berumen Covarrubias et al. Stanford-CIDE Coronavirus Simulation Model (SC-COSMO)–Technical Description Document, Version 2.0. (2020).
7 COVIDActNow. U.S. COVID Risk & Vaccine Tracker. https://covidactnow.org/?s=22231149
8 https://www.imperial.ac.uk/media/imperial-college/medicine/sph/ide/gida-fellowships/Imperial-College-COVID19-NPI-modelling-16-03-2020.pdf
9 Wu (Lancet): https://www.thelancet.com/journals/lancet/article/PIIS0140-6736(20)30260-9/fulltext
10 Wu (JAMA): https://jamanetwork.com/journals/jama/fullarticle/2762130
11 Guan (NEJM): https://www.nejm.org/doi/full/10.1056/NEJMoa2002032
12 Italy (Washington Post): https://www.washingtonpost.com/world/europe/coronavirus-in-italy-fills-hospital-beds-and-turns-doctors-into-patients/2020/03/03/60a723a2-5c9e-11ea-ac50-18701e14e06d_story.html
13 Stata (https://www.statnews.com/2020/03/10/simple-math-alarming-answers-covid-19/)
14 "WHO": https://www.who.int/docs/default-source/coronaviruse/who-china-joint-mission-on-covid-19-final-report.pdf
15 Wang (JAMA, based on Wuhan experience): https://jamanetwork.com/journals/jama/fullarticle/2761044
16 Reddit: https://www.reddit.com/r/Coronavirus/comments/fgdc0d/critical_care_beds_per_100000_people/
17 Florence Nightingale as Statistician. 1916. JSTOR. Publications of the American Statistical Association. Vol. 15: 116. https://doi.org/10.2307/2965763
18 https://www.imperial.ac.uk/media/imperial-college/medicine/sph/ide/gida-fellowships/Imperial-College-COVID19-NPI-modelling-16-03-2020.pdf
19 CDC: https://www.cdc.gov/nchs/data/nhsr/nhsr116.pdf
20 Klein, M. G., Cheng, C. J., Lii, E., Mao, K., Mesbahi, H., Zhu, T., Muckstadt, J. A., et al. (2020). COVID-19 Models for Hospital Surge Capacity Planning: A Systematic Review. Disaster Medicine and Public Health Preparedness, 1–8. Cambridge University Press.
21 Locey, K., Khan, J., Webb, T. and Hota, B.N. *Rush Center for Quality, Safety & Value Analytics*. Chicago, IL.
22 Mullner, R. & Rafalski, E. 2020. *Healthcare Analytics, Foundations and Frontiers*. Abingdon, Oxon. Taylor & Francis Group, LLC.
23 Wasden, C. & Wasden, M. 2014. *Tension, The Energy of Innovation*. Midway, Utah. Scipio Press.
24 Rafalski, E. 2002. Using data mining/data repository methods to identify marketing opportunities in healthcare. *Journal of Consumer Marketing*. 19(7), 607–613. https://doi.org/10.1108/07363760210451429.

25 https://emsa.ca.gov/disaster-medical-services-division-hospital-incident-command-system-resources/

26 Hawkins, Devan, Letitia Davis, and David Kriebel. 2021. COVID-19 deaths by occupation, Massachusetts, March 1–July 31, 2020. *American Journal of Industrial Medicine*, 64(4), 238–244.

27 Romagnolo, Alberto, Roberta Balestrino, Gabriele Imbalzano, Giovannino Ciccone, Franco Riccardini, Carlo Alberto Artusi, Marco Bozzali et al. 2021. Neurological comorbidity and severity of COVID-19. *Journal of Neurology* 268(3), 762–769.

28 Kodera, Sachiko, Essam A. Rashed, and Akimasa Hirata. 2020. Correlation between COVID-19 morbidity and mortality rates in Japan and local population density, temperature, and absolute humidity. *International Journal of Environmental Research and Public Health* 17(15), 5477.

29 Skinner, R. 2010. *GIS in Hospital and Healthcare Emergency Management.* Boca Raton, FL. CRC Press.

Chapter 6

Quantifying and responding to COVID's financial and operational impact

Mark Grube
JMP Ventures
Delray Beach, FL, USA

Rob Fromberg
Kaufman Hall
Chicago, IL, USA

CONTENTS

An approach to modeling..62
The state of play...63
Strategic goals for an uncertain future...65
    Live to fight another day...66
    Rethink the future in a post-COVID world 66
    Manage the shift to outpatient settings 66
    Aggressively pursue no-regrets strategies..................................67
Conclusion: Regaining lost balance 68

At the time of this writing, 18 months into the COVID-19 pandemic, America's hospitals still faced significant, ongoing financial instability. With cases and hospitalizations once again on the rise with the rapid spread of the Delta variant, physicians, nurses, and other hospital personnel continued working tirelessly to care for COVID-19 patients. At the same time, hospitals were experiencing profound net income losses likely to continue throughout the rest of 2021.

For the entire pandemic period, hospitals and health system leaders have needed to confront unprecedented uncertainty while at the same time guiding their organizations toward long-term strategic and operational visions into a hard-to-understand future.

This task requires demand modeling, data analysis, and financial planning that is very likely more sophisticated than any most hospital organizations have ever undertaken. At the same time, it requires leadership that is focused not on returning to a pre-pandemic comfort zone, but on a truly new and largely unknown environment.

DOI: 10.1201/9781003204138-8

AN APPROACH TO MODELING

A recommended approach to modeling the future impact of the COVID-19 pandemic and other external factors affecting hospital performance should focus on three key elements: market context, volume recovery, and impact scenarios.

Those three elements can be thought of in terms of the following three questions:

1. What market forces will affect volume and financial recovery? Those factors could include:
   - Unemployment and payer mix shifts
   - Consumer price sensitivity and delays in care due to cost
   - Patients' willingness to return
   - Reduced travel and tourism

2. What are the anticipated volume recovery trends across forecast groups? Those trends could include:
   - Lag in return to hospital vs. ambulatory
   - Required capacity and resource constraints
   - COVID-19 hospitalization scenarios

3. How do we anticipate impact across the healthcare provider land-scape? Answering this question involves:
   - Linking model outputs to global drivers
   - Developing potential scenarios and sensitivity analyses

The model should include assumptions of rate of volume recovery based on consumer surveys, volume recovery based on COVID-19 archetypes, and revenue recovery based on payer mix and patient population shifts. Optimistic and pessimistic scenarios should be modeled to understand range in performance.

Once the model is developed, it needs to be loaded with the best available data from as large a pool of sources as possible. That data should include performance before the pandemic, during the pandemic, and most current performance.

Key metrics to track include at a minimum:

- Total operating revenue per patient day
- Total operating expense per patient day
- Total volume
- Total revenue
- Total expense
- Operating margin

THE STATE OF PLAY

What has actual data and model shown us about the current and possible future state of play? As of the summer of 2021, hospitals were still struggling to regain pre-pandemic performance levels (Kaufman Hall National Hospital Flash Report, August 2021). Volumes remained significantly below pre-pandemic levels, with results suggesting that some healthcare consumers once again may be postponing non-urgent procedures and other outpatient care due to COVID-19 concerns. Although revenues were higher than pre-pandemic levels, margins were lower due to escalating expenses (see Figure 6.1).

A forecast using the methodology outlined above showed that as of mid-2021, hospitals were poised to lose an estimated $54 billion in net income over the course of the year, even taking into account federal Coronavirus Aid, Relief, and Economic Security (CARES) Act funding from 2020 (see Figure 6.2).

An increase in high-acuity patients contributed to the forecast losses. The median length of stay was up 8% as of mid-2021 date compared to 2019 for most hospitals, indicating higher-acuity patients, and up as high as 18% for some hospitals with 500 beds or more.

One-time Provider Relief Fund payments contributed to a temporary growth in revenues. Also, most hospitals continued to see a shift in revenue, with higher cost inpatient services making up a larger share of overall revenue than prior to the pandemic. However, the higher expenses associated with those patients put downward pressure on income.

Meanwhile, although outpatient revenue was slightly up compared to 2019, the accompanying increase in inpatient services was such that the portion of outpatient revenue to total revenue is down for many organizations.

Median Change in Hospital Performance: January-July 2021

Median Change Jan.-July 2021		From YTD 2020	From YTD 2019
Margin	Operating Margin (w/out CARES)	5.6 percentage points	(0.6 percentage point)
	Operating Margin (w/CARES)	2.4 percentage points	0.2 percentage point
Volume	Adjusted Discharges	9%	(4%)
	OR Minutes	17%	0%
	ED Visits	5%	(13%)
Revenue	Gross IP Revenue	11%	4%
	Gross OP Revenue	22%	10%
Expenses	Total Expense per Adjusted Discharge	0%	14%

- The median Kaufman Hall hospital Operating Margin Index was 3.2% in July, not including federal Key Observations CARES aid. With the funding, it was 4.1%. The median Operating EBITDA Margin for the month was 7.7% without CARES and 8.9% with CARES.

- Adjusted Discharges fell 3.9% below 2019 YTD results, but were up 8.7% compared to January-July 2020. ED Visits fell 13.1% YTD below 2019 levels but were up 5% YTD versus the same period in 2020.

- Outpatient Revenue increased 10% YTD versus 2019 and 21.6% YTD versus 2020. Compared to June, however, Outpatient Revenue was down nearly 2%.

- Total Expense per Adjusted Discharge rose 14.1% versus January-July 2019, but was essentially flat (down just 0.2%) compared to the same period in 2020.

* Note: The Kaufman Hall Hospital Operating Margin and Operating EBITDA Margin indices are comprised of the national median of our dataset adjusted for allocations to hospitals from corporate, physician, and other entities.

Figure 6.1 Median change in hospital performance: January–July 2021.

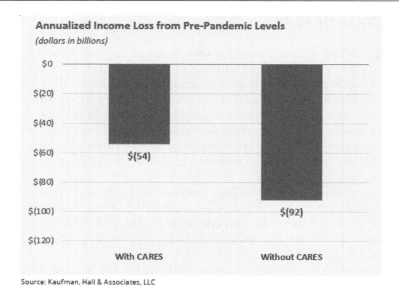

Source: Kaufman, Hall & Associates, LLC

Figure 6.2 Annualized income loss from pre-pandemic levels.

This suggested that patients as of mid-2021 continued to delay outpatient services due to pandemic concerns. At the worst-hit hospitals for this trend, the share of outpatient revenue dropped 20% compared to pre-pandemic levels.

The forecast also showed that hospital margins would likely remain below pre-pandemic levels throughout 2021 (see Figure 6.3).

Hospital margins are expected to remain close to Q2 performance, shifting only slightly to 10% and 11% below pre-pandemic levels in Q3 and Q4, respectively. However, it is important to note that these projections do not factor in recent increases in COVID-19 cases from the Delta variant, which could drive margins even lower in the second half of the year. More than a third of U.S. hospitals were expected to have negative operating margins through year's end.

This forecast reflects margin deficits that would inhibit hospitals' ability to invest in growth or additional community services throughout 2021.

This slow performance recovery was driven by several contributing factors.

Sicker patients. Hospitals were seeing more high acuity, inpatient cases—including COVID-19 patients—requiring longer lengths of stay than prior to the pandemic in 2019. While such cases contributed to revenue increases, any gains were offset by higher care costs for treating patients with more severe conditions.

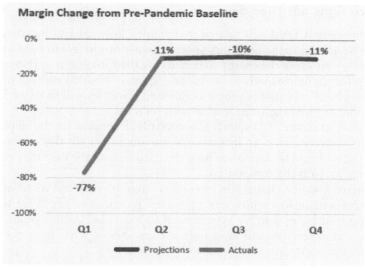

Margin Change from Pre-Pandemic Baseline

Source: Kaufman, Hall & Associates, LLC

Figure 6.3 Margin change from pre-pandemic baseline.

Higher expenses. Expenses rose across the board, as hospitals faced increasing costs for labor, drugs, purchased services, personal protective equipment (PPE), and other medical and safety supplies needed to care for higher acuity patients.

Fewer outpatient visits. Hospital outpatient visits—which tend to have lower expenses and higher margins—remained depressed compared to 2019 levels. As of mid-2021, they had not yet fully recovered after plummeting with nationwide shutdowns and COVID-19 mitigation efforts in the early months of the pandemic in 2020.

STRATEGIC GOALS FOR AN UNCERTAIN FUTURE

Hospitals and health systems face uncertainty regarding several key factors that will influence the future delivery system. These factors include (1) the pace of hospital inpatient, outpatient, and emergency department volumes return to pre-pandemic levels; (2) the ways in which post-COVID America, its economy, and its culture will affect the relative strengths of traditional healthcare provider organizations; and (3) the ways in which COVID-19, having greatly accelerated the growth of virtual business models, will effect basic patient care delivery and the encroachment of non-traditional competitors on that traditional delivery system.

Live to fight another day

Amid lingering COVID-19 related uncertainty, hospital and health system leaders need to take the necessary short-term actions to live to fight another day, while mustering the energy to recalibrate their long-term trajectory and prepare for an increasingly value-based payment model. Leadership teams with the ability to multitask those competing priorities will have the broadest options for blazing a sustainable path forward.

The cost structure of hospitals is necessarily dependent on the slope of its revenue recovery curve, an increasingly moving target. To this end, organizations must begin to determine how the total cost of the care they provide measures up with the competition.

Ultimately, major changes in operations may be required to adjust to a long-term revenue loss whose exact level still remains unclear. What will the resulting healthcare delivery system need to look like? At this point, many boards and executives still have only a hazy idea of what their organization's new cost structure will need to be.

Rethink the future in a post-COVID world

Beyond the immediate financial and operational challenges of the pandemic, healthcare executives must also decide how to best steer their organizations toward a successful long-term operating model.

For hospitals and health systems, future success will depend on how well they can respond to customer needs at "purchasing events," when employees select health plans from their employers or consumers with non-acute issues decide where to access care.

At the same time, the technology sector's economic dominance significantly accelerated since the start of the pandemic. Verticals with a face-to-face orientation (e.g., retail, hospitality, and live entertainment) have been devastated by COVID-19. Within healthcare, access on demand is a new requirement for success.

More than ever, scale is critical to achieve these goals. Signs suggest that health systems are moving beyond their traditional geographies in new merger activity, as the pandemic has accelerated the need to transform care delivery models and reimagine health system configuration. Systems also are restructuring their portfolios to monetize or exit underperforming assets and strengthen their financial viability.

Manage the shift to outpatient settings

The COVID-19 pandemic is likely to intensify decades-long movement from inpatient to outpatient care delivery settings. As shown in Figure 6.4, as of 2020 the long-time dominance of inpatient over outpatient revenue has flipped, with outpatient services constituting 60% of total revenue for hospitals (AHA, Kaufman Hall).

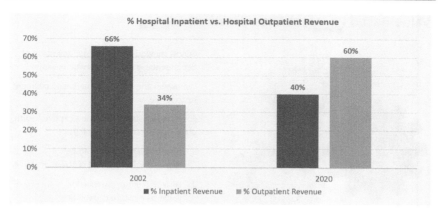

Source: American Hospital Association and Kaufman Hall proprietary data

Figure 6.4 Percentage of hospital inpatient vs. hospital outpatient revenue.

Hospitals and health systems also must be able to compete in an environment where patients are cared for in the home by physicians, nurse practitioners, therapists, and home health aides—*instead* of inpatient care or *after* hospital discharge. The Centers for Medicare & Medicaid Services' Acute Care at Home Waiver, launched during COVID-19, is expected to be permanent, providing reimbursement for Medicare patients in this setting. Almost 200 health systems are taking advantage of this waiver, including the largest systems in the country. And a coalition called Moving Health Home includes Amazon Care, CVS Health, large integrated systems such as Ascension and Advocate Aurora, and many companies providing therapeutic services.

Aggressively pursue no-regrets strategies

The financial challenges brought on by COVID-19 will likely only increase the need for vertical alignment and readiness for value-based care. At the same time, health plans and providers will have a greater incentive to integrate and maximize performance in value-based arrangements (Figure 6.5), a growing proportion of total revenue. This may involve expanding existing relationships or developing new partnerships to increase the number of covered lives across the most profitable lines of business, such as commercial and Medicare Advantage plans.

Rebalancing asset allocation across the service delivery system can help reduce operating risk as external risks remain high. This might include converting short-term financing to permanent financing, and scrubbing operating models for accumulated assets that have increased operating risk but are not positively contributing to operating performance.

Value-Based Payment Considerations

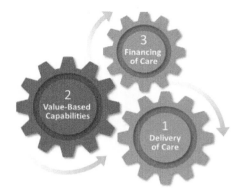

COVID showed the economic downside of dependence on fee-for-service revenue

We expect the shift to value-based payment to continue

For health systems without a captive health plan, that means determining:

1. How delivery of care can be more coordinated and efficient

2. How to build or partner for value-based care capabilities

3. Whether and how to partner with purchasers/payers

Figure 6.5 Value-based payment considerations.

CONCLUSION: REGAINING LOST BALANCE

Current analyses and future projections underscore the ways in which COVID-19 has continued to create not only clinical but also financial challenges for hospitals. Even as overall hospital revenues are improving, they are offset by mounting expenses in caring for greater numbers of sicker, high-acuity patients who require longer hospital stays, more supplies and staff time, and more resources overall.

While many hospital leaders hoped 2021 would provide an opportunity to return their organizations to greater financial stability after the severe losses seen in 2020, those hopes are dimming as the virus continues to circulate throughout the population. As of this writing, the surge in COVID-19 patients driven by spread of the highly contagious Delta variant threatened to set hospitals back even more—heightening the need for thoughtful, responsive strategies for both short-term and long-term recovery.

Organizations with weak capitalization pre-COVID are likely to face significant short- and long-term viability concerns, and their leaders may need to consider partnering with other organizations in the near future.

Moderately affected organizations with median liquidity, leverage, and profitability prior to the pandemic will likely face more short-term COVID-related pressures and have an opportunity to reinvigorate their operating models moving forward.

Organizations with limited COVID-related balance sheet and operating damage have a significant, once-in-a-generation opportunity to allocate capital and leadership toward their long-term strategic goals.

For providers, the healthcare environment has never been static, but change has been incremental and to a great extent predictable. The COVID-19 pandemic has brought new, unpredictable external forces to healthcare that have already begun to affect the nature of healthcare's competitive dynamic and accelerate the pace of change. To weather this new environment, healthcare organizations need to achieve a new basis of stability. And they will need financial, strategic, and human resources to pivot to an environment that demands innovation in the face of new and intensified competitive pressures.

Section 2

State case studies

Chapter 7

Measuring and addressing healthcare employee well-being in an Alabama health system during COVID-19

Katherine A. Meese
The University of Alabama at Birmingham
Birmingham, AL, USA

Alejandra Colon-Lopez
The University of Alabama at Birmingham
Birmingham, AL, USA

Ashleigh M. Allgood
The University of Alabama at Birmingham
Birmingham, AL, USA

Davis A. Rogers
The University of Alabama at Birmingham
Birmingham, AL, USA

CONTENTS

Introduction 74
Before the crisis 74
Measuring well-being 74
Maintaining well-being in crisis 76
Assessing well-being during the pandemic 77
    Data collection 77
    Results 78
Employee considerations for pandemic preparedness 80
    Staffing 80
    Well-being 82
    Healthy teams 82
    Perceived organizational support 82
    Ability to solicit rapid and frequent feedback 83
The recovery period 83
References 84

DOI: 10.1201/9781003204138-10

INTRODUCTION

The COVID-19 pandemic brought a unique constellation of stressors to the doorstep of almost every person on the planet. Across the globe, few were exempt from its physical, social, and economic impacts (Pfefferbaum and North 2020; Wren-Lewis 2020). In the United States, hospitals and health systems faced supply shortages and demand overload (Solomon, Wynia, and Gostin 2020). Additionally, due to the unknowns surrounding virus transmission and treatment early in the pandemic, and the severity of the virus, both patients and healthcare workers were susceptible to infection, complications, and death (Ashcroft et al. 2020). A parallel crisis also began to emerge as healthcare workers, a highly resilient segment of the population, dealt with mounting pressures at home and at work leading to distress and deteriorating mental health (Bradley and Chahar 2020). Within the healthcare setting, clinicians were burdened by the barrage of COVID-19 patients, understaffing due to sick or quarantining colleagues, frequent deaths, and their own exposures and infection with the virus. In many cases, they were also dealing with pay cuts and furloughs (Carroll and Smith 2020; Collins and Haigh 2020; Paavola 2020), closed daycares and schools (Donohue and Miller 2020), job losses of spouses or partners, and illness and death of family members (Thomeer, Yahirun, and Colón-López 2020). While healthcare systems had many priorities ranging from public health, securing supplies, and implementing COVID-19 protocols, the focus of this chapter will be on the wellness of the healthcare workforce as a condition of emergency preparedness and how to measure it. The chapter will use a case study from UAB Medicine, a large academic hospital system in Alabama affiliated with the University of Alabama at Birmingham (UAB).

BEFORE THE CRISIS

Long before the pandemic, the well-being of healthcare workers has been a serious problem. Physicians, nurses, and Advanced Practice Providers (APPs) suffer high rates of burnout (Berg 2020; King and Leigh 2019; Wittkieffer 2019). Physician suicide rates are nearly twice that of the same age adjusted population (Lindeman et al. 1996). As a result, many healthcare organizations appointed a Chief Wellness Officer (CWO) in an attempt to identify and mitigate sources of employee burnout (Ripp and Shanafelt 2020). Several strategies have been suggested to mitigate burnout within the healthcare context. A critical component of managing employee well-being is to ensure that there is a routine way to measure it and to identify its correlates.

MEASURING WELL-BEING

To measure well-being, UAB Medicine implemented a tool called the Well-Being Index (WBI). This tool includes a validated measure of distress and a

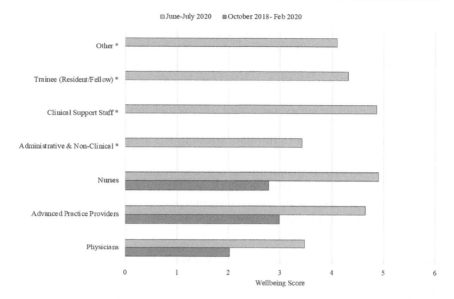

Figure 7.1 Change in WBI distress score from pre-pandemic to early pandemic phases.

confidential self-assessment tool for individuals to better understand their own well-being (Dyrbye et al. 2013, 2019; Dyrbye, Satele, and Shanafelt 2016). This tool was first implemented with physicians, APPs, residents, and medical students, and then had been extended to nurses and finally all UAB Medicine employees right as the pandemic was beginning in February 2020.

The online assessment tool allows UAB Medicine to provide periodic reports to leaders with the aggregate results of WBI scores across various employee sub-populations.

Consistent with national trends, many employees were experiencing high distress prior to the pandemic. A WBI> = 2 is considered "high distress" for the general population and is associated with increased risk of burnout, suicidal ideation, and turnover intentions (Beresin et al. 2016; Dyrbye et al. 2013, 2019, 2016; Menon et al. 2020; Tawfik et al. 2018) (Figure 7.1).

Based on these pre-pandemic levels, UAB Medicine Office of Wellness was actively involved in trying to mitigate sources of distress. These efforts were based on the Jobs Demands-Resources (JD-R) model of well-being, which suggests that well-being occurs when an individual has sufficient resources to meet their demands (Bakker and Demerouti 2007). Changes to achieve this balance can either be made to the demands or resources side of the equation. Improving job-related resources had two components. The first was to improve and develop support programs. To that end, resources were expanded to include additional counseling and coaching support and to connect employees to existing resources such as the Employee Assistance Program (Joseph, Walker, and Fuller-Tyszkiewicz

2018), and lobbying for expanded childcare resources (Blake et al. 2020). The other area of focus was in reducing demands and this element of the program included two areas (Demerouti et al. 2001). The first was to develop objective measures of the work of teams using industrial engineering processes combined with validated measures of engagement and burnout. These measures would be used to better understand the relationship of work processes to engagement and to consider this relationship before change was undertaken. These measures were also used by leadership to thoughtfully plan change to mitigate stress to the greatest degree possible and to aspire to improve wellness and burnout.

When the COVID-19 pandemic struck, the health system had to drastically pivot and rapidly adapt to changing conditions. Additionally, efforts to support employee well-being had to metamorphosize to meet the myriad of challenges facing the healthcare workforce.

MAINTAINING WELL-BEING IN CRISIS

The pandemic changed the focus of wellness efforts and was informed through the JD-R model (Bakker and Demerouti 2007). This pandemic brought a massive increase in demands that included physical, psychological, and social elements (Britt et al. 2021). Our initial efforts were related to physical demands in the form of threats to safety of frontline providers and their families. News from other parts of the country shed light on the dire situations where providers were compelled to deliver care with inadequate, improvised or no professional protective equipment (Beusekom 2020). The main area of focus of the health system was in developing alternatives to the N-95 masks given the fact that COVID-19 was predominately spread via respiratory droplets. There were several groups that were working on alternatives and began connecting these groups. A re-sterilization process for N-95 masks was developed and implemented while the health system awaited additional supplies.

A second area of initial emphasis was advocating for housing and meals for providers who had been exposed to COVID-19. Housing was emphasized because providers would be anxious between the exposure to an infected patient and testing and would not want to expose people living with them to the virus (Bekele, Mechessa, and Sefera 2021; Thomeer et al. 2020). This illustrates that this new job-related demand had physical, psychological, and social dimensions. Housing alternatives were brought online in several days using nearby hotels and empty dormitories. Fortunately, the community expressed their desire to appreciate frontline providers with donations of food and a community-based initiative was developed in partnership to distribute meals to the front line.

Simultaneously, the organization was grappling with the uncertainty of the financial impact due to the cancellation of elective surgeries (Carroll and

Smith 2020). Initially, it was unknown when surgeries would be able to resume and whether or how much federal funding would arrive to help keep hospitals afloat, which resulted in pay cuts and layoffs across the country. As a result, UAB Medicine prioritized keeping as many employees as possible and had minimal furloughs. However, in order to do this, they needed to implement pay cuts, which were graduated based on income with administration taking the largest percentage cut.

ASSESSING WELL-BEING DURING THE PANDEMIC

A limitation of the existing WBI self-assessment tool is that there are restrictions on how the data can be accessed or analyzed (Dyrbye et al. 2016). While this ensures absolute anonymity, it also precludes more sophisticated analytic techniques. This is a similar problem with many vendor-offered solutions around measuring employee engagement. The opacity of the measures and constructs and the inability to analyze the raw data has the potential to occlude the details of the story the data can tell. Additionally, while the WBI tool allowed us to add a few open-ended questions, this did not seem sufficient to capture the diversity and quantity of unique stressors affecting different employee sub-groups.

Data collection

As the pandemic marched slowly to Alabama's doorstep, responses from the rest of the country made it clear that UAB Medicine's healthcare workers would be under tremendous stress. UAB Medicine Office of Wellness wanted a way to hear voices from the front line, distill important trends and concerns, and provide actionable data to leadership in a methodologically rigorous and statistically valid way. An all-employee survey would allow for rapid data collection. However, there was some debate about the appropriateness of an employee survey as the pandemic pressures mounted. On one hand, some viewed it to be insensitive to ask stressed and burdened employees to complete a survey. On the other hand, some viewed it as insensitive *not* to ask all employees how they were doing and to give them a chance to share feedback given the stressful environment. The communication surrounding the survey positioned it as a way for the UAB Medicine Office of Wellness to hear every employee's voice and input and to identify areas of high distress that might need urgent or immediate intervention.

A survey was rapidly developed, largely using existing validated measures. The WBI questions were used to assess distress, as UAB Medicine had already some baseline, pre-pandemic data from physicians, nurses, and APPs. In addition to the WBI, we also used measures from the Veteran's Affairs annual employee survey which contains items such as psychological safety, moral distress, and civility. We also asked employees to select their major general work, clinical, and non-work-related stressors from a multiple selection list. This list of potential stressors was developed in collaboration with a multi-disciplinary team including nurses, an APP, physicians, a psychologist, wellness champions, and administration. General work stressors included things like heavy workload and long hours, increased job demands and responsibilities, rapid changes in workflows and policies, fear of exposure to COVID-19 while at work, and discrimination. Clinical stressors included lack of PPE, difficulty accessing testing, COVID-19 exposure, uncertainty about how to treat COVID-19 patients, patients receiving poor treatment, and adaptation to telemedicine. Non-work stressors included items such as ill family members, social isolation and loneliness, childcare, eldercare, strained relationships, and fear of infecting family. A fill-in-the-blank option was also included in each category. Lastly, we partnered with the leadership of the inpatient and outpatient telemedicine effort to ask a few targeted questions of telemedicine users. This included their perceptions of inpatient and/or outpatient telemedicine for patient care, their own satisfaction with it, major benefits and frustrations.

We had to carefully balance our two goals with the survey: (1) Help inform leadership decision-making with timely and actionable data and (2) collect data in such a way that it could be used for scholarship and to effect broader changes within the industry. Generally, a short survey would garner greater responses, pose less of a burden to our workforce, and would be sufficient for leadership decision-making. However, this would preclude us from using validated instruments that would allow us to generate rigorous scholarly work. We aimed to find the shortest possible measures for constructs of interest that had also been previously used and validated. While this prevented the use of certain "gold standard" instruments, it allowed us to balance our operational and scholarly aims.

Results

We expected a low response rate, given the pressure everyone was under both at work and outside of work, rapidly adapting to pandemic life. Surprisingly, over 1,130 people responded, for a response rate of 18%. Given the immense pressure and length of the survey, we considered this a success. We received positive feedback that getting the survey made people feel seen, heard, and that their opinion mattered. Receiving such a survey seemed to validate that there was an understanding that things were uniquely stressful for everyone.

Interestingly, the survey provided detailed insight into what factors were driving distress among various employee sub-groups. It also highlighted that the entire care team was at risk for high distress (Meese et al. 2021) (see Figure 7.2), despite the disproportionate share of attention on physician and nurse burnout in the media and in prior research.

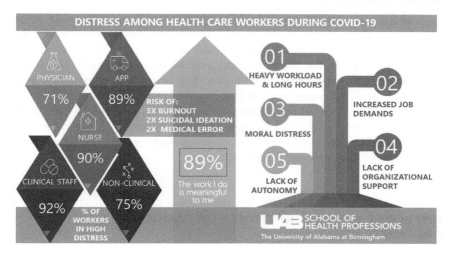

Figure 7.2 Key results from all employee survey during COVID-19. (Adapted from Meese, K. A., Colón-López, A., Singh, J. A., Burkholder, G. A., & Rogers, D. A. (2021). Healthcare is a Team Sport: Stress, Resilience, and Correlates of Well-Being Among Health System Employees in a Crisis. *Journal of Healthcare Management/American College of Healthcare Executives*, 66(4), 304–322. https://doi.org/10.1097/JHM-D-20-00288.)

There were several overarching themes and concepts that arose from the data:

1. <u>It is the work</u> – Despite collecting a variety of general work, clinical and non-work stressors when we conducted dominance analysis of the regression model on distress, the top items that contributed to overall distress were work-related. Additionally, they were general work stressors, not clinical stressors. This was surprising given the number of unique and intense clinical stressors such as PPE and testing shortages. However, our interpretation is that many of our clinicians were well trained and equipped to deal with other infectious diseases, and thus the stress of a new one was not the core driver of distress. While we know that non-work stressors were considerable during this time, very few were significantly associated with distress, except for social isolation and loneliness and fear of exposing one's family.
2. <u>All groups are at risk</u> – Despite the focus on physicians and nurses in the burnout literature and the news media, we found that all healthcare employees are at risk for high distress. Clinical support staff, nurses, and APPs had the highest distress, followed by administrative and non-clinical employees and physicians.
3. <u>Positive changes for one group may mean negative changes for another</u> – We found that inpatient telemedicine was generally positively

received by physicians and APPs, but that this was perceived of coming at the expense of the nurse. Nurses felt they were entering the patient's room more to help patients use the inpatient telemedicine technology so that the physician could be more protected. This highlighted the importance of understanding how an intervention affects the entire care team, not just one group of end users.

4. Staffing – Given the staffing shortages brought about by employee illness, early retirement or exit from the workforce, and departure for higher-paying traveler jobs, understaffing appeared to be the root cause of the top three drivers of distress.

EMPLOYEE CONSIDERATIONS FOR PANDEMIC PREPAREDNESS

Staffing

Staffing for a hospital is generally the most expensive item on the income statement (Zhao et al. 2008). As financial pressures have mounted amid declining reimbursements to hospitals, CEO's have also cited financial concerns in challenges and shortages of healthcare providers the two top concerns facing health care (American College of Healthcare 2020). Thus, it logically follows that hospital leaders face both financial and supply pressures which might result in lean staffing in the clinical enterprise (Kumar, Subramanian, and Strandholm 2002). Clinician-to-patient ratios are often kept as low as possible while ensuring a specified standard of quality that ensures financial survival and performance. Prior to the pandemic, these lean staffing ratios led to increased expectations for physicians to see more patients during shorter visits, adding to the burnout epidemic (Army and Cantonment 2019).

However, an even more serious complication of these lean staffing practices came to light during the pandemic. Staffing just enough to handle current volumes leaves very little capacity for drastic changes in supply of clinicians or demand from patients, leaving the hospital, and more broadly, the nation's healthcare infrastructure, vulnerable (Weissman et al. 2020). The COVID-19 pandemic brought this weakness in infrastructure to light in a way that prior disasters could not – by a surge of patients happening concurrently with an exodus of clinicians.

In other types of disasters such as a tornado, flood, or hurricane, the hospital will often designate a "ride-out" team of staff and clinicians to ensure that the hospital is able to protect its critical workers and handle an influx of patients that is expected to arrive immediately after (Labdi 2006; Smith 2019). While this leads to a surge in patients, the hospital can also ensure that they are staffed at maximum capacity in response. However, with COVID-19, the patients surged, and clinicians were scarce for several reasons, including:

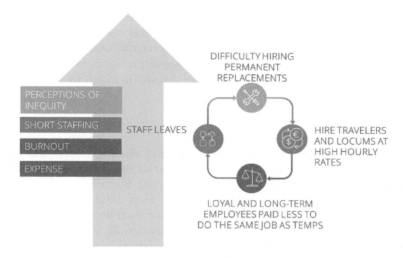

DIFFICULTY HIRING
PERMANENT
REPLACEMENTS

PERCEPTIONS OF
INEQUITY

SHORT STAFFING   STAFF LEAVES   HIRE TRAVELERS
                                              AND LOCUMS AT
BURNOUT   HIGH HOURLY
                                              RATES
EXPENSE

LOYAL AND LONG-TERM
EMPLOYEES PAID LESS TO
DO THE SAME JOB AS TEMPS

Figure 7.3 The curious case of traveling nurses.

- Awaiting testing after a potential exposure
- Quarantining after an exposure or positive result
- Higher risk of COVID infection due exposure risk from patients and colleagues
- Exiting the workforce or early retirement due to fears and concerns about contracting COVID
- Leaving the hospital for higher paying traveler/locum jobs or hazard pay
- Furlough or job loss typically due to financial pressures

What resulted from lean staffing ratios before the pandemic was a workforce drastically understaffed to handle to surge of patients during the pandemic, resulting in taxing and unsustainable workloads for the remaining staff (Long et al. 2020). The acute shortages in staffing have led to somewhat of a downward spiral involving travel nurses and staff or locum tenens clinicians. Specifically for nurses, many hospitals and travel agencies offered high wages and hazard pay for staffing COVID units. Nurses left to take traveling jobs, while others chose to exit the workforce to care for children at home (with daycares closed) or to take an early retirement (as the risk of exposure outweighed the rewards of the job). This led to drastic workforce shortages, which required the hospital to fill needed spots with expensive traveling nurses. However, the end result was that the nurses that showed loyalty to the organization and stayed ended up getting paid less than travel nurses doing the same or similar jobs. This caused discontentment which led to further departures from the workforce, resulting in an ongoing cycle (see Figure 7.3). While strategies are underway to break this cycle, the long -term effects of using travelers for surge staffing need to be considered as a condition of preparedness.

In order to create more resilient hospitals and health systems in the face of future pandemics, norms around staffing and clinician–patient ratios must be challenged (Aiken et al. 2002). However, this cannot be done effectively without addressing the intense financial pressures hospitals face. If hospitals are to be staffed with a potential disaster in mind, we must be willing to pay for it.

Well-being

Maintaining a healthy work environment and tending to the well-being of healthcare workers is a critical component of organizational resilience. Simply put, when an individual is in distress or burned out, their ability to handle a massive crisis is diminished (De Hert 2020). They simply do not have enough excess emotional capacity for such an event, particularly an extended event. Taking a physically and emotionally exhausted, burned-out clinician and drastically increasing their patient load with severely ill patients with a high likelihood of death is a recipe for disaster. If a healthcare worker is in a state of well-being under the normal conditions of their job, they are more likely to have the physical, emotional, and mental stamina to withstand a crisis.

Healthy teams

In addition to maintaining the health and well-being of its workers, hospitals have a responsibility to maintain the health of their teams. Teams that have cultivated trust, belonging, and psychological safety may offer a more supportive environment and protective effects against external crises (Kessel, Kratzer, and Schultz 2012). When the pandemic hit, UAB Medicine was in the early stages of implementing an Accountable Care Team (ACT) intervention. This intervention is aimed at flattening the traditional physician hierarchy by creating a leadership triad and developing healthy team functioning behaviors and systems thinking. The preliminary survey results showed that ACT team members felt a greater sense of community at work and perceived greater support from the organization. Ensuring healthy teams may be an important condition of helping individuals withstand prolonged crises.

Perceived organizational support

Maintaining a high level of organizational support for employees is a crucial element of preparedness (Panaccio and Vandenberghe 2009). The data collected on employee well-being during COVID-19 at UAB Medicine showed that perceived organizational support was associated with lower distress (Meese et al. 2021). Perceived organizational support measured specifically, the degree to which employees felt that UAB medicine cared about them and valued their extra efforts and contributions.

Additionally, those with greater perceived organizational support were less likely to view the pay cuts as inequitable and were less likely to report concerns about PPE. Perceived organizational support is something that is developed over time and accumulates (or diminishes) as an employee spends more time in the organization. This is not something that can be developed during a crisis but must be strengthened prior to a crisis to create a buffer to protect employees' well-being. Showing high concern for people during a crisis can further serve to increase perceptions of support. One example was UAB Medicine's goal to keep as many people in their jobs as possible, even amid great financial uncertainty. This resulted in broad pay cuts, including the highest percentage decrease in compensation for senior leaders. Efforts to procure additional PPE and rapidly develop alternative and safe PPE solutions further helped to increase feelings of organizational support. This element is critical to buffering increased distress during a crisis.

Ability to solicit rapid and frequent feedback

Lastly, organizations must be ready and able to rapidly gather employee feedback. During a crisis, rapid decisions must often be made. However, gathering feedback from those most affected by the changes will likely result in better outcomes. The people on the front lines often have the best solutions for how to fix problems at the front lines, but their voices are not always heard. The nature of crisis decision-making does not always allow time for committee meetings, focus groups, or slow methods of soliciting feedback.

Organizations must have both a mechanism for rapid data collection and input, as well as a culture of soliciting and incorporating feedback from all levels of the organization. Rapid pulse surveys on specific issues can help meet this aim, but people will disengage from these types of surveys over time if they feel that their input and feedback is not incorporated or considered. Therefore, organizations must also have a mechanism in place to share results and explain how decisions have been influenced or changed by those results.

THE RECOVERY PERIOD

Traditional models of disaster recovery suggest that emotional recovery after a disaster really starts to steadily improve at or just after the one-year anniversary of the event (DeWolfe 2000). This model has been used to understand recovery after discrete events such as hurricanes, earthquakes and tornadoes. However, the difference with the COVID-19 pandemic is that the acute crisis – particularly for healthcare workers – did not even start to subside until over a year after it began with the introduction and dissemination of vaccines. As a result, the healthcare industry should expect a prolonged period of mental and emotional recovery given the duration and intensity of the crisis.

There will likely be vestiges of damage for some time. First of all, clinicians had to provide care with minimal information, equipment, and resources at the beginning of the pandemic, undoubtedly leading to unnecessary death and human suffering for their patients (Kakemam et al. 2021; Litam and Balkin 2021). Secondly, there are likely to be remnants of crisis decision-making and behavior on individual and team well-being and trust (Bernstein 2020; Guzzo et al. 2021). The COVID-19 pandemic brought many unknowns in terms of transmission, treatment, navigating shocks to the supply chain, and financial pressures. Generally speaking, just as clinicians were making the best decisions possible with limited information and resources and under stress, so were healthcare leaders. As such, some of the decisions made during the crisis were likely suboptimal in retrospect, yet still inflicted inadvertent damage to employee well-being.

An early example is regarding the provision of PPE or lack thereof. Across the country, clinicians struggled to access appropriate PPE, particularly in areas where the pandemic hit early. In some instances, Nurses went on strike (Collins and Haigh 2020). People described this as "feeling led to the slaughter," and these feelings are unlikely to easily subside despite adequate access to PPE in the present (Mroziak 2020).

Another example that is likely to have a lasting impact is the many pay cuts and furloughs that were implemented for clinicians during COVID-19 (Paavola 2020). At the same time clinicians were being asked to risk their lives with minimal PPE and high risk of exposure, they were also having their sacrifices devalued financially and their job stability threatened.

Additionally, feelings of inequity in the vaccine distribution process will likely have a lasting impact on healthcare workers. While the vaccine rollout was complex involving numerous logistical challenges and uncertainty in quantity and timing of supply, organizations differed vastly in their approach to deciding who should get the vaccine first. Feelings of inequity in this selection process led to protests and a further feeling of devaluation (Bernstein 2020).

As the healthcare workforce begins to recover, leaders must acknowledge the lasting effects of these decisions and work to build, restore, and repair trust. Failure to do so will leave us more vulnerable for the next pandemic.

REFERENCES

Aiken, Linda H., Sean P. Clarke, Douglas M. Sloane, Julie Sochalski, and Jeffrey H. Silber. 2002. "Hospital Nurse Staffing and Patient Mortality, Nurse Burnout, and Job Dissatisfaction." *Journal of the American Medical Association* 288(16):1987–93. doi: 10.1001/jama.288.16.1987.

American College of Healthcare. 2020. "ACHE's Most Resent Top Issues Confronting Hospitals Survey Identified the Following Top Challenges for Hospitals in

2019." Retrieved (https://www.ache.org/learning-center/research/about-the-field/top-issues-confronting-hospitals).

Army, Nigerian, and Adekunle Fajuyi Cantonment. 2019. "Physician Burnout: An Overview." *J Res Bas Clin Sci* [Internet]. 1(1): 111–14. Retrieved (https://jrbcs.org/index.php/jrbcs/article/view/9)

Ashcroft, Peter, Jana S. Huisman, Sonja Lehtinen, Judith A. Bouman, Christian L. Althaus, Roland R. Regoes, and Sebastian Bonhoeffer. 2020. "COVID-19 Infectivity Profile Correction." *Swiss Medical Weekly* 150(32): 1–5. doi: 10.4414/smw.2020.20336.

Bakker, Arnold B., and Evangelia Demerouti. 2007. "The Job Demands-Resources Model: State of the Art." *Journal of Managerial Psychology* 22(3): 309–28. doi: 10.1108/02683940710733115.

Bekele, Firomsa, Desalegn Feyissa Mechessa, and Birbirsa Sefera. 2021. "Prevalence and Associated Factors of the Psychological Impact of COVID-19 among Communities, Health Care Workers and Patients in Ethiopia: A Systematic Review." *Annals of Medicine and Surgery* 66: 102403. doi: 10.1016/j.amsu.2021.102403.

Beresin, Eugene V, Tracey A. Milligan, Richard Balon, John H. Coverdale, Alan K. Louie, and Laura Weiss Roberts. 2016. "Physician Wellbeing: A Critical Deficiency in Resilience Education and Training." *Academic Psychiatry* 40(1): 9–12.

Berg, Sara. 2020. "Physician Burnout: Which Medical Specialties Feel the Most Stress." *AMA: Physician Health*. Retrieved (https://www.ama-assn.org/practice-management/physician-health/physician-burnout-which-medical-specialties-feel-most-stress).

Bernstein, Lenny. 2020. "Stanford Apologizes for Coronavirus Vaccine Plan That Left out Many Front-Line Doctors." *The Washington Post*. Retrieved (https://www.washingtonpost.com/health/2020/12/18/stanford-hospital-protest-covid-vaccine/).

Beusekom, Mary Van. 2020. "Hospitals Improvise to Address COVID-19 PPE Shortage." *Center for Infectious Disease Research and Policy*. Retrieved (https://www.cidrap.umn.edu/news-perspective/2020/06/hospitals-improvise-address-covid-19-ppe-shortage).

Blake, Holly, Fiona Bermingham, Graham Johnson, and Andrew Tabner. 2020. "Mitigating the Psychological Impact of COVID-19 on Healthcare Workers: A Digital Learning Package." *International Journal of Environmental Research and Public Health* 17(9): 2997. doi: 10.3390/ijerph17092997.

Bradley, Meredith, and Praveen Chahar. 2020. "Burnout of Healthcare Providers during COVID-19." *Cleveland Clinic Journal of Medicine*. doi: 10.3949/ccjm.87a.ccc051.

Britt, Thomas W., Marissa L. Shuffler, Riley L. Pegram, Phoebe Xoxakos, Patrick J. Rosopa, Emily Hirsh, and William Jackson. 2021. "Job Demands and Resources among Healthcare Professionals during Virus Pandemics: A Review and Examination of Fluctuations in Mental Health Strain during COVID-19." *Applied Psychology* 70(1): 120–49. doi: 10.1111/apps.12304.

Carroll, Nathaniel W., and Dean G. Smith. 2020. "Financial Implications of the CoviD-19 Epidemic for Hospitals: A Case Study." *Journal of Health Care Finance* 46(4): 11–22.

Collins, Dave, and Susan Haigh. 2020. "Nurses Go on Stick over Protective Gear, Pay in Connecticut." *AP News*. Retrieved (https://apnews.com/article/virus-outbreak-connecticut-strikes-norwich-7db8a7a43bb22a436d02cd345477544c).

Demerouti, E., F. Nachreiner, A. B. Bakker, and W. B. Schaufeli. 2001. "The Job Demands–Resources Model of Burnout." *Journal of Applied Psychology* 86(3): 499–512.

DeWolfe, Debora J. 2000. *Training Manual for Mental Health and Human Service Workers in Major Disasters.* 2nd ed. Rockville, MD: US Department of health and Human Services, Substance Abuse and Mental Health Services Administration, Center for Mental Health Services.

Donohue, Julie M., and Elizabeth Miller. 2020. "COVID-19 and School Closures." *JAMA–Journal of the American Medical Association* 324(9): 845–47. doi: 10.1001/jama.2020.13092.

Dyrbye, Liselotte N., Pamela O. Johnson, LeAnn M. Johnson, Michael P. Halasy, Andrea A. Gossard, Daniel Satele, and Tait Shanafelt. 2019. "Efficacy of the Well-Being Index to Identify Distress and Stratify Well-Being in Nurse Practitioners and Physician Assistants." *Journal of the American Association of Nurse Practitioners* 31(7): 403–12. doi: 10.1097/JXX.0000000000000179.

Dyrbye, Liselotte N., Daniel Satele, and Tait Shanafelt. 2016. "Ability of a 9-Item Well-Being Index to Identify Distress and Stratify Quality of Life in US Workers." *Journal of Occupational and Environmental Medicine* 58(8): 810–17. doi: 10.1097/JOM.0000000000000798.

Dyrbye, Liselotte N., Daniel Satele, Jeff Sloan, and Tait D. Shanafelt. 2013. "Utility of a Brief Screening Tool to Identify Physicians in Distress." *Journal of General Internal Medicine* 28(3): 421–27. doi: 10.1007/s11606-012-2252-9.

Guzzo, Renata F., Xingyu Wang, Juan M. Madera, and JéAnna Abbott. 2021. "Organizational Trust in Times of COVID-19: Hospitality Employees' Affective Responses to Managers' Communication." *International Journal of Hospitality Management* 93: 102778. doi: 10.1016/j.ijhm.2020.102778.

De Hert, Stefan. 2020. "Burnout in Healthcare Workers: Prevalence, Impact and Preventative Strategies." *Local and Regional Anesthesia* 13: 171–83. doi: 10.2147/LRA.S240564.

Joseph, Beulah, Arlene Walker, and Matthew Fuller-Tyszkiewicz. 2018. "Evaluating the Effectiveness of Employee Assistance Programmes: A Systematic Review." *European Journal of Work and Organizational Psychology* 27(1): 1–15. doi:10.1080/1359432X.2017.1374245.

Kakemam, Edris, Zahra Chegini, Amin Rouhi, Forouzan Ahmadi, and Soheila Majidi. 2021. "Burnout and Its Relationship to Self-reported Quality of Patient Care and Adverse Events during COVID-19: A Cross-sectional Online Survey among Nurses." *Journal of Nursing Management* 29(7): 1974–1982. doi: 10.1111/jonm.13359.

Kessel, Maura, Jan Kratzer, and Carsten Schultz. 2012. "Psychological Safety, Knowledge Sharing, and Creative Performance in Healthcare Teams." *Creativity and Innovation Management* 21(2):147–57. doi: 10.1111/j.1467-8691.2012.00635.x.

King, Cynthia, and Bradley Ann Leigh. 2019. "Trends and Implications with Nursing Engagement PRC National Nursing Engagement Report Utilizing the PRC Nursing Quality Assessment Inventory." *PRCCustom Research Research* 1–15. Retrieved (http://prccustomresearch.com)

Kumar, Kamalesh, Ram Subramanian, and Karen Strandholm. 2002. "Market and Efficiency-Based Strategic Responses to Environmental Changes in the Health Care Industry." *Health Care Management Review* 27(3): 21–31. doi: 10.1097/00004010-200207000-00003.

Labdi, Bonnie A. 2006. "Working with Hurricane Rita." *American Journal of Health-System Pharmacy* 63(21): 2053–54. doi: 10.2146/ajhp060266.

Lindeman, Sari, Esa Läärä, Helinä Hakko, and Jouko Lönnqvist. 1996. "A Systematic Review on Gender-Specific Suicide Mortality in Medical Doctors." *British Journal of Psychiatry* 168(3): 274–79. doi: 10.1192/bjp.168.3.274.

Litam, Stacey Diane Arañez, and Richard S. Balkin. 2021. "Moral Injury in Health-Care Workers during COVID-19 Pandemic." *Traumatology* 27(1): 14–19. doi: 10.1037/trm0000290.

Long, Dustin, Dustin Long, Wesli Turner, Crystal Chapman Lambert, Thomas Creger, Michael J. Mugavero, and Greer A. Burkholder. 2020. "LB-13. Economic and Workload Impact of COVID-19 Pandemic on Physicians in the United States: Results of a National Survey." *Open Forum Infectious Diseases* 7(Supplement_1): S850–S850. doi: 10.1093/ofid/ofaa515.1910.

Meese, Katherine A., Alejandra Colón-López, Jasvinder A. Singh, Greer A. Burkholder, and David A. Rogers. 2021. "Healthcare Is a Team Sport: Stress, Resilience, and Correlates of Well-Being Among Health System Employees in a Crisis." *Journal of Healthcare Management* 66(4): 304–22. doi: 10.1097/JHM-D-20-00288.

Menon, Nikitha K., Tait D. Shanafelt, Christine A. Sinsky, Mark Linzer, Lindsey Carlasare, Keri J. S. Brady, Martin J. Stillman, and Mickey T. Trockel. 2020. "Association of Physician Burnout With Suicidal Ideation and Medical Errors." *JAMA Network Open* 3(12): e2028780. doi: 10.1001/jamanetworkopen.2020.28780.

Mroziak, Michael. 2020. "Doctors Draft Own Bill Seeking Physical, Financial Protections While Battling COVID-19." *WXXI News*. Retrieved (http://wxxinews.org)

Paavola, Alia. 2020. "1 in 5 Physicians Hit with Pay Cut or Furlough Due to COVID-19, Survey Says." *Becker's Hospital Review*. Retrieved 7 May, 2022 (http://beckershospitalreview.com)

Panaccio, Alexandra, and Christian Vandenberghe. 2009. "Perceived Organizational Support, Organizational Commitment and Psychological Well-Being: A Longitudinal Study." *Journal of Vocational Behavior* 75(2): 224–36. doi: 10.1016/j.jvb.2009.06.002.

Pfefferbaum, Betty, and Carol S. North. 2020. "Mental Health and the Covid-19 Pandemic." *New England Journal of Medicine* 383(6): 510–12. doi: 10.1056/NEJMp2008017.

Ripp, Jonathan, and Tait Shanafelt. 2020. "The Health Care Chief Wellness Officer: What the Role Is and Is Not." *Academic Medicine* 95(9): 1354–58. doi: 10.1097/ACM.0000000000003433.

Smith, Uniqua. 2019. "The Calm before the Storm: Staffing during Times of Disaster." *Nursing Economic$* 37(5): 250–54.

Solomon, Mildred Z., Matthew Wynia, and Lawrence O. Gostin. 2020. "Scarcity in the Covid-19 Pandemic." *Hastings Center Report* 50(2): 3–3. doi: 10.1002/hast.1093.

Tawfik, Daniel S., Jochen Profit, Timothy I. Morgenthaler, Daniel V. Satele, Christine A. Sinsky, Liselotte N. Dyrbye, Michael A. Tutty, Colin P. West, and Tait D. Shanafelt. 2018. "Physician Burnout, Well-Being, and Work Unit Safety Grades in Relationship to Reported Medical Errors." *Mayo Clinic Proceedings* 93(11): 1571–80. doi: 10.1016/j.mayocp.2018.05.014.

Thomeer, Mieke Beth, Jenjira Yahirun, and Alejandra Colón-López. 2020. "How Families Matter for Health Inequality during the COVID-19 Pandemic." *Journal of Family Theory and Review* 12(4): 448–63. doi: 10.1111/jftr.12398.

Weissman, Gary E., Andrew Crane-Droesch, Corey Chivers, ThaiBinh Luong, Asaf Hanish, Michael Z. Levy, Jason Lubken, Michael Becker, Michael E. Draugelis, George L. Anesi, Patrick J. Brennan, Jason D. Christie, C. William Hanson, Mark E. Mikkelsen, and Scott D. Halpern. 2020. "Locally Informed Simulation to Predict Hospital Capacity Needs During the COVID-19 Pandemic." *Annals of Internal Medicine* 173(1): 21–28. doi: 10.7326/M20-1260.

Wittkieffer. 2019. *The Impact of Burnout on Healthcare Executives: A WittKieffer Study*.

Wren-Lewis, Simon. 2020. *The Economic Effects of a Pandemic*. Social Europe. Retrieved (https://socialeurope.eu/the-economic-effects-of-a-pandemic)

Zhao, Mei, Gloria J. Bazzoli, Jan P. Clement, Richard C. Lindrooth, Joann M. Nolin, and Askar S. Chukmaitov. 2008. "Hospital Staffing Decisions: Does Financial Performance Matter?" *Inquiry* 45(3): 293–307. doi: 10.5034/inquiryjrnl_45. 03.293.

Chapter 8

Colorado state case study

Adom Netsanet
University of Colorado School of Medicine
Denver, CO, USA

Sera Sempson
University of Colorado School of Medicine
Denver, CO, USA

William Choe
South Denver Cardiology Associates
Aurora, CO, USA

CONTENTS

Introduction 90
COVID-19 case summary, Colorado, United States 90
COVID-19 response in Colorado, United States 91
Geographic patterns of COVID-19 cases in Colorado 92
Mask protests in Colorado 93
Differences in COVID compliance and outcomes by race 94
Reports of cardiac events decrease amidst rise of the coronavirus
    pandemic in Colorado and nationally 96
Denver EMS runs decreased amidst coronavirus
    pandemic, while out-of-hospital cardiac arrests increased 97
Cardiac alert activations decrease in Denver amidst coronavirus
    pandemic 98
Clinicians urge patients not to delay medical interventions 98
Responses among different hospital systems in the Denver metro area 99
Telehealth 100
The impact of elective procedure cancellation on cardiac morbidity,
    sequela and mortality in Colorado 101

DOI: 10.1201/9781003204138-11

Heart disease and COVID-19 – A rocky tale from the
    rocky mountains 101
Conclusion 102
References 102

INTRODUCTION

The rise of the novel Coronavirus-19 (COVID-19) pandemic shook healthcare systems internationally; even the largest and most robust hospitals were overwhelmed with patients contracting this nebulous virus, including the healthcare providers working to fight it. With little being known about the spread of this virus, local communities and the greater public scrambled to effectively combat it. Many individuals held conflicting views about how to best contain the spread of this disease and how to attenuate the heavy impact that it imparted on both public health and public relations. Individuals and government entities frantically juggled their personal health considerations, those of their loved ones, and extraneous considerations, like maintaining economic stability amidst the devastating impact of a global pandemic on the public sector.

The rise and patterns of COVID-19 cases impacted patients and the general public in various, and sometimes unexpected, ways. This chapter will address the impacts of the novel Coronavirus-19 pandemic on Colorado residents, with emphases on the impact among cardiovascular patients and differences in health outcomes between demographic groups within the state.

COVID-19 CASE SUMMARY, COLORADO, UNITED STATES

On March 5, 2020, the first official case of Coronavirus in Colorado was recorded from a skier who traversed the slopes of Summit County following a trip to Italy. [22] Shortly after, a case was reported in the Denver metro area from a woman who had traveled on an international cruise before returning to Colorado and seeking care for flu-like symptoms.[11] Both cases were confirmed through a positive result on a state-administered test, although neither result was sent to the Center for Disease Control (CDC) for confirmation.[8] Soon after, on March 11, 2020, the World Health Organization officially declared COVID-19 as a pandemic.

In Colorado, COVID-19 cases rose throughout the months of March and April, then decreased considerably in May and the early weeks of June. Then, July 2020 saw a considerable spike in cases that experts speculated to be the result of various social factors, which will be discussed throughout this chapter. Cases began to rise again in Fall 2020, concurrent with the beginning of the regular flu season. These case trends in Colorado mirrored that of national averages.[3, 6] Figure 8.1 demonstrates new COVID-19 cases in Colorado, as reported by the CDC, starting on March 31, 2020 and measured at every 4-week interval through September 2020.

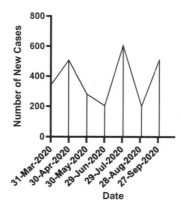

Figure 8.1 New COVID-19 cases in Colorado from March to September 2020.

Importantly, gender identity did not appear to impact the probability of contracting COVID-19 in Colorado. According to the Colorado Department of Public Health and Environment and the United States Census Bureau, females accounted for 49.79% of the COVID-19 cases in Colorado, while making up 49.96% of the total state population. Males accounted for 49.01% of cases in Colorado while making up 50.04% of the population.[6, 4]

The trends of COVID-19 case transmission in the early months of this pandemic offer vital insight into social trends, which subsequently impact public health, patient safety, the extent of government interventions, and highlight structurally engrained medical disparities that disproportionately ravage the health of underserved communities.

COVID-19 RESPONSE IN COLORADO, UNITED STATES

Colorado entered a statewide declaration of emergency on March 8, 2020. During this time period and the following months, various public health orders emerged from the office of Governor Jared Polis.[5] All in-person instruction at primary and secondary schools were suspended in Colorado on March 18, 2020. March 19 saw the closure of gyms, bars, restaurants, and other public gathering locations that were considered "nonessential" work. Many healthcare workers were given official letters stating the essential work of their medical work in case these would need to be presented in the instance of a public security stop. Due to the economic burden placed by these necessary public health measures, the office of Governor Polis amended many executive orders in the following weeks to provide reasonable leniency for small businesses and Colorado communities. For instance, the statute suspending all nonessential operations was modified on May 2, 2020 to allow for food trucks to support commercial vehicle activities, many of whom were small businesses. An infamous mandate was the initial closure of liquor stores and marijuana shops which, after public outcry and long lines at the stores, were swiftly permitted to reopen.

During a global health emergency, government interventions undeniably impact social relations. The different regions and demographics within Colorado responded differently to this virus, subsequent government mandates, and innovations in medical research. This impacted the frequency of virus outbreak, while imparting significant and long-lasting impacts on public health and economic recovery.

GEOGRAPHIC PATTERNS OF COVID-19 CASES IN COLORADO

Colorado counties that were notable for relatively large numbers of COVID-19 outbreaks were generally rural areas, including Mesa and Pueblo.[7] After being flagged during the initial months of the pandemic, Mesa County was identified again in July 2021 as being a "hotspot" for the new Delta variant of COVID-19.[12] Rural counties boasted the highest case fatality rates from COVID-19, along with El Paso County (which includes Colorado Spring with a politically conservative population), while urban areas held the highest percentage of deaths from COVID-19. This means that, in these mostly rural areas, an individual diagnosed with COVID-19 would have a lower chance of survival when compared to individuals diagnosed with COVID-19 in areas with relatively low case fatality rates.[1] According to the Multidisciplinary Digital Publishing Institute, population density was associated with COVID-19 deaths in urban areas while poverty and unemployment were associated with COVID-19 deaths reported from rural areas.[13] The populations in rural Colorado areas tend to be more politically conservative and report higher rates of resistance to vaccination against COVID-19 when compared to the rest of the state. Resistance to vaccination as well as other unique factors of rural areas, including older populations and lack of healthcare resources, impacted COVID-19 transmission patterns throughout Colorado. This pattern between political tendencies and vaccine hesitance in Colorado is similar to that of the United States as a whole, as depicted in Figure 8.2.[17]

Additional geographic areas that were notable for initial COVID-19 outbreaks included Fort Collins and Boulder, cities which host two of Colorado's largest undergraduate universities: Colorado State University and the University of Colorado at Boulder, respectively. Potential causes for the markedly disproportionate pattern of outbreaks in these cities are subject to speculation as associated factors do not always show clear correlations. Furthermore, even correlations do not always impart a causal relationship; therefore, it is important to assess reported data with scrutiny. However,

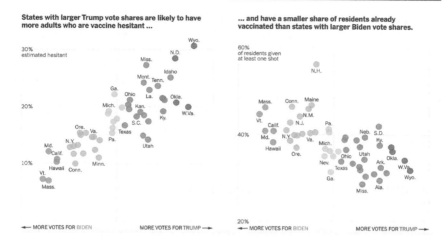

States with larger Trump vote shares are likely to have more adults who are vaccine hesitant ... and have a smaller share of residents already vaccinated than states with larger Biden vote shares.

Figure 8.2 Image source: The New York Times.[17]

case tracking from the CDC indicates that relatively young adults accounted for a higher proportion of reported cases during the summer of 2020 compared to previous months, starting around late June 2020. For instance, 20–39-year-olds accounted for 47.31% of total COVID-19 cases in Colorado in the first week of July, a swift and marked increase from the final week of June, during which they accounted for 39.1% of cases.[7]

Many experts speculated that virus fatigue, opportunistic travel as travel costs decreased, and misinformation leading to individuals not treating the spread of COVID-19 seriously may have contributed to these initial case outbreaks.[7]

MASK PROTESTS IN COLORADO

The impact of the contemporary political climate and misinformation allowed to spread on social and cable news media cannot be separated from COVID-19 infection and vaccination rates. Colorado is politically considered a "purple state", with more liberal leaning (blue) urban counties and more conservative (red) rural counties. At the height of the Coronavirus pandemic, in May 2020, the county with the highest COVID-19 infection rate was a rural area known as Morgan County.[9] Outbreaks in other rural counties like Gunnison County and Weld County also contributed to disproportionately high infection rates. Several counties, including Weld Gunnison Counties, rejected state mask mandates, pushing for local mandates that opposed state, federal, and national health guidelines.[2] Officials from the Gunnison County Department of Health reported threats to their lives over public health precautions enacted to attenuate the spread of the virus.[11]

Various Colorado cities, like Colorado Springs, which is politically conservative, faced challenges with several contentious protests opposing the use of protective masks.[22] These protests were met with counter-protests from community members as well as physicians, nurses, and other hospital staff who were fighting on the front lines to treat patients while also facing the challenge posed by the politicization of a global pandemic and the incivility that followed. These incidents were referred to as "super-spreader" events, so nicknamed for the disproportionate lack of safety measures upheld and the resulting sizable spikes of cases.[6, 4]

DIFFERENCES IN COVID COMPLIANCE AND OUTCOMES BY RACE

According to the National Library of Medicine, Black, Latina/o, and Asian populations were more likely to wear masks in response to efforts to reduce the spread of the Coronavirus pandemic compared to White US respondents. White respondents, and particularly White men, were reported as the least likely to comply with mask-wearing protocols in response to this pandemic.[12] This observation was prominent from April 2020 to June 2020, some of the most severe months of this pandemic. Ironically, despite greater compliance with public health orders, minorities in Colorado were the most severely impacted by COVID-19. This is due to various systemic factors, social factors, and racism.[10]

An overwhelmingly large number of published studies have shown that structural and individual racism contribute to minorities facing higher levels of stress, poorer health, and being more likely to have low socioeconomic status (SES).[23] A global pandemic, like COVID-19, exacerbates the healthcare disparities caused by these historic and structural trends. Social factors that more commonly impact minorities are also notable, such as being more likely to work low-wage, essential jobs, rendering them unable to isolate at home, as well as being more likely to live in multigenerational households causing them to be more susceptible to infections from family members. This non-exhaustive list of complex, interconnected factors helped facilitate the disproportionately adverse impact of COVID-19 among racial or ethnic minorities.

Despite being among the most adherent groups to COVID-19 mask mandates,[12] Black Coloradans had the highest mortality rates from COVID-19. In the early months of this pandemic, the World Medical and Health Policy (WMHP) recorded that Black Americans accounted for 8.24% of deaths but only 3.82% of the population.[31] Many factors collectively contributed to this shocking statistic, including structural racism leading to poorer baseline health, limited access to COVID testing compared to White counterparts, and the reduced ability to shelter at home insofar as Black Coloradans maintain a larger proportion of "essential" job roles in comparison to their

White counterparts. There were more COVID testing centers in the suburbs compared to the densely populated city centers.

Unfortunately, as stated by the Center for American Progress, among other scholarly sources, this too is intimately tied to historical racism, specifically, how racism precludes wealth accumulation and social mobility.[14, 10, 17] When faced with large structural gaps, the delivery of healthcare becomes inherently unequal. Dr. Alexandra Smart, M.D., a pulmonary and critical care physician in the Denver metro area, described her experience seeing healthcare disparities unfold while working in Intensive Care Units (ICUs) in the Denver metro area throughout the COVID-19 pandemic:

> We absolutely noticed that minority patients were overrepresented in terms of being hospitalized in the ICU and how sick they became. Our COVID ICU was predominantly filled with Latino patients, and they tended to become more critically ill than their Caucasian counterparts. Additionally, we had more African American patients in the ICU than you would expect per-capita for the population. It was all so distressing to our teams to witness.

On the other hand, White and Asian Coloradans had death rates from COVID-19 that were comparable to their respective populations, while Hispanics had a notably low mortality rate from COVID-19 (16.49%) compared to their overall population (21.62%), as depicted in Figure 8.3.[31] This positive trend among the Hispanic population in Colorado tapered over time, and the Hispanic population later experienced large increases in reported rates of death from COVID-19.[25]

Some of the dilemmas many minorities, immigrants, and low SES Coloradans were placed in were exemplified in the outbreak observed at a Greeley meatpacking plant in April 2020, one of Colorado's largest workplace outbreaks of COVID-19. Meatpacking plants employ many immigrant workers including, but not limited to, those from African and Latin American countries. Despite local union efforts to close this plant as COVID-19 cases were rising and devastating communities they were deemed essential and kept open. Vice-President Mike Pence and national leaders declared meat packing plants to be a national security priority and its workers frontline workers since it was vital in providing stable food supply for the

State	Percent COVID-19 deaths[a] | Percent population[b]					Ratio[c]	Date[d]
	White	Black	Hispanic	Asian	Other		
Colorado	70.21 |	8.24	16.49	3.99	1.07	2.16	4/18/2020
	67.95	| 3.82	| 21.62	| 3.27	| 3.34		

Figure 8.3 Percent of overall population deaths by race. Data source: World Medical and Health Policy (WMHP).[31]

country. Workers continued to work in close quarters with suboptimal protective gear which were in short supply at the time.[1, 20] This plant officially closed on April 10, 2020, and although it reopened eight days later, the impact of this super spreader event would permanently impact the families of the workers affected.[9] By May 2020 reports of over 300 confirmed cases of COVID-19 among workers were documented at this plant.

In addition to some minorities being more likely to contract COVID-19 compared to their relative population, they also experienced worse outcomes for various cardiac morbidities, including out-of-hospital cardiac arrests (OHCAs).[14] The Coronavirus pandemic undeniably hit cardiovascular patients hard throughout Colorado. Although factors like financial resources and access to care impact the outcomes of cardiovascular patients, this virus and its sequelae did not discriminate on infecting individuals based on race, class, or anything else.

REPORTS OF CARDIAC EVENTS DECREASE AMIDST RISE OF THE CORONAVIRUS PANDEMIC IN COLORADO AND NATIONALLY

The rise of the Coronavirus pandemic (COVID-19) was accompanied by increased anxiety and uncertainty among patients over the risk of virus exposure that could come with pursuing medical care for pre-existing and emerging conditions. An additional reason for patients' delay in seeking medical attention during the early months of the pandemic may have been a fear that going to the hospital could lead to exposure and infection from the virus. Several cases of frontline workers exposed were highlighted in the media despite their adequate protection. During the initial weeks of the pandemic, the testing resources were not available, and testing was only performed if the patient met the clinical criteria. Other patients were asked to isolate at home. In addition, stories of patients arriving and being placed in isolation without further family contact may have delayed patients to seek medical attention until they were extremely ill. The messages that you should not seek medical attention unless you were very ill may have confused the general public. This is problematic because delaying intervention for necessary medical treatments leads to poorer outcomes, reduced survival rates, and a higher risk of long-term complication. The resulting inverse relationship between the increase of COVID-19 cases and decreased access to, or confidence in, seeking care for emergent or existing cardiac conditions resulted in the development of public health patterns with adverse impacts on Colorado's cardiac patients.

The result of this concerning trend was a decrease in reported cardiac events in Colorado during the early and exceedingly uncertain times of the Coronavirus pandemic in 2020. According to a survey from Healthier Colorado conducted in April 2020, the two most frequently reported concerns from Coloradans about the impact of COVID-19 were: (1) the potential negative impacts that this pandemic would have on their health, and (2) their financial stability.[13] Another measure of the public's overall anxiety about the spread of Coronavirus was determined by investigating whether Coloradans believed that local regulations, enacted to reduce spread of the pandemic were necessary, not harsh enough, or too harsh. On April 27, 2020, 64% of Colorado residents reported that states should continue enforcing public safety regulations, including keeping businesses closed, to attenuate the spread of the virus. 29% of Coloradans said that states should ease up on public health regulations to help re-stimulate the economy, 6% of respondents reported being unsure or having no opinion, and 1% of respondents refused to answer. This report from Healthier Colorado also indicated that 89% of respondents were insured, so the marked decrease in reported cardiac events during this time is less likely due to patients delaying care due to lack or loss of insurance coverage.

Another outcome was a spike in reported cases of cardiac events during the summer of 2020 as COVID-19 reports decreased in Colorado and patients were more confident in their ability to safely seek care for cardiac events. The spike in reported cardiac events in Colorado during the summer of 2020 may also have been caused by patients seeking care for symptoms that were exacerbated during the rise of the pandemic, symptoms that became worse after waiting for cardiac procedures that were deemed "elective" while hospitals were initially saturated with COVID-19 patients, and/or cardiac symptoms that arose from complications of previous COVID-19 infection.

DENVER EMS RUNS DECREASED AMIDST CORONAVIRUS PANDEMIC, WHILE OUT-OF-HOSPITAL CARDIAC ARRESTS INCREASED

A survey by Dr. Matthew Holland et al. found that the total number of EMS runs by the Denver Health Paramedic Division, which covers the city and county of Denver, decreased during the periods of peri-mandate (between the Colorado statewide declaration of emergency, 3/8/2020, through 3/28/2020) and post-mandate (the two-week period following the Colorado shelter-in-place order; 3/29/2020–4/11/2020). Interestingly, the total number of OHCAs in the Denver metro area skyrocketed during this post-mandate period, increasing by a factor of 2.2 compared to average historical controls from the same two-week period from the years 2011–2019. Of note, Holland et al. indicated that the 2.2-fold increase in OHCAs exceeded the number of patients who died with COVID-19 diagnoses over the same time period. This suggests that the increase in OHCAs cannot solely be accounted for by patients experiencing OHCAs after contracting COVID-19, and that there are likely additional considerations that led to the increase in OHCAs. One potential explanation, supported by the decrease in EMS runs by the Denver Health Paramedic Division, is that patients were less likely to seek emergency care during the height of the Coronavirus pandemic for any number of reasons.[9] These trends of OHCAs in Denver mirror national observations. During the height of the Coronavirus pandemic, instances of OHCSs in the United States rose, while mortality rates also rose, and rates of successful resuscitation declined.[14]

CARDIAC ALERT ACTIVATIONS DECREASE IN DENVER AMIDST CORONAVIRUS PANDEMIC

The Denver metro area also experienced a decline in the number of Cardiac Alert activations for acute myocardial infarction (MI) emergencies during the initial months of the pandemic. At a large medical center in Denver, there were large declines in Cardiac alert activations in March–May 2020 when compared to the same time period in 2019. There were 16 total Cardiac Alert activations from March–May 2020; far fewer than the 34 activations during the same time period in 2019. In contrast, June had more activations in 2020 than in 2019 by 142.9%. In June 2020 alone, there was a surge to 20 total activations, in contrast to June 2019 which only saw 7 activations. Cardiac alerts at this medical center began to normalize after August 2019. Cardiac Alert activation data at this medical center from January 2019 to March 2021 is depicted in Figure 8.4.

Figure 8.4 demonstrates that the rise in COVID-19 cases during the spring of 2020 (March–May 2020) is paralleled by a decrease in reported Cardiac Alerts at a major medical center in Denver during the same time period. June 2020 also had the lowest number of COVID-19 cases in Colorado compared to any other month in 2020, which bears a strikingly predictable and inversely related pattern with the spike of Cardiac Alerts in June 2020.[6] These patterns align with the hypothesis that increasing COVID-19 cases and heightened public anxiety surrounding the Coronavirus pandemic may have contributed to lower rates of patients seeking care for their cardiac conditions.

CLINICIANS URGE PATIENTS NOT TO DELAY MEDICAL INTERVENTIONS

As clinicians began to notice the concerning trend of decreasing reported cardiac events amidst increasing COVID-19 reports in the spring of 2020, influential medical associations like the American College of Cardiology urged patients to seek medical attention for life-threatening conditions despite patients' fear of virus infection in order to avoid delaying critical treatments, exacerbating existing chronic conditions, or death. Overall deaths from non-coronavirus causes, like heart disease, diabetes, and overdoses rose by about 22% across Colorado during the early months of the pandemic.[31] As hospitals were taking the utmost precautions, with protocols being frequently updated to reflect the most recent and reliable knowledge of the epidemiology of the novel COVID-19, clinicians urged patients to safely seek care rather than delaying treatment. Initiatives like CardioSmart from the American College of Cardiology provided accurate information for patients regarding which cardiac symptoms are appropriate for telehealth consultations and which symptoms necessitate 911 calls. These initiatives also urged patients to not delay seeking care for cardiac symptoms due to fears related to the Coronavirus pandemic.[30]

RESPONSES AMONG DIFFERENT HOSPITAL SYSTEMS IN THE DENVER METRO AREA

Hospital leaders were faced with the concern of patients delaying care for pre-existing or emergent conditions due to the fear of virus transmission at hospitals and clinics. The Denver Metro area has four large healthcare systems; from the onset of the pandemic the systems did communicate and work together. However, each system communicated with their respective physicians differently. One system was proactive and engaged the physicians early, allowing physician leaders to develop protocols for the constantly changing epidemiologic circumstances then disseminate these protocols to the medical staff. This system was also transparent in reporting the number of patients who were seen and admitted to their hospital. They held weekly town hall meetings led by physicians which facilitated frequent, effective communication as well as collaboration between providers. The other system was more private about their patient numbers, concerned that reported cases would influence patients' decisions about whether or not to seek care.

In the early phase of the pandemic, there was a shortage of personal protective equipment (PPE) and possible lack of resources such as ventilators, medications, and even IV tubing. Once the PPE supply stabilized and ICU staff became experienced in treating the sick patients, semi elective procedures were slowly approved by the state and hospitals. Having real-time data helped determine the true impact of the spread in our local community and plan our patient care appropriately. Daily COVID-19 data updates at hospitals impacted real-time physician decision-making regarding whether or not they would perform semi elective cardiac procedures that day, based on the perceived safety of performing such procedures along with PPE supplies.

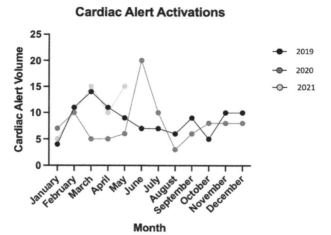

Figure 8.4 Cardiac alert activations at a large medical center in the Denver metro area.

TELEHEALTH

Telehealth visits prior to the COVID pandemic were mostly confined to patient interactions in rural areas. Without Medicare approval and therefore no billing code, telehealth visits were not a financially viable way to deliver healthcare. In the past couple of years, with the rise in acceptance by the public of video conferencing software programs such as Zoom, the pandemic was able to advance telemedicine in a way not possible in normal times. Within a few weeks, most medical practices were able to convert their inpatient appointments to video conferencing calls. By the end of the summer when most of the public and medical practices were comfortable with mask protocols, in person visits slowly resumed. Most patients now prefer inpatient visits over telehealth visits.

In the beginning of the pandemic, it was unclear if the virus was transmitted via airborne droplets or by contact as well. Without rapid testing capabilities, all patients had to be assumed to be positive when presenting to the emergency room. With limited stock of N95 respirator masks, prioritization of allocated supplies was given to the high-risk hospital personnel. Hospital rooms had to be converted to negative airflow rooms. These rooms bring air into the patient room from the hallways thus not spreading any of the airborne contaminants that the patient may have into the general hallways. HVAC units were placed into the windows and directly vented outside. Since all surgical suites including catheter labs are positive airflow (pushing the air from within the room out into the hallways), these rooms had to have their airflow converted into negative airflow to reduce the risk of inadvertently spreading the virus within the hospital. Reuse of N95 masks was required until the mask shortage abated.

THE IMPACT OF ELECTIVE PROCEDURE CANCELLATION ON CARDIAC MORBIDITY, SEQUELA AND MORTALITY IN COLORADO

On March 19, 2020, Colorado Governor Jared Polis announced an executive order suspending elective procedures to attenuate the spread of COVID-19 and preserve precious medical resources that were becoming scarce in the midst of the Coronavirus pandemic.[5] Cost–benefit analyses elicited this difficult decision, as state leadership weighed the risk of exacerbating cardiac symptoms against increasing patients' susceptibility to COVID-19 during both the pre- and post-procedure period.

This mandate also removed the responsibility (and power) of decision-making from physicians regarding whether or not elective procedures should proceed. However, physicians still had to decide whether patients needed a semi-urgent procedure such as pacemaker generator replacements, how long these patients could wait for these life-altering procedures, and what risks hospitalizations posed to these cardiac patients during the dynamic rise of the Coronavirus pandemic. By diminishing elective procedures, this mandate impacted the ability of patients with valvular and structural heart disease to receive treatment, even if the treatment was desired.[32]

Researchers from the American Journal of Cardiology (ACC) found a 42% reduction in cardiac procedure volumes nationally between March 2019 and March 2020, and a further 64% reduction between March 2020 and April 2020. These recorded reductions were broken down by procedure: Coronary angiographies, either invasive or by computed tomography (CT), were reduced by 55%, (cardiac) stress tests by 78%, transesophageal echocardiography was reduced by 76%, transthoracic echocardiography by 59%, and transesophageal echocardiography by 76%. These diagnostic and treatment procedures are among the most impactful in a cardiologist's toolbox when it comes to treating and diagnosing heart conditions, and the lack of access to these procedures during the Coronavirus pandemic surely left an epidemiological impact in Colorado, as well as nationally and globally.[22]

HEART DISEASE AND COVID-19 – A ROCKY TALE FROM THE ROCKY MOUNTAINS

Due to the reduction in procedures that were considered elective, like cardiac catheterizations, cardiac patients in Colorado who suffered from the morbidities associated with these life-altering procedures were acutely at risk for medical decompensation. Due to this relationship, one could reasonably hypothesize that there would be higher mortality rates among cardiac patients with ischemic or hypertensive diseases in 2020 (concurrent with the Coronavirus pandemic and the mandate suspending elective procedures) compared to previous years, while cardiac deaths from morbidities that were not directly impacted by this mandate would not show such a trend. According to the ACC, deaths from hypertensive and ischemic heart diseases increased during the early rise of the Coronavirus pandemic, which is the time associated with the Colorado mandate against elective procedures in March 2020, compared to the same time period in 2019. However, the deaths from cerebrovascular diseases, other circulatory system diseases, or heart failure did not change between 2019 and 2020.[22]

Furthermore, the ACC alleges that the COVID-19 pandemic caused disruptions in the diagnosis and acutely available treatment for cardiovascular diseases, which have outcomes that are highly dependent on early diagnosis intervention. As the cardiologists say, "*Time is muscle*". This is especially significant at a population level because heart disease is the leading killer worldwide and the second leading killer in Colorado. In 2017, 18.5% of deaths in Colorado were from heart disease, closely following Colorado's leading killer, Cancer, which accounted for 20.6% of deaths in the same year.[1, 4]

CONCLUSION

With the epidemiology of COVID-19 being heavily influenced by so many factors, it is no surprise that there is great debate over how to best combat and control its spread. Ethical decisions are abundant, and community members are forced, almost daily, to make individual decisions that stand to create rippling effects across the nation. As a result, there is no definitive solution to controlling a contagious virus within a population influenced by so many personal, interpersonal, and political factors. However, there are many steps that can be taken over time to reduce the long-term impact of COVID on the Colorado population. These include, but are surely not limited to, acknowledging and combating structures that give rise to differences in COVID-19 outcomes and encouraging flexibility on the familial, communal, state, and national level to quickly modify and change policy as COVID-19 evolves. That being said, the pandemic is still ongoing and, as we have seen through changing policy and mandates, what works today could potentially not suffice tomorrow.

REFERENCES

1 American Heart Association. (n.d.). *Colorado State Fact Sheet [Infographic]*. Retrieved July 12, 2021 from https://www.heart.org/-/media/files/about-us/policy-research/fact-sheets/quality-systems-of-care/quality-systems-of-care-colorado.pdf?la=en
2 Bloom, M. (2021, May 14). Following CDC, Colorado To Drop Statewide Mask Mandate For Vaccinated Residents. *KUNC*. https://www.kunc.org/news/2021-05-14/following-cdc-colorado-plans-to-ease-mask-mandate-for-vaccinated-residents

3 Centers for Disease Control and Prevention. (n.d.). *Trends in Number of COVID-10 Cases and Deaths in the US Reported to CDC, by State/ Territory [Infographic]*. Retrieved July 12, 2021, from https://covid.cdc.gov/ covid-data-tracker/#trends_dailytrendscases

4 Centers for Disease Control and Prevention. (n.d.). *National Center for Health Statistics Colorado [Infographic]*. Retrieved July 11, 2021 from https://www. cdc.gov/nchs/pressroom/states/colorado/co.htm

5 Colorado Continues to Take Action in Response to COVID-19. (2020, March 19). *Colorado Governor Jared Polis*. Retrieved July 11, 2021 from https://www.col- orado.gov/governor/news/colorado-continues-take-action-response-covid-19

6 Colorado Department of Public Health and Environment. (n.d.). Retrieved from https://covid19.colorado.gov/data

7 Colorado Department of Public Health & Environment. (n.d.). *CDPHE COVID-19 Outbreak Map [Interactive map]*. Retrieved July 12, 2021, from https://cdphe.maps.arcgis.com/apps/webappviewer/index.html?id=dcc0b9936 32a4bc68dc7b9a1dd015cfe

8 COVID-19 pandemic in Colorado. (n.d.). *In Wikipedia*. Retrieved July 10, 2021, from https://en.wikipedia.org/wiki/COVID-19_pandemic_in_Colorado

9 Daley, J. (2020, September 10). The Coronavirus Exposed Colorado's Racial Inequalities in Health Care. Community Health Centers are Trying to Help. *CPR*. https://www.cpr.org/2020/09/10/communities-of-color-hit-hard-by-coronavirus- step-in-to-fill-the-gaps-in-the-governments-response/

10 Dickinson, K. L., Roberts, J. D., Banacos, N., Neuberger, L., Koebele, E., Blanch-Hartigan, D., & Shanahan, E. A. (2021). Structural Racism and the COVID-19 Experience in the United States. *Health Security*, 19(S1). [Abstract]. doi. 10.1089/hs.2021.0031

11 Dukakis, A., Birkeland, B., & Daley, J. (2021, January 25). Attacked in Public, Threatened at Work, Picketed at Home: Public Health Leaders Have Seen it All in the Pandemic. *CPR*. https://www.cpr.org/2021/01/25/attacked-in-public- threatened-at-work-picketed-at-home-public-health-leaders-have-seen-it-all- in-the-pandemic/

12 Ellen Bichell, R. (2021, July 8). Colorado's Mesa County Emerges as Hot Spot for COVID Delta Variant. https://www.aspentimes.com/news/ colorados-mesa-county-emerges-as-hot-spot-for-covid-delta-variant/

13 Flaherty, D., & Sievers, C. (2020, April 27). April 27th, 2020 Memorandum Colorado Coronavirus Opinion Survey Summary Part 1. *Magellan Strategies*. https://healthiercolorado.org/wp-content/uploads/2020/04/Colorado- Coronavirus-Opinion-Survey-Summary-Release-One-042720-1-3.pdf

14 Hanks, A., Solomon, D., & Weller, C. (2018, February 21). Systematic Inequality. *American Progress*. https://www.americanprogress.org/issues/race/ reports/2018/02/21/447051/systematic-inequality/

15 Hearne, B. N., & Niño, M. D. (2021). Understanding How Race, Ethnicity, and Gender Shape Mask-Wearing Adherence During the COVID-19 Pandemic: Evidence from the COVID Impact Survey. *Journal of Racial and Ethnic Health Disparities*, 9, 176–183. Advance online publication. doi. 10.1007/ s40615-020-00941-1

16 Holland, M., Burke, J., Hulac, S., Morris, M., Bryskiewicz, G., Goold, A., McVaney, K., Rappaport, L., & Stauffer, B. L. (2020). Excess Cardiac Arrest in the Community During the COVID-19 Pandemic. *JACC. Cardiovascular Interventions*, 13(16), 1968–1969. doi. 10.1016/j.jcin.2020.06.022

17 Ivory, D., Leatherby, L., & Gebeloff, R.. Least Vaccinated U.S. Counties Have Something in Common: Trump Voters. *The New York Times*. Retrieved July 30, 2021 from https://www.nytimes.com/interactive/2021/04/17/us/vaccine-hesitancy-politics.html?referringSource=articleShare. Published April 17, 2021. Accessed.

18 Johnson, D., & Powell, E. (2020, March 6). Man Visiting Colorado, Woman in DougCO Test Positive for Coronavirus. *9 News*. https://www.9news.com/article/news/health/coronavirus/colorado-has-first-case-of-coronavirus-covid-19/73-3d2f21d8-7969-45bc-b172-a6b0d1a1516f

19 Kerwin McCrimmon, K. (2020, December 15). The First COVID-19 Case Likely in Colorado Long Before March. *UC Health*. https://www.uchealth.org/today/covid-19-likely-in-colorado-way-before-march/#:~:text=The%20first%20person%20to%20receive,29

20 Klemko, R., & Kindy, K. (2020, August 6). He Fled Congo to Work in a U.S. Meat Plant. Then He- and Hundreds of His Co-Workers- Got the Coronavirus. *The Washington Post*. https://www.washingtonpost.com/national/he-fled-the-congo-to-work-in-a-us-meat-plant-then-he--and-hun-dreds-of-his-co-workers--got-the-coronavirus/2020/08/06/11e7e13e-c526-11ea-8ffe-372be8d82298_story.html

21 Kovach, C. P., & Perman, S. M. (2021). Impact of the COVID-19 Pandemic on Cardiac Arrest Systems of Care. *Current Opinion in Critical Care*, 27(3), 239–245. doi. 10.1097/MCC.0000000000000817

22 Napoli, N. (2020, January 11) COVID-19 Pandemic Indirectly Disrupted Heart Disease Care. (2021, January 11). *American College of Cardiology*. Retrieved July 12, 2021 from https://www.acc.org/about-acc/press-releases/2021/01/11/16/40/covid19-pandemic-indirectly-disrupted-heart-disease-care

23 National Academies of Sciences, Engineering, and Medicine; Health and Medicine Division; Board on Population Health and Public Health Practice; Committee on Community-Based Solutions to Promote Health Equity in the United States; Baciu, A., Negussie, Y., Geller, A., et al., editors. *Communities in Action: Pathways to Health Equity*. Washington (DC): National Academies Press (US); 2017 Jan 11. 3, The Root Causes of Health Inequity. Available from: https://www.ncbi.nlm.nih.gov/books/NBK425845/

24 Paul, J. (2020, May 7). The Colorado Country with the Highest Coronavirus Infection Rate is Now on the Eastern Plains. *The Colorado Sun*. https://coloradosun.com/2020/05/07/morgan-county-colorado-coronavirus-outbreak/

25 Podewils, L. J., Burket, T. L., Mettenbrink, C., Streiner, A., Seidel, A., Scott, K., Cervantes, L., & Hasnain-Wynia, R. (2020, December 4). Disproportionate Incidence of COVID-19 Infection, Hospitalizations, and Deaths Among Persons Identifying as Hispanic or Latino—Denver, Colorado March–October 2020. *US Department of Health and Human Services/Centers for Disease Control and Prevention*. https://www.cdc.gov/mmwr/volumes/69/wr/pdfs/mm6948a3-H.pdf

26 Powers, M., Brown, P., Poudrier, G., Ohayon, J. L., Cordner, A., Alder, C., & Atlas, M. G. (2021). COVID-19 as Eco-Pandemic Injustice: Opportunities for Collective and Antiracist Approaches to Environmental Health. *Journal of Health and Social Behavior*, 62(2), 222–229. doi. 10.1177/00221465211005704

27 Public Health & Executive Orders. (2021). Colorado Department of Public Health & Environment, Colorado State Emergency Operations Center. Retrieved July 12, 2021 from https://covid19.colorado.gov/public-health-executive-orders

28 Ramírez, I. J., & Lee, J. (2020). COVID-19 Emergence and Social and Health Determinants in Colorado: A Rapid Spatial Analysis. *International Journal of Environmental Research and Public Health*, *17*(11), 3856. doi. 10.3390/ijerph17113856

29 Rogers, T. N., Rogers, C. R., VanSant-Webb, E., Gu, L. Y., Yan, B., & Qeadan, F. (2020). Racial Disparities in COVID-19 Mortality Among Essential Workers in the United States. *World Medical & Health Policy*. Advance online publication. doi. 10.1002/wmh3.358

30 Roth, S. (2020, April 14) American College of Cardiology Urges Heart Attack, Stroke Patients to Seek Medical Help. (2020, April 14). *American College of Cardiology*. Retrieved July 11, 2021 from https://www.acc.org/about-acc/press-releases/2020/04/14/10/17/american-college-of-cardiology-urges-heart-attack-stroke-patients-to-seek-medical-help

31 Seaman, J. (2020, August 8). Deaths From Heart Disease, Overdoses Increased in Colorado During Pandemic, Data Shows. *The Denver Post*. https://www.denverpost.com/2020/08/08/colorado-deaths-heart-disease-overdose-covid-pandemic/

32 Shah, P. B., Welt, F. G. P., Mahmud, E. Phillips, A., Kleiman, N. S., Young, M. N., Sherwood, M., Batchelor, W., Wang, D. D., Davidson, L., Wyman, J., Kadavath, S., Szerlip, M., Hermiller, J., Fullerton, D., & Anwaruddinon, S. (2020). Triage Considerations for Patients Referred for Structural Heart Disease Intervention During the COVID-19 Pandemic: An ACC/SCAI Position Statement. *JACC Journals: Cardiovascular Interventions*, *13*(12), 1484–1488. https://www.jacc.org/doi/full/10.1016/j.jcin.2020.04.001

33 Snouwaert, J. (2020, July 13). WATCH|Protesters Oppose Colorado Springs' Potential Mask Requirement. *The Gazette*. https://gazette.com/news/watch-protesters-oppose-colorado-springs-potential-mask-requirement/article_c9f628d0-c526-11ea-b861-6ba8c83b9fa9.html

34 Udell, E. (2020, April 23). After Coronavirus Outbreak, Greeley Meat Plant to Reopen Under New Restrictions. *Coloradoan*. https://www.coloradoan.com/story/news/2020/04/23/greeley-meat-plant-reopen-after-coronavirus-outbreak-infects-dozens/3015531001/

35 United States Census Bureau. (n.d.). Quick Facts Colorado. Retrieved July 12, 2021 from https://www.census.gov/quickfacts/fact/table/CO/RHI825219

36 Yearby, R., & Mohapatra, S. (2020). Law, Structural Racism, and the COVID-19 Pandemic. *Law and Biosciences*, *7*(1). doi. 10.1093/jlb/lsaa036

Chapter 9

Case study
A Florida COVID-19 dashboard

Zachary Pruitt
College of Public Health University of South Florida
Tampa, FL, USA

Jason L. Salemi
College of Public Health University of South Florida
Tampa, FL, USA

CONTENTS

Introduction 107
Summary of case study 109
Common concerns with COVID-19 dashboards 109
    Can the public trust the COVID-19 data from the FDOH? 109
    Were the rising COVID-19 cases in the summer of 2020
        simply due to increased testing? 110
    Which date should be used for reflecting the temporal
        progression of COVID-19 cases on an epidemic curve? 118
    Are COVID-19 case positivity rates enough to fully convey
        the changes pandemic severity? 123
    Were vaccinations effective at decreasing COVID-19 cases,
        hospitalizations and death in Florida? 127
    Why would the FDOH change the way it reports cases and
        deaths to CDC? 132
Lessons learned 134
Looking ahead 138
Conclusion 138
References 139

INTRODUCTION

During the COVID-19 pandemic, state and federal government public health agencies collected data on a variety of metrics, including cases, testing, hospitalizations, vaccinations, virus variants, and deaths. In Florida, the official Florida Department of Health (FDOH) COVID-19 Data and Surveillance

Dashboard provided this important public service for stakeholders of all types (e.g., public, media, scientists, clinicians, politicians, public servants). Crucially, the dashboard showed the epidemic curve – the number of new cases reported every day – so that stakeholders could monitor the outbreak. In fact, for much of the pandemic, the FDOH made available one of the largest assortments of downloadable electronic files and related reports in the country (Florida Department of Health, 2020).

However, the FDOH COVID-19 Data and Surveillance Dashboard lacked key elements, such as interactivity, queryability, and granularity, which hindered the ability to fully leverage the abundant publicly released data. This means that simply publishing the data in a COVID-19 tracker website did not convey optimal meaning for key stakeholders. Without further explanation, the public could not make sound judgments about how to protect themselves and their families from COVID-19. Without context, public messaging from public health professionals became more complicated. Without clarification, public health policy suffered from miscalculations and unnecessary conflict proliferated in the media. Moreover, misleading information – unintentional or nefarious – fueled widespread societal discord that challenged Florida's effort to control the coronavirus pandemic.

To improve decision-making, stakeholders needed data analytics that could only be accomplished by posing important questions, skillfully interpreting data, and clearly presenting the analyses. One of the authors of this chapter, Jason Salemi, PhD, MPH, an epidemiologist and biostatistician at the University of South Florida created a widely cited statewide Florida COVID-19 dashboard with interactive graphs, maps, animations, sociodemographic and geospatial filters, and explanatory tooltips (Salemi, 2021; USF Health News, 2021). In addition to data from the FDOH, the dashboard incorporated publicly available files from the Florida Agency for Health Care Administration (AHCA), the federal Department of Health and Human Services (DHHS), the Centers for Disease Control and Prevention (CDC), and the United States Census Bureau.

The dashboard provided a public service to Florida stakeholders by performing data analytics, such as data extraction, cleaning, linkage, analysis, and visualization. However, the presentation of the data was not derivative. Rather, the dashboard presented data more expansively by creating different visualizations than those government sources. The independent and free COVID-19 dashboard website became a highly valued and cited resource (Akhtar et al., 2020; Gamio, Mervosh, & Collins, 2020; Levin & Querolo, 2021). When creating the COVID-19 dashboard, the following questions were asked in order to enhance the utility for stakeholders:

- Granularity of the information – What is the state of the pandemic according to time, geographies, age groups, or gender?
- Visual appeal – How easy is it to illustrate the essence of COVID-19 data metrics in a visualization?

- Value-added analyses – Do the data extend beyond static figures and tables to provide important pre-calculated information when someone interacts with (i.e., hovers over) a visualization?
- Provide context – Does the analysis put the data into perspective? How do the metrics compare to other subgroups, such as geographies, age groups, or gender, and to other points in time? For example, are county-level comparisons of COVID-19 death rates age-adjusted? Have these comparisons changed over time?
- Highlight important methodological issues – Do the data support understanding of various COVID-19 data metrics, such as lag in death reporting and how that lag changes over time?

SUMMARY OF CASE STUDY

As the coronavirus pandemic unfolded, a number of central concerns emerged that could be clarified using data analytics and visualizations on Salemi's Florida COVID-19 dashboard. The questions posed here reflect the oft-expressed concerns of a variety of stakeholders, including the public, media, scientists, clinicians, politicians, and public servants.

1. Can the public trust the COVID-19 data from the FDOH?
2. Were the rising COVID-19 cases in the summer of 2020 simply due to increased testing?
3. Which date should be used for reflecting the temporal progression of COVID-19 cases on an epidemic curve?
4. Are COVID-19 case positivity rates enough to fully convey the changes in pandemic severity?
5. Were vaccinations effective at decreasing COVID-19 cases, hospitalizations, and death in Florida?
6. Why would the FDOH change the way it reports cases and deaths to CDC?

COMMON CONCERNS WITH COVID-19 DASHBOARDS

Can the public trust the COVID-19 data from the FDOH?

To maintain trust of the stakeholders and act as a steward of the data, data analysts must conduct due diligence on the data to every extent possible. While the "truth" in the data cannot be known by those external to the agencies that "own" the data, epidemiologists and data analysts reporting on diseases should scrutinize the data to every extent possible. Best practices in data analytics hold that, if errors are discovered, assistance should be provided to the source entity. For example, Florida hospitals and AHCA employees worked diligently during the pandemic to make data on pediatric hospitalization rates in Florida publicly available through routine submissions to the federal government. When errors were discovered, the potential mistakes were communicated to state officials with professionalism and humility, which allowed for a deeper investigation and timely correction of the erroneous data. These understaffed agencies have an immense responsibility and workload, making simple but consequential mistakes almost inevitable. Combining ongoing data scrutiny with clear, expert feedback is of immense value to public health agencies.

How should data analysts vet the data? One important step is to ask questions, such as, "How do these data compare?" For example, there were considerable suggestions that Florida was underreporting COVID-19 deaths (Downey, 2021; Tatar, 2021). In response, prudence requires a detailed assessment regarding how each state reported the total percent excess deaths and the percent of all deaths that were attributable to COVID-19. As illustrated in Figure 9.1, a correlation of those two metrics was created using a scatter plot. So, when asking, "Does Florida or any other state stand out?," the answer, even using simple visualizations like a correlation plot, is "no." Regarding the relationship between percent excess deaths and percent of all deaths attributable to COVID-19, Florida is plotted in the middle and close to the national average (labeled as United States).

However, some data need additional context to evaluate trustworthiness. For example, a news article reported that the Institute for Health Metrics and Evaluation (IHME) presented new calculations for COVID-19 death estimates, accounting for underreporting across jurisdictions (Downey, 2021). Irrespective of whether one possesses confidence in the IHME death estimation methodology or not, the news report highlighted that the death toll in Florida was estimated to be 41% higher than what the FDOH had officially reported to the public. Without context, the reporting in the media about IHME estimate and the discrepancy from the Florida reported deaths led FDOH officials to dismiss the use of statistical modeling (Downey, 2021). However, when the IHME death estimates for all states were compared to each state's COVID-19 reported deaths, just about every state has underreported COVID-19 deaths (Colombini, 2021). In fact, among the five most populous states, Florida landed in the middle with New York and Illinois having slightly less underreporting and Texas and California having slightly larger underreporting, compared to the IHME estimates. Also, compared to the national average, Florida had less estimated underreporting. Without context, or perhaps with a biased view of the analysis, useful data analytics can be readily (and unfortunately) dismissed, discredited, or misconstrued.

Were the rising COVID-19 cases in the summer of 2020 simply due to increased testing?

On June 25, 2020 Florida experienced a second day in a row of 5,000 COVID-19 cases per day, the highest reported number of cases to that point since the FDOH began COVID-19 tracking. Figure 9.2 shows the Florida

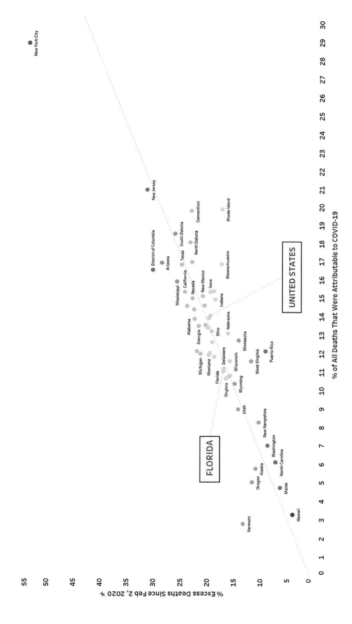

Figure 9.1 Scatter plot of all-cause deaths to deaths attributable to COVID-19 in 2020.

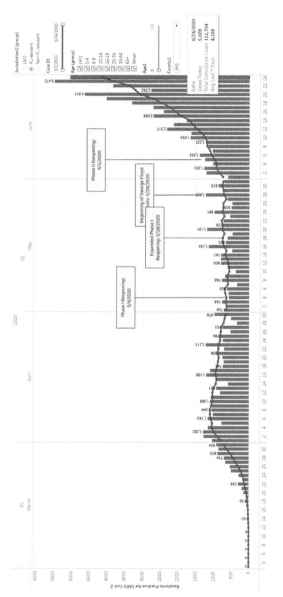

Figure 9.2 Florida COVID-19 epidemic curve March 1, 2020 through June 24, 2020.

epidemic curve among the entire resident population in Florida from March 1, 2020 through June 24, 2020. What was thought to be a massive increase in cases occurring in early April was far overshadowed by an increase in the number of COVID-19 cases that really began at the beginning of June. This led to a number of concerns.

First, it stands to reason that if more people are tested for SARS-COV-2, then more people will test positive. Perhaps the June increase in COVID-19 cases was due to just more testing? Figure 9.3 shows the number of viral lab tests per day from the beginning of March 2020 through June 23, 2020. While there was an ebb and flow in cases on a daily basis, the red line undoubtedly demonstrates the overall pattern of the increase. So, this data chart alone might indicate that the increase in COVID-19 cases was due to increased testing.

However, another question that data analysts needed to ask during the pandemic was "What proportion of all people who are being tested are testing positive?" Figure 9.4 shows the daily case positivity from March 1, 2020 through June 24, 2020. In late March and early April 2020, Florida saw the proportion of people who received a COVID-19 test and tested positive exceeded 10%. Then throughout May, the case positivity declined to below 10%. Then again in late June, Florida experienced a COVID-19 positivity rate above 10%.

So, the claim that more cases are due to more testing is plausible. Figures 9.2 and 9.3 seem to be correlated, and the increase in daily case positivity in June 2020 shown in Figure 9.4 also seems to support this claim. But, what if additional data analyses were performed?

In Figure 9.5, each dot represents a different date with coloring of the dots ranging from dark green in early March, lighter green is April, light red in early June, and dark red in June. The X axis shows the daily volume in testing or "how many tests were performed?" The Y axis indicates the case positivity rate, or "what proportion of all people tested that are testing positive?" The descending trend line suggests that as Florida performed more testing, the proportion of people who tested positive went down. This means that as Florida expanded testing availability, more people were getting tested. But the positivity rate went down as fewer people actually had the virus and healthy people were also tested along with sick people. However, if the savvy data analyst noted deep red at the top-center of Figure 9.5, then they would see high case positivity (Y axis), but only moderate daily testing volume. In other words, the highest case positivity rate (18%) occurred later in the period (June 23, 2020), even though the daily testing volume was about half of the highest volume. Still, there is certainly a negative correlation between testing volume and the percent that tests positive, that is, the higher the testing volume, the lower the case positivity. However, this analysis does not tell the complete story.

Additional analysis reveals the answer to the question of whether increase in cases is due to more testing. Note that Figure 9.6 illustrates the same

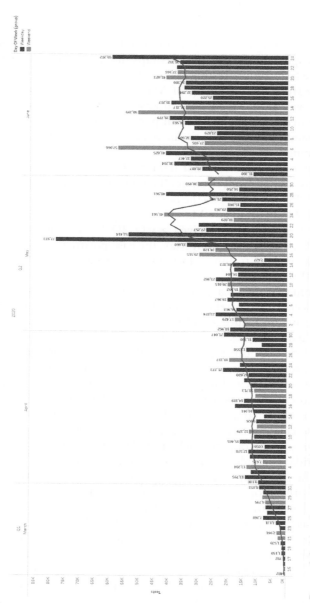

Figure 9.3 Number of viral lab tests per day through June 23, 2020.

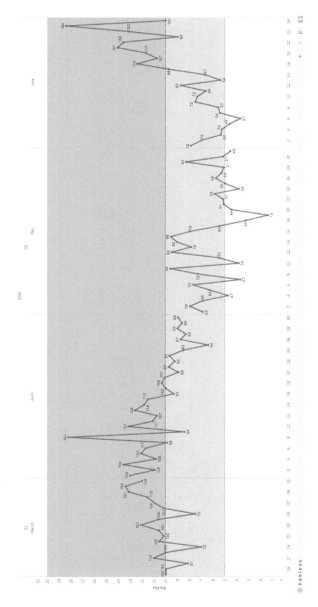

Figure 9.4 Daily case positivity from March 1, 2020 through June 24, 2020.

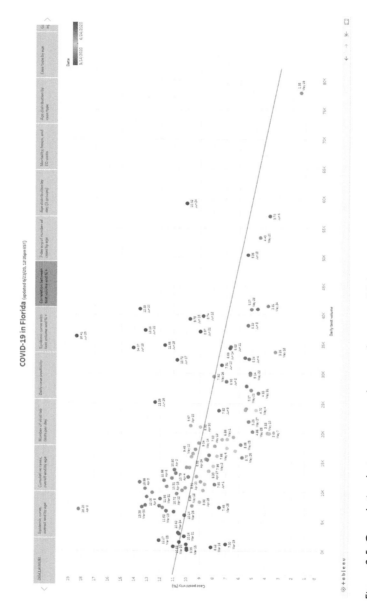

Figure 9.5 Correlation between test volume and case positivity percentage.

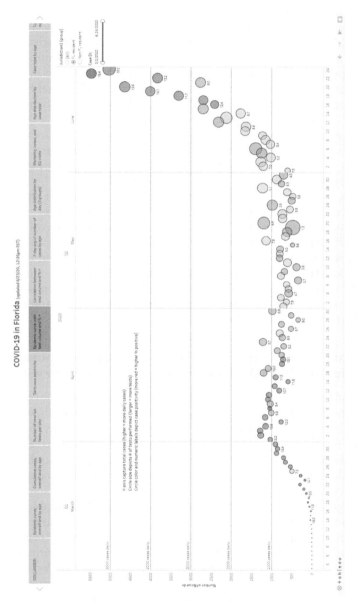

Figure 9.6 Epidemic curve with test volume and case positivity percentage.

shape as the epidemic curve showing the number of daily COVID-19 cases over time on the Y axis. In contrast to Figure 9.2 that uses dots instead of bars and a line, the size of each dot pertains to daily testing volume – the bigger the bubble, the more the number of tests performed. The color of the dots represents case positivity rates from green (low) to yellow (moderate) to red (high). The visualization of Figure 9.6 shows that in early April the number of positive tests was low, but the dots are shaded red, meaning that a high proportion of people were testing positive. At this time in the pandemic, fewer tests were available, so the small red dots reflect that Floridians were probably only getting tested when they demonstrated symptoms of COVID-19. In late April, the yellow dots with larger size show a decreasing case positivity rate and increasing testing volume, relative to March. In May, Florida was testing more individuals (larger dots), but the case positivity relates were low (green); that is, the big green dots indicate that Florida was testing many people, but getting fewer positive results.

However, by the middle to late part of June, as the number of cases of COVID-19 increased rapidly (the Y axis), the dots were similar in size as late May but turning darker red, which means a higher case positivity rate. Therefore, Figure 9.6 clearly demonstrates that the epidemic curve shown in Figure 9.2 is not just due to the fact that Florida was conducting more tests but that Florida actually experienced a marked increase in numbers of COVID-19 infections in June. If the rising epidemic curve was in fact due to increased testing, then the visualization would show much larger dots in mid- and late June, compared to May 2020.

Which date should be used for reflecting the temporal progression of COVID-19 cases on an epidemic curve?

When Florida stakeholders see an epidemic curve that shows 5,409 COVID-19 cases reported on a single day, as they did on Tuesday June 29, what does that actually mean? Is that based on the date that these individuals were exposed to the virus? Is that the date that they became infectious? Is that the date they showed signs or symptoms? Is that the date they tested positive? Is that the date the case was reported and what is reported missing? Or is it something else?

During the coronavirus pandemic, the FDOH publicly available data file contained multiple date variables. In terms of the epidemic curve, the two most important dates provided were the "case date" and the "event date." The case date means the date that the COVID-19 case was confirmed by the FDOH through a positive test reported by a laboratory or by a contact tracer who spoke to the individual. The event date is the date that symptoms began for the person who reported positive for COVID-19. Both of these dates are available in the publicly available data file.

More often than not, these two dates were different for COVID-19. Why? Imagine that a healthy individual was exposed to the SARS-COV-2 virus.

At the beginning, the virus is "latent" (sleeping) within their body. After a certain period, the virus starts to replicate and the individual enters the infectious state, meaning that they can pass this virus to others. However, infection and viral replication do not necessarily mean the person feels sick. Many people get infected and may infect others with the coronavirus without having any symptoms, called "asymptomatic" transmission (Kimball, et al., 2020).

Eventually, some individuals infected with the SARS-COV-2 virus would display signs and symptoms. The time period between when an individual was exposed to the virus, to when they actually started to show signs and symptoms is called the "incubation period." Of course, what prompts most people to get tested are those signs and symptoms. Although there can be considerable variability, individuals usually get tested a week or so after exposure, typically after they begin to feel ill.

For example, if a person was exposed to the virus on June 1st, he/she might develop signs and symptoms on June 6th. In this example, the incubation period is five days, which was approximately the median incubation period for the original strain of the SARS-COV-2 virus (Wassie et al., 2020). So, individuals suffer through the mild signs and symptoms at the beginning, but eventually they go to the emergency department because the effects of the virus worsen. After being tested in the emergency department, a COVID-19 positive test comes back on June 9th. Suppose there is no lag in reporting, so what actually gets documented for that case date by the FDOH is June 9th. Notice that there is a difference between that case date on June 9th and when the individual developed symptoms, which was three days before that, and it was eight days before that, they were actually exposed to the virus.

Now, let's consider another scenario: an individual who was exposed to the virus but never developed symptoms. Maybe they socially engaged with people who have actually developed symptoms and tested positive for COVID-19. So, they decide to get tested on June 9th. In this case, the individual was confirmed positive for COVID-19 on June 9th. What about the event date, which is supposed to be the date of symptom onset? In this example, the documentation, in the absence of symptoms, will show the event date equal to the case date (June 9th). That is, the FDOH just knows when the person tested positive not when they were exposed, so the event date is documented as the same date as the case date.

Finally, there is a scenario when individuals develop signs and symptoms the day after they test positive. The time period between exposure to the virus and when a person actually develops signs and symptoms can extend to as long as 14 days (Wassie et al., 2020). In this example, the time between June 1st (exposure) and June 10th (event date) is 10 days (latent period).

Figure 9.7 demonstrates that these scenarios exist in the June 2020 publicly available data sample from the FDOH. The gray bar shows that the case date and event date are exactly the same (34.7%). For 45% of this, the event date/symptoms onset comes between 1 and 7 days before the case

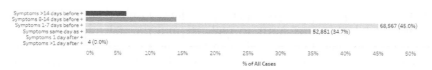

Figure 9.7 Difference between case date (COVID-19 test positive) and event date (symptoms onset).

		Cases	%
Infected	Symptoms >14 days before +	7,097	5.7%
	Symptoms 8-14 days before +	15,555	12.4%
	Symptoms 1-7 days before +	53,487	42.6%
	Symptoms same day as +	49,368	39.3%
	Symptoms 1 day after +	41	0.0%
	Symptoms >1 day after +	3	0.0%
ED Visit	Symptoms >14 days before +	1,103	9.9%
	Symptoms 8-14 days before +	2,695	24.1%
	Symptoms 1-7 days before +	6,455	57.8%
	Symptoms same day as +	916	8.2%
Hosp	Symptoms >14 days before +	1,147	9.5%
	Symptoms 8-14 days before +	2,555	21.1%
	Symptoms 1-7 days before +	6,661	55.0%
	Symptoms same day as +	1,747	14.4%
Died	Symptoms >14 days before +	293	8.1%
	Symptoms 8-14 days before +	526	14.6%
	Symptoms 1-7 days before +	1,964	54.5%
	Symptoms same day as +	820	22.8%
	Symptoms >1 day after +	1	0.0%
Grand Total		152,434	100.0%

Figure 9.8 Location of COVID-19 test: difference between case date (COVID-19 test positive) and event date (symptoms onset).

date/positive test. Smaller proportions of individuals developed symptoms between 8 and 14 days before testing positive, and an even smaller proportion developed symptoms more than 14 days before testing positive. A very small number developed symptoms after testing positive.

Figure 9.8 breaks out the difference between case date (COVID-19 test positive) and event date (symptoms onset) by location at which the person was tested for COVID-19. In the top category, "Infected" means that the person did not seek healthcare services, such as in the emergency department, which most people visited in June 2020. Among this group, 39.3% show the case date (COVID-19 test positive) and event date (symptoms) as the same. That is, if a person is asymptomatic, then both case and event positive dates are equal. However, as soon as individuals seek healthcare services, a much lower proportion shows that these two dates are the same. More often, the COVID-19 symptoms became worse for week and up to two weeks before that.

So, does it really matter whether we use the case date or the event date in the epidemic curve? While the publicly available data from the FDOH contains both variables, the epidemic curve that on the FDOH COVID-19 Data and Surveillance Dashboard is based on the case date (COVID-19 test positive), not the event date (symptom). However, if *cumulative* case count epidemic curve charts were created for each of the case date (COVID-19 test confirmed) and event date (symptom onset) data variables, then the difference becomes apparent. (Note: the two axes are not aligned because there were no confirmed cases based on that case date before March.) Figure 9.9 uses a case date as the cumulative case count. In this instance it would be 6,829 at the end of March 2020. If the epidemic curve charts were based on when symptoms began (event date), then the count would be more than double at 16,208. As the pandemic progressed through the end of June 2020, the difference was not as dramatic, compared to the numbers earlier in the epidemic.

What this means is that the case date lags behind event date. By the time 6,829 cases were counted at the end of March 2020, more than two times that number of people were already infected with COVID-19 and were developing the symptoms. And yet, these individuals would not test positive counted later. This is important to understand because early in a pandemic, stakeholders need to know when the numbers are increasing. If the decision-making is not based on symptom onset, then any take action may be taken too late. Ideally, you would have a curve that shows when people were exposed to the virus, but of course that would be impossible to know. Therefore, the best date available to epidemiologists for identifying cases and controlling outbreaks is the date of symptom onset (event date).

During a pandemic, the ultimate public health goal is to identify and isolate positive cases. If the time frame between symptom and onset can be shortened, then the outbreak can be controlled. This is a challenge. Nevertheless, if the data analytics do not present the epidemic curve based on event date/symptom onset, then additional people may be exposed and infected during the delay.

However, this is not a criticism of the FDOH COVID-19 Data and Surveillance Dashboard. Plausibly, the reasons that the FDOH used case date-based epidemic curve were justifiable. Perhaps public health officials were concerned about recall bias tainting the data. For example, during the COVID-19 pandemic, some people reported that they were sick in early January, when they actually tested positive in March. While improbable, this recall bias would introduce inconsistency in the data. In addition, the decision to use case date could be related to the time it takes to conduct contact tracing. That is, it could be that the FDOH would not have been able to update symptom onset (event date) until too much time had passed. So for consistency and timeliness sake, the FDOH may have decided to use the date individual tested positive (case date).

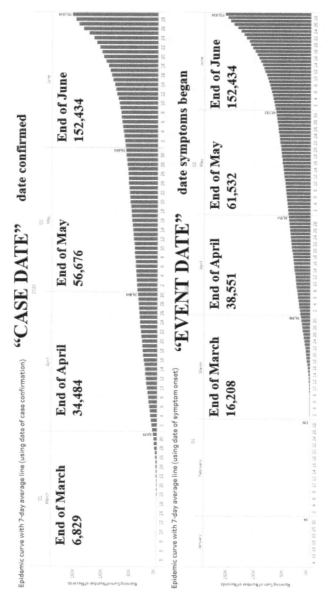

Figure 9.9 Cumulative case count epidemic curve charts for case date (COVID-19 test confirmed) event date (symptom onset).

Are COVID-19 case positivity rates enough to fully convey the changes pandemic severity?

Florida experienced a steady decrease in COVID-19 cases in the fall of 2020, after the stressful summer peak. Then, in the month of October 2020, the case positivity increased again. During this time, stakeholders again asked, "Are increases in COVID-19 cases really just due to more testing?" Figure 9.10 shows that in October 2020, the case positivity rate increased from 4.6% to 7.2%.

There are nine different testing scenarios that can provide an answer to this question. Each of these calculations requires using seven-day rolling averages with two variables: (1) testing volume and (2) case positivity. Both of these variables were made publicly available by the FDOH. The case positivity measure is the weekly average percent positivity among all people tested on a given day that removes duplicates (repeat testers within the given week) from the numerator and the denominator. While none of the mathematics are complicated, there are basic calculations that data analysts must consider to understand the relative changes in cases versus testing volume during the pandemic.

For "Time 1" of each of these nine scenarios, each of the variables remains constant; that is, the calculated 7-day average of positive cases is 7,000 and the calculated 7-day average of the volume of people tested daily is 1,00,000, which equals an average of 7% case positivity for past 7 days. In Figure 9.11, the case positivity is 7% in both time point one ("Time 1") and time point two ("Time 2").

In Testing Scenario 1 (Figure 9.11), if testing volume stayed the same from Time 1 to Time 2, then the number of cases will be the same. Of course, this in Scenario 1 both testing volume and case positivity will show 0% change.

In Testing Scenario 2 (Figure 9.11), what happens if there were 1,00,000 daily tests Time 1 and then 80,000 tests in Time 2. Because case positivity remains constant, both testing volume and case positivity decrease by 20%.

In Testing Scenario 3 (Figure 9.11), what happens if testing increases? In this Testing Scenario, testing increased from 1,00,000 people tested each day to 1,20,000 a day. Because case positivity has remained at 7%, a concomitant increase in cases at 20%. Therefore, when positivity does not change, testing volume and case positivity track together.

In Figure 9.12, each of the following three testing scenarios, the case positivity decreases from 7% to 6% and the testing volume changes. In Testing Scenario 4 (Figure 9.12 in yellow), there is no change in the number of tests, but because of the decreased case positivity (from 7% to 6%), there is a reduction in the number of cases (−14.3%). The reduction in cases is because a smaller proportion of people who were tested had positive test results.

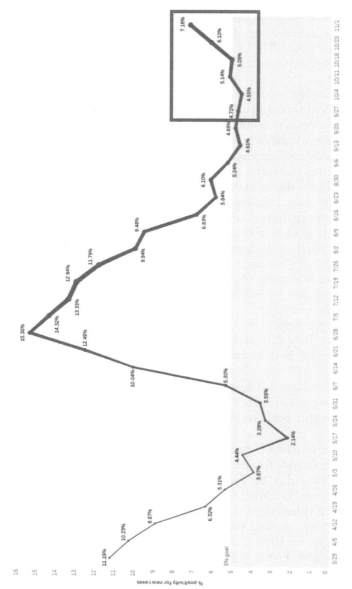

Figure 9.10 Percent positivity for new cases from March 29, 2020 to November 1, 2020.

Testing Scenario	Metric	Report released "TIME 1"	Report released "TIME 2"	% change
Testing stays the same	People Tested	100,000	100,000	**0.0**
	New Positive Tests (Cases)	7,000	7,000	**0.0**
	% pos (among all people tested)	7.0	7.0	0.0

Testing Scenario	Metric	Report released "TIME 1"	Report released "TIME 2"	% change
Testing decreases 20%	People Tested	100,000	80,000	-20.0
	New Positive Tests (Cases)	7,000	5,600	-20.0
	% pos (among all people tested)	7.0	7.0	0.0

Testing Scenario	Metric	Report released "TIME 1"	Report released "TIME 2"	% change
Testing increases 20%	People Tested	100,000	120,000	20.0
	New Positive Tests (Cases)	7,000	8,400	20.0
	% pos (among all people tested)	7.0	7.0	0.0

Figure 9.11 Case positivity remains constant at 7%.

In Testing Scenario 5 (Figure 9.12), testing volume decreased from an average 1,00,000 to 80,000 per day and the case positivity decreased from 7% to 6% over the 7-day period. In this scenario, the decrease in testing volume and decrease in case positivity results in a pronounced reduction in cases (−31.4%).

In Testing Scenario 6 (Figure 9.12), an increase in average testing volume from 1,00,000 per day to 1,20,000 per day along with the decrease in case positivity (7%–6%) results in an increase number of cases, but not nearly as pronounced (only a 3% increase). Therefore, Scenario 6 shows an increase in cases due to substantial increases in testing, despite a decrease in case positivity.

Finally, Figure 9.13 illustrates the three scenarios where the case positivity increased from 7% to 8%. In Scenario 7 (Figure 9.13), the testing volume is constant at 1,00,000 for Time 1 and Time 2. With no change in testing volume, there is an increase in cases from 7,000 cases to 8,000 cases because of the increase in case positivity from 7% to 8%. Therefore, the 14.3% increase in cases was not due to increases in testing volume, but due to an increase in case positivity.

In Scenario 8 (Figure 9.13), there is a decrease in the number of tests, from 1,00,000 to 80,000 (a 20% reduction). Even though case positivity has actually increased from 7% to 8%, the relative decrease in cases (−8.6%) is less than the decrease in testing volume (−20.0%).

Scenario 9 (Figure 9.13), shows the scenario similar to what happened in the summer of 2020, when Florida conducted more testing. This scenario illustrates a case positivity increase from 7% to 8% and testing volume increase from 1,00,000 to 1,20,000 per day on average. The proportionate increase in testing volume (20% increase) does not explain all of the increase in cases (37.1% increase), only a portion.

Testing Scenario	Metric	Report released "TIME 1"	Report released "TIME 2"	% change
Testing stays the same	People Tested	100,000	100,000	0.0
	New Positive Tests (Cases)	7,000	6,000	-14.3
	% pos (among all people tested)	7.0	6.0	-14.3

Testing Scenario	Metric	Report released "TIME 1"	Report released "TIME 2"	% change
Testing decreases 20%	People Tested	100,000	80,000	-20.0
	New Positive Tests (Cases)	7,000	4,800	-31.4
	% pos (among all people tested)	7.0	6.0	-14.3

Testing Scenario	Metric	Report released "TIME 1"	Report released "TIME 2"	% change
Testing Increases 20%	People Tested	100,000	120,000	20.0
	New Positive Tests (Cases)	7,000	7,200	2.9
	% pos (among all people tested)	7.0	6.0	-14.3

Figure 9.12 Case positivity decreases from 7% to 6%.

Testing Scenario	Metric	Report released "TIME 1"	Report released "TIME 2"	% change
Testing stays the same	People Tested	100,000	100,000	0.0
	New Positive Tests (Cases)	7,000	8,000	14.3
	% pos (among all people tested)	7.0	8.0	14.3

Testing Scenario	Metric	Report released "TIME 1"	Report released "TIME 2"	% change
Testing decreases 20%	People Tested	100,000	80,000	-20.0
	New Positive Tests (Cases)	7,000	6,400	-8.6
	% pos (among all people tested)	7.0	8.0	14.3

Testing Scenario	Metric	Report released "TIME 1"	Report released "TIME 2"	% change
Testing increases 20%	People Tested	100,000	120,000	20.0
	New Positive Tests (Cases)	7,000	9,600	37.1
	% pos (among all people tested)	7.0	8.0	14.3

Figure 9.13 Case positivity increases from 7% to 8%.

In summary, case positivity rates alone do not fully convey the changes pandemic severity. For example, if case positivity is staying the same over time, then testing volume and cases will track together at approximately the same rate. However, if case positivity is changing along with testing volume, then both metrics are required to convey changes to the pandemic severity. For example, when case positivity increases over time, cases will increase when testing volume is constant. However, if case positivity increases over time and there is a decrease in testing volume, case numbers may increase, stay the same, or may actually even be decreasing. Therefore, it is insufficient to report case positivity rates without test volumes in ever-changing pandemic scenarios.

Were vaccinations effective at decreasing COVID-19 cases, hospitalizations and death in Florida?

As of May 4, 2021 over 14 million doses had been administered to Florida residents, nearly 9 million people with at least one dose of one of the three major COVID-19 vaccines and over 6 million people who had been fully vaccinated (Salemi, 2021). Figure 9.14 shows how Florida vaccinations changed by age group over time. The elderly in Florida experienced pronounced vaccination growth early in 2021. By May 2021 more than four in five people aged 65 and over had been vaccinated in Florida, nearly 1 million elderly people. In addition, as soon as some of the younger age groups became eligible to get vaccinated in Florida, these age groups demonstrated an immediate increase in vaccination rates. However, by April, Florida vaccination rates plateaued for almost every age group.

Figure 9.15 shows the 7-day average COVID-19 cases from April 1, 2020 to May 1, 2021. The black line represents the number of all COVID-19 cases per day (the typical epidemic curve). In Florida, people over 65 years of age were prioritized for vaccines ahead of those under 18 (cite). By March 2020, COVID-19 cases among Florida's senior population dipped below the cases in the pediatric population, largely due to vaccinations.

Figure 9.15 also shows the percent of daily cases occurring among people 65 and older in the gray-shaded area curve in the background, which represents the proportion of daily cases that is occurring among seniors. Early in 2020, a high percentage of cases –mainly because testing was not widespread – occurred in seniors. By summer 2020, the proportion of seniors who tested positive for COVID-19 remained constant at about 16%–17% until widespread vaccinations in the senior population in mid- to late January. By May 1, 2021, the proportion of seniors testing positive for COVID-19 had fallen to about 7%.

Vaccinations seemed to have impacted COVID-19-related hospitalizations in Florida as well. This is information based on a report that comes from the federal DHHS, a report publically available since the end of February 2021. Figure 9.16 shows that in Florida at the end of February, about 41% of new admissions to the hospital for COVID-19 were among people aged 70 or older, a group at high risk for severe illness and mortality. Since the administration of COVID-19 vaccinations increased (see Figure 9.16), the proportion of new hospital admissions of people in Florida who were 70 and over fell from 41% to less than 30%. So the age distribution of people who were hospitalized for COVID-19 shifted to younger, less vulnerable age groups.

Figure 9.17 shows why reducing hospitalizations for groups vulnerable to mortality related to COVID-19 was so important in Florida. COVID-19 hospitalization is highly predictive of actual deaths. Figure 9.17 shows the relationship of hospitalizations COVID-19 (red line on right vertical axis) and mortality (gray bars on left vertical axis). The three gray bars are deaths

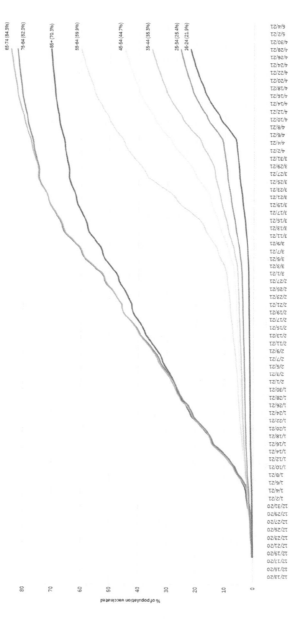

Figure 9.14 Florida vaccinations by age group from December 13, 2021 to May 4, 2021.

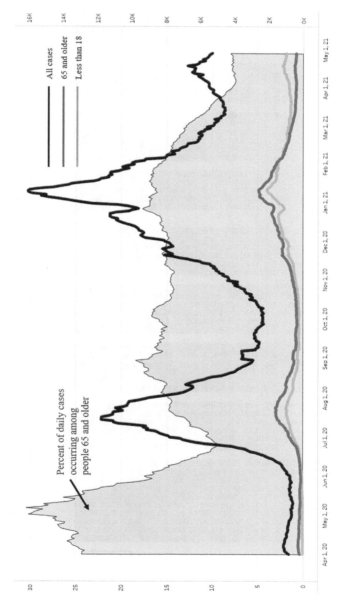

Figure 9.15 Seven-day average COVID-19 cases from April 1, 2020 to May 1, 2021.

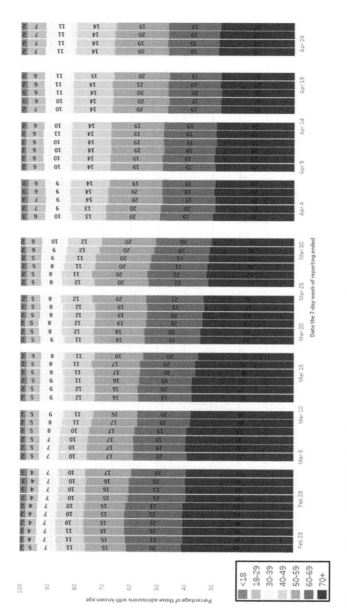

Figure 9.16 New COVID-19 hospitalizations by age group, February 23, 2021 to April 24, 2021.

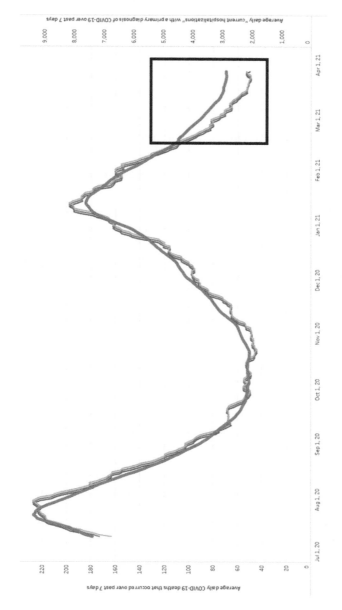

Figure 9.17 COVID-19 hospitalizations as a predictor of COVID-19 deaths 5–7 days later.

that actually occurred five to seven days later. This figure clearly illustrates that the shapes of these curves were almost identical throughout this time period. The black box highlights the separation of these lines wherein the same number of hospitalizations is now predictive of fewer deaths. This phenomenon is likely due in large part to the fact that a significant number of elderly people, who are most vulnerable to mortality, were fully vaccinated.

Obviously, zero deaths are the goal, but the fact that the same number of hospitalizations are resulting in fewer deaths is certainly a positive result related to vaccinations. These few visualizations underscore the importance of our progress on vaccines and how it can make a difference in cases among vulnerable age groups and current hospitalizations and in mortality.

Why would the FDOH change the way it reports cases and deaths to CDC?

In August 2021, CDC published data on the federal COVID-19 tracker that showed that Florida experienced over 28,300 new COVID-19 cases for both the 7th and 8th of August, record highs for the State. Local news organizations, which meticulously monitor the CDC website, quickly announced that "Florida Again Breaks Record" (Associated Press, 2021; Neal, 2021). However, the FDOH official Twitter account (@HealthyFla) soon disputed the numbers stating, "The daily case counts for Florida currently posted on the CDC COVID Tracker are incorrect," and the FDOH posted the correct numbers for August 6th, 7th, and 8th (Florida Department of Health, 2021).

In the hyper-charged political environment surrounding COVID-19, citizens and media outlets speculated whether the CDC was intentionally making the Florida pandemic conditions look worse than it was, or whether Florida was hiding COVID-19 cases and deaths (Musgrave, 2021). Neither of the two extremes was correct. In instances like this, independent data analysts must thoroughly investigate all reasons that may underlie seeming discrepancies between government agency reporting. Accusations of nefarious behavior may be explained by simple mathematical errors.

What happened? Earlier in the pandemic, the FDOH and AHCA made a myriad of detailed reports and comprehensive datasets publicly available on a daily basis. That changed in early June 2021, when the Florida agencies decreased how frequently data were released to the public – from daily comprehensive reports to weekly summary reports. However, the FDOH and AHCA continued to send the detailed data to the CDC. The mistake occurred when the CDC misinterpreted the detailed Florida data.

In the past, Florida reported an updated cumulative case and death counts (among other elements) to the CDC. However, over weekends, the FDOH did not provide daily updates of the cumulative numbers. On data covering weekends, the CDC reconciliation process required dividing the multi-day total (the weekend) by the number of days to estimate the daily number of cases and deaths reported each day during that time. The mistake was likely due to timing; perhaps the data came to the CDC a little earlier than usual, and the CDC assumed it pertained to a two-day instead of a three-day window. This simple mistake led to public speculation and acrimony.

The following two scenarios explain how this misunderstanding occurred. In the simpler "weekday" scenario, Florida may report a total of 2,020,000 resident COVID-19 cases to date on a Tuesday. If the cumulative total on the previous day was 2,000,000, then CDC would subtract the two numbers and report 20,000 new cases reported on Tuesday. However, in the second more complicated "weekend" scenario, Florida would send the cumulative case and death count to the CDC on Monday. So, if Florida's previous numbers to the CDC equaled 2,000,000, and the latest report sent on Monday at 5:30pm updated the number to 2,060,000, then that represents 60,000 new cases reported. However, since these 60,000 new cases actually included Friday, Saturday, and Sunday, CDC should have divided 60,000 by 3 to compute an average of 20,000 newly reported cases for each of the three days. Unfortunately, CDC divided the three-day total by two days, making the daily average of 30,000 cases per day, a 50% increase over the reality.

Once the mistake was identified, the data processing procedures were improved so that every few days the entire time series would be updated and reported to the CDC with daily COVID-19 cases and deaths dating back to the beginning of the pandemic. This important change resulted in another benefit – more accurately reporting daily COVID-19 deaths based on when they occurred instead of based on date the deaths were reported. Unfortunately, some accused Florida public health officials of using this change as a way to underreport COVID-19 deaths (Sidorowicz, 2021). First a mathematical mistake produced misunderstanding, and then the data processing change created controversy.

However, the FDOH was not engaging in chicanery. A closer examination of the data revealed that the revised reporting process actually enabled Florida to more accurately reflect the daily deaths based on when they occurred. The old procedure was problematic because of the time lag associated with reporting deaths. As described above, when a person dies from COVID-19, it can take from days to months for the death certificate to be certified and reported in the official numbers. Skilled data analysts should always sufficiently explore data to understand the different ways in which data, even on the same metric, may be reported, and provide the necessary context so that various stakeholder groups are capable of deriving meaningful and actionable evidence from what is being reported.

Despite the initial animosity and confusion caused by change how the FDOH reported to CDC, Florida's revised reporting approach actually allowed for a more thorough investigation of recent trends in deaths. During the pandemic, the media commonly reported the number of COVID-19 deaths reported on a particular day without any information on when those people actually died. However, the date on which a death was reported does not help public health officials to track severe outcomes of the pandemic. Figures 9.18 and 9.19 illustrate the difference between charting the date in which deaths are reported and when deaths occurred. First, Figure 9.18 shows the Florida epidemic curve for COVID-19 deaths by date reported. During the week of August 6 to August 12, 2021, Florida reported 1,071 deaths, but only 286 (27%) people actually died during that week (see blue arrow). It is not known when the other 785 people died based on the report alone (in the red rectangle or in the blue rectangle?) because the epidemic curve adds all 1,071 COVID-19 deaths to the date when they were reported (far right bar).

In contrast, Figure 9.19 illustrates the reporting of COVID-19 deaths for on the date the deaths occurred for the dates of July 1 through August 25, 2021. The different lines reflect different reporting dates. The vertical line marks the deaths that occurred on one date, August 12. As of August 13 ((a) curve), the 7-day average daily deaths were 36. With each subsequent update of the time series file – August 17 ((b) curve), August 19 ((c) curve), August 23 ((d) curve), and August 26 ((e) curve) – more COVID-19 deaths had been reported to the FDOH so each subsequent curve demonstrates increasingly more deaths that occurred on August 12. As a result of the updates between August 13 and August 26, the 7-day average of deaths that occurred on August 12 increased from 36 to 200.

Parenthetically, another source of confusion for stakeholders was the downturn of the COVID-19 deaths for the most recent time period, as shown in Figure 9.19 from August 13 to August 26. This downward trending curve on the right side of the figure should not be interpreted to mean that COVID-19 deaths were decreasing. Rather, the characteristic decline in when the deaths occurred for the most recent period happens because it can take a few weeks before all COVID-19 deaths are reported for a particular date (i.e., reporting lag).

LESSONS LEARNED

For much of the pandemic, the FDOH dashboard made Florida's basic epidemic curve available to the public. However, the public website lacked the in-depth data analysis for effective decision-making. In response to the need for more information, several independent dashboards were created, including Salemi's statewide Florida COVID-19 dashboard, to serve Florida's stakeholders (Salemi, 2021). Salemi's interactive data visualization dashboard supported comprehensive examination of the coronavirus pandemic with visual appeal and functional flexibility. Stakeholders could query the Tableau-based visualizations along many dimensions, including Florida counties, age groups, and gender. Moreover, users could interactively investigate additional COVID-19 data metrics linked from other publicly available files (e.g., AHCA, DHHS, CDC) that were linked to the FDOH data.

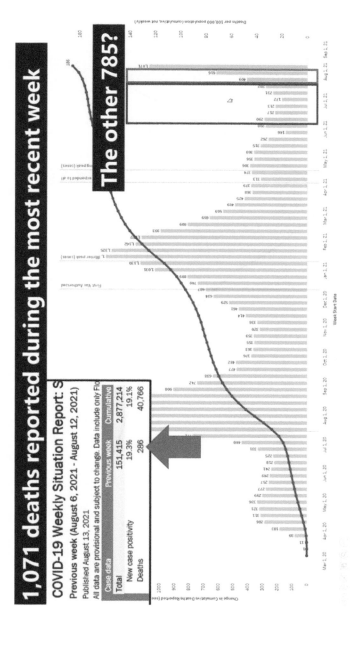

Figure 9.18 Florida epidemic curve for COVID-19 deaths by date reported.

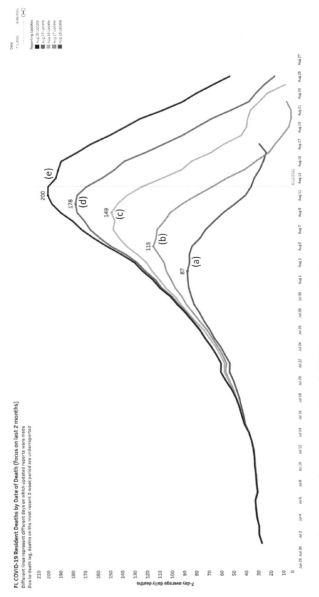

Figure 9.19 Florida epidemic curve for COVID-19 deaths by date occurred.

Despite the advanced data analytics supplied by Salemi's Florida COVID-19 dashboard, additional concerns were raised by stakeholders that required additional explanation. Multiple lessons emerged from answering stakeholder questions.

- Independent data analysts can support government officials who supply publicly available data – Data should be thoroughly vetted and, if errors are discovered, assistance should be provided to the government entities with professionalism and humility. Data analysts who act as a "second set of eyes" and provide non-judgmental feedback to public servants can improve data accuracy and increase value to all stakeholders during public health crises, such as the coronavirus pandemic.
- Data without context can be dismissed, discredited, or misinterpreted – Data analysts should make comparisons, standardize data elements, or identify incongruences so as to the evaluate the data's trustworthiness. While this can be difficult and time consuming for data analysts, the additional effort can prevent inadvertent or disreputable interpretation of the data that can lead to misinformation and serious health consequences.
- Data analysts can combat misinformation through data visualization – Simple data presentation, such as tables or linear trend lines, may not clarify misunderstandings regarding disease conditions. Data visualization tools, such as Tableau, can add value to stakeholders by highlighting important methodological issues or providing critical context.
- Data analysts can enable more timely decisions from stakeholders – In a public health crisis, stakeholders need to know as soon as possible when disease case numbers are increasing so that they quickly can implement interventions. Selection of the most appropriate metric is crucial for timely and effective decision-making. Lagging data variables, misinterpreted data, or misconstrued conclusions can lead to erroneous decisions with serious consequences.
- Data analysts can assist stakeholders to reduce complexity of disease tracking metrics – A single variable may not be enough to track disease outbreak severity. Oftentimes, a constellation of metrics will be needed to describe the state of a public health crisis. Data analyst can play a key role in definition, selection, and contextualization of disease data.
- Data analysts provide a public service when objectively evaluating the success or failures of public health interventions – Trust in government institutions may be in decline due to politicization of public health issues. As such, independent assessment of public health interventions during a health crisis, such as community mitigation strategies (e.g., masks) or vaccine effectiveness, can provide a trustworthy source of information for the public, media, and policymakers.

LOOKING AHEAD

These lessons from the coronavirus pandemic can empower data analysts to provide a valuable service to stakeholders as they contemplate the data analytics required for the next public health crisis. First, while the FDOH provided data to the public on a daily basis for much of the pandemic, in the summer of 2021 the State of Florida officials decided to move to weekly release of a limited dataset (Funk 2021; Paz, 2021). This lack of transparency generated uncertainty regarding public health interventions and impeded decisions for local government officials, the media, and the public (Glassman & Ladyzhets, 2020). Without data, stakeholders turned to anecdotes to describe the state of the pandemic without objective assessment by data analysts, which can lead to misinformation spread through social media (Bergquist, Otten, & Sarich, 2020; Suarez-Lledo & Alvarez-Galvez, 2021). In the future, data should be made publicly available throughout the course of the health crisis.

Furthermore, future health crises should avoid politicization of data collection and dissemination. During the coronavirus pandemic, the official Florida COVID-19 dashboard became fodder for accusations of data manipulation, employee recrimination, and conspiracy (Blaskey, 2021; Desai, 2020; Shankar, 2021). Irrespective of the facts behind the maelstrom, the politicization of the COVID-19 dashboard detracted from the public health aims of data transparency and public accountability. Even COVID-19 dashboards created by independent epidemiologists and data analysts attracted controversy fueled by political partisanship and media coverage (Oh, 2020). The politicization of the public health dashboards weakened the perception of objectivity of the COVID-19 dashboards, which hampered the ability to enact public health measures to control the pandemic (Jones, 2020; Persaud, 2020).

Finally, the COVID-19 pandemic has exposed weaknesses inherent in the disease surveillance data collection and reporting in the United States. While data analysts should recognize data limitations inherent of the decentralized collection of data by the states and coordination by the federal government, improvements in data can be made (Xu, 2020). As a part of the federal government's support and coordination of states' public health disease surveillance systems, a national standard should be created that prescribes detailed data documentation for data collection and reporting. Such documentation should prioritize data variables and define key metrics and calculations that would assure data uniformity and consistency across states.

CONCLUSION

Supplied with publicly available data files from various states and federal government public health agencies, data analysts can improve decision-making for stakeholders during any future public health crisis. Professional and collaborative data analysts can add value to the official government dashboards through scrutinizing the data, understanding the important methodological issues, and providing comprehensive and visually appealing tools for a variety of stakeholders, including the public, media, scientists, clinicians, politicians, and public servants.

REFERENCES

Akhtar, N., Tabassum, N., Perwej, A., & Perwej, Y. (2020). Data Analytics and Visualization using Tableau Utilitarian for COVID-19 (Coronavirus). *Global Journal of Engineering and Technology Advances*, 3(2), 28–50. doi: 10.30574/gjeta.2020.3.2.0029

Associated Press. (2021, August 7). Florida Again Breaks Record in Number of Single-Day COVID-19 Cases Reported Saturday. *NBC 6 South Florida*. Retrieved from https://www.nbcmiami.com/news/coronavirus/florida-again-breaks-record-in-number-of-single-day-covid-19-cases-reported-saturday/2524030/

Bergquist, S., Otten, T., & Sarich, N. (2020). COVID-19 Pandemic in the United States. *Health Policy and Technology*, 9(4), 623–638.

Blaskey, S. (2021, June 4). Records in Rebekah Jones Case Give Peek at Florida COVID-19 Response. *The Tampa Bay Times*. https://www.tampabay.com/news/health/2021/06/04/florida-whistleblower-rebekah-jones-gives-a-look-behind-the-scenes/

Colombini, S., (2021, May 20). Institute Estimates 40% More Florida COVID Deaths Than State Data. *Health News Florida from WUSF Public Media*. https://wusfnews.wusf.usf.edu/health-news-florida/2021-05-20/ihme-estimates-51-000-covid-19-deaths-in-florida

Desai, J. (2020, December 8). Who is Rebekah Jones? Former Florida COVID-19 Data Scientist Had Home Raided by Authorities. *Tallahassee Democrat*. https://www.usatoday.com/story/news/nation/2020/12/08/rebekah-jones-coronavirus-scientist-dashboard-ron-desantis-florida-covid-19/6488291002/

Downey, R. (2021, May 11). 50,000 Floridians have Died from COVID-19, Health Institute Estimates. *Florida Politics*. https://floridapolitics.com/archives/428196-50000-floridians-have-died-from-covid-19-health-institute-estimates/

Florida Department of Health. (2020). Florida COVID19 Case Line Data. https://open-fdoh.hub.arcgis.com/datasets/florida-covid19-case-line-data/about

Florida Department of Health. [@HealthyFla]. (2021, August 9). *The daily case counts for Florida currently posted on the CDC COVID Tracker are incorrect. The current listing states 28,317. The accurate data are as follows: Friday, August 6: 21,500 Saturday August 7: 19,567 Sunday, August 8: 15,319 The 3 day average: 18,795.* [Tweet]. Twitter. https://twitter.com/HealthyFla/status/1424918312748822547

Funk, J. (2021, July 26). States Scale Back Virus Reporting Just as Cases Surge. *Associated Press*.https://apnews.com/article/health-coronavirus-pandemic-f9c58c50f565e707be9bedfa9a82319e

Gamio, L., Mervosh S., & Collins, K. (2020, July 23). Where the Virus Is Sending People to Hospitals. *The New York Times*. https://www.nytimes.com/interactive/2020/07/23/us/coronavirus-hospitalizations-us.html

Glassman, R. & Ladyzhets B. (2020, August 11). The COVID Tracking Project at the Atlantic. Hospitalization Data Reported by the HHS vs. the States: Jumps, Drops, and Other Unexplained Phenomena. https://covidtracking.com/analysis-updates/hospitalization-data-reported-by-the-hhs-vs-the-states-jumps-drops-and-other

Jones, R. (2020, July 8). Rebekah Jones: Florida's COVID-19 Data Unreliable, Raises Too Many Questions. *Treasure Coast News*. Retrieved from https://www.tcpalm.com/story/opinion/readers/2020/07/08/covid-19-data-reporting-florida-unreliable-opinion/5393098002/

Kimball, A., Hatfield, K. M., Arons, M., James, A., Taylor, J., Spicer, K., ... & Zane, S. (2020). Asymptomatic and Presymptomatic SARS-CoV-2 Infections in Residents of a Long-term Care Skilled Nursing Facility – King County, Washington, March 2020. *Morbidity and Mortality Weekly Report*, 69(13), 377.

Levin, J. & Querolo, N. (2021, April 20). Covid Shows Polarized U.S. Politics Kills, Delays Pandemic Exit. *Bloomberg*. Retrieved from https://www.bloomberg.com/news/articles/2021-04-20/covid-shows-polarized-politics-can-kill-delaying-pandemic-exit

Musgrave, J. (2021, August 11). Florida Accuses CDC of Inflating COVID Numbers in Apparent CDC Mistake. *Palm Beach Post*. https://www.palmbeachpost.com/story/news/coronavirus/2021/08/10/florida-accuses-cdc-inflating-covid-numbers-cdc-changes-tally/5558411001/

Neal, D.J. (2021, August 9). Florida COVID Update: More than 28,000 Cases per day Over the Weekend, Another Record. *Miami Herald*. Retrieved from https://www.miamiherald.com/news/coronavirus/article253368768.html

Oh, I. (2020, May 5). As States Reopen, Concern Grows Over Data Manipulation. *Mother Jones*. https://www.motherjones.com/coronavirus-updates/2020/05/georgia-florida-coronavirus-data/

Paz, I.G. (2021, June 23). Covid News: Florida Will Stop Releasing Daily Virus Data. *The New York Times*. https://www.nytimes.com/live/2021/06/04/world/covid-vaccine-coronavirus-mask

Persaud, C. (2020, August 14). FAU Pushes Coronavirus Skeptic as 'Expert' Even as Scientists Pan his Views. *Palm Beach Post*. https://www.palmbeachpost.com/story/news/local/2020/08/14/fau-pushes-coronavirus-skeptic-as-rsquoexpertrsquo-even-as-scientists-pan-his-views/42209087/

Salemi, J. (2021). COVID-19 Dashboard. *A Focus on Florida with State & National Comparisons*. https://covid19florida.mystrikingly.com/

Shankar, K., Jeng, W., Thomer, A., Weber, N., & Yoon, A. (2021). Data Curation as Collective Action During COVID-19. *Journal of the Association for Information Science and Technology*, 72(3), 280–284.

Sidorowicz, J. (2021, August 7). No, Florida was not 'Caught Underreporting' COVID-19 Deaths in Latest Report. WTSP Tampa Bay 10 News. Retrieved from https://www.wtsp.com/article/news/verify/florida-covid19-deaths-report/67-60964c73-5c2b-4492-a2f1-03b0fc55bf3d

Suarez-Lledo, V., & Alvarez-Galvez, J. (2021). Prevalence of Health Misinformation on Social Media: Systematic Review. *Journal of Medical Internet Research*, 23(1), e17187.

Tatar, M., Habibdoust, A., & Wilson, F. A. (2021). Analysis of Excess Deaths during the COVID-19 Pandemic in the State of Florida. *American Journal of Public Health*, 111(4), 704–707.

USF Health News. (2021, January 22). Dr. Jason Salemi uses Online Dashboards to Explain the Spread of Covid-19. https://hscweb3.hsc.usf.edu/blog/2021/01/15/dr-jason-salemi-uses-online-dashboards-to-explain-the-spread-of-covid-19/

Wassie, G. T., Azene, A. G., Bantie, G. M., Dessie, G., & Aragaw, A. M. (2020). Incubation Period of SARS-CoV-2: A Systematic Review and Meta-Analysis. *Current Therapeutic Research*, 93, 100607.

Xu, H. D., & Basu, R. (2020). How the United States Flunked the COVID-19 Test: Some Observations and Several Lessons. *The American Review of Public Administration*, 50(6–7), 568–576.

Chapter 10

State case study
Illinois

Helen Margellos-Anast
Sinai Urban Health Institute
Chicago, IL, USA

Fernando De Maio
American Medical Association; DePaul University
Chicago, IL, USA

C. Scott Smith
DePaul University
Chicago, IL, USA

Pamela Roesch
Sinai Urban Health Institute
Chicago, IL, USA

Emily Laflamme
American Medical Association
Chicago, IL, USA

Eve Shapiro
West Side United
Chicago, IL, USA

CONTENTS

Introduction 144
    COVID-19: First signs.. 145
Chicago's COVID-19 experience, March 1, 2020 to July 6, 2021 145
    Five periods of the COVID-19 pandemic 146
    Citywide variations in COVID-19 burden.................................... 147
    Neighborhood-level variations in COVID-19 burden.................... 149
Data to action 149
    Racial Equity Rapid Response Team (RERRT) 149
    Making data accessible and usable... 152
    Progressive collaboration 153

DOI: 10.1201/9781003204138-13

Lessons learned 155
Looking forward 157
Notes 158
References 159

INTRODUCTION

In 1901, a full 20 years before Chicago's official community areas were drawn, a striking map displayed the inequities of infant mortality between the city's burgeoning neighborhoods (Bushnell, 1901). Since then, health data mapped across Chicago's neighborhoods have told a striking story. By the 1930s, detailed maps illustrated geospatial inequities in mental health (Faris and Dunham, 1939), and in the subsequent decades, a plethora of analyses examined geographic inequities across a range of health indicators (De Maio et al., 2019). Over the past 120 years, our data have become more refined and our analytics more sophisticated, but arguably, the fundamental problem has remained the same. The spatial patterns we have seen in life expectancy, infant mortality, and other health outcomes are now echoed in our COVID-19 data, a reflection of the inequitable systems of power that underlie the distribution of health and wellbeing in Chicago.

At present, Chicago remains a starkly divided city, ranking near the top in most demographic studies of residential segregation (Huang, 2021; Sampson, 2012). The effects of racial segregation manifest clearly in our epidemiological profile. Between 2012 and 2017, life expectancy fell for everyone except White (non-Latinx) Chicagoans. In that time period, Latinx Chicagoans experienced a 3.1-year drop in life expectancy, from 83.1 to 80.0. Black (non-Latinx) life expectancy fell from 72.6 to 71.4, with a gap of 8.8 years between Black and White life expectancy (CDPH, 2021). Chicago is one of the only six large US cities with growing gaps in mortality rates between Black and White populations (Benjamins et al., 2021).

These inequities exist across the city, but they are most pronounced – and best understood – with hyper-local data. Across Chicago's officially designated 77 community areas, there were profuse inequities in our most important epidemiological indicators *before* COVID-19 (see Table 10.1).

Across Chicago's community areas, life expectancy varies from 66.3 to 83.2 years, a gap of almost 17 years. Other key indicators, including infant, heart disease, and cancer mortality show similar patterns. While similar to inequities found across US cities, Chicago's pre-COVID health inequities help us meaningfully understand the impact of COVID-19 on the health of the city's population. Like in other cities, the burden of COVID-19 fell on Chicago communities in predictable ways that reflected the city's inequitable distribution of power and resources. The data reveal a heavy toll. It is a testament to the work and activism of a remarkable group of people and institutions – who collaborated in new and profound ways – that the numbers are not even worse.

Table 10.1 Summary of Chicago inequities before COVID-19

Outcome	Overall	Minimum	Maximum	Gap
Life expectancy[a]	77.3 years	66.3 years	83.2 years	16.9 years
Infant mortality rate[b]	6.6	1.5	22.3	20.8
Heart disease mortality rate[c]	201.3	79.3	381.8	302.5
Cancer mortality rate[d]	179.2	88.6	313.5	224.9
Rent-burdened[e]	46.0%	23.4%	76.7%	53.3%
Median household income[f]	$55,703	$14,877	$1,21,287	$1,06,410

Source: Chicago Health Atlas, https://chicagohealthatlas.org/

[a] Life expectancy at birth in years; reported from 2019
[b] Rate of infant deaths in first year of life per 1,000 live births; 2013–2017
[c] Age-adjusted rate of people who died due to heart disease per 1,00,000 total population; 2013–2017
[d] Age-adjusted rate of people who died due to cancer per 1,00,000 total population; 2013–2017
[e] Percent of renter-occupied housing units where households spend more than 30% of income on rent (rent costs do not include utilities, insurance, or building fees); 2015–2019
[f] Income in the past 12 months, in inflation-adjusted 2017 dollars; 2015–2019

COVID-19: First signs

The first reports of COVID-19 deaths in Chicago echoed the city's historical fault lines: of the first 100 deaths, 70% were Black (despite only one-third of the city's population being Black). One of the most powerful analyses of these data was published in *ProPublica Illinois*: "70 of the city's 100 first recorded victims of COVID-19 were Black. Their lives were rich, and their deaths cannot be dismissed as inevitable. Immediate factors could – and should – have been addressed" (Eldeib et al., 2020).[1] Eldeib et al. reached out to families and friends of these first victims, painting an ethnographic sketch of their lives – in the process, reminding all of us that data on health inequities *always* represent the lives and struggles of individuals, families, and communities. These data are never abstract numbers or math. Underneath the models, underneath the regressions and coefficients, are people like Larry Arnold, one of the first people in Chicago to succumb to COVID-19 at age 70, who took an Uber from his south side apartment with a 103-degree fever to a hospital 30 minutes away because he did not trust the hospital that was less than a mile from his home. As told by Eldeib et al., Larry Arnold's story is both a tragic tale of an individual's personal troubles and also a warning of the harmful consequences of systems that unfairly concentrate access and privilege in some communities while disadvantaging others.

CHICAGO'S COVID-19 EXPERIENCE, MARCH 1, 2020 TO JULY 6, 2021

Chicago was the first city in the United States to report a person-to-person transmission of COVID-19 (Ghinai et al. 2020) and, by spring 2020, it was experiencing infection and death rates rivaling many other large metropolitan areas around the world that had dealt with earlier outbreaks (Stier, Berman,

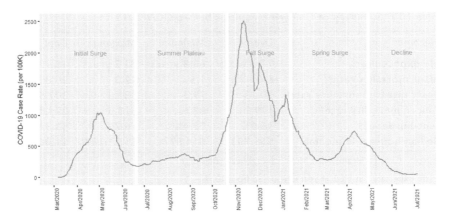

Figure 10.1 Seven-day moving average COVID-19 daily case rates for Chicago, Illinois, 3/1/2020 to 7/6/2021.

and Bettencourt 2021). After this initial surge, which peaked in early May 2020, the city would endure another two waves in the autumn/winter of 2020/2021 and spring of 2021, culminating in 285,394 total reported infections, 28,615 hospitalizations, and 5,622 deaths due to COVID-19 by July 6, 2021. On July 4, 2021, the city's 7-day average daily death rate dropped to less than one for the first time since March 18 the prior year. On July 6, 2021 Mayor Lori E. Lightfoot announced that, after 16 months, the city had entered Phase 5 of the pandemic and Chicago's City Hall was reopened to the public. Figure 10.1 plots 7-day moving average daily COVID-19 case rates between March 1, 2020 and July 6, 2021.

Five periods of the COVID-19 pandemic

To explore how Chicago's racial and ethnic inequities in COVID-19 changed over the course of the pandemic, the 492-day span represented in Figure 10.1 was divided into five periods. The five periods were identified by endogenously computing structural breakpoints in the city's 7-day moving average case rates using a dynamic programming approach (Bai and Perron 2003). The first period of the pandemic represents the *initial surge* of COVID-19 infections, which occurred between March 1 and June 1, 2020. It was during this first period that public health providers began mobilizing vast resources to combat the pandemic, including formation of the Racial Equity Rapid Response Team (described below). It was also when the State of Illinois and the City of Chicago implemented a wide range of policies – such as the closure of public schools (3/13/2020), a social distancing mandate (3/16/2020), and suspension of the City of Chicago's debt-collection practices (3/18/2020) – designed to slow infection rates and ease economic hardship among the city's hardest-hit communities. Within this period alone, the City adopted 30 of its eventual 63 COVID-19 local policy responses to mitigate the deleterious effects of the pandemic (NLC, 2021).

The second period, the *summer plateau*, represents a span of 142 days between June 2 and October 21, 2020 when case rates stabilized averaging approximately 250–750 new reported infections per day (9.3–27.8 cases per 100,000 per day). Case rates remained low despite multiple social protests across the city – some exceeding 30,000 in number – in response to the May 25th killing of George Floyd, and the easing of social distancing mandates. On June 3, Chicago entered Phase 3 of its reopening plan which included the opening of childcare facilities, non-lakefront public parks, and restaurants (outdoor dining only). Twenty-three days later, the city would enter Phase 4, extending its reopening to additional business sectors and lifting capacity restrictions with appropriate safeguards. On October 19, CDPH Commissioner Dr. Arwady sounded the alarm of a second COVID-19 wave.

The third period covers the second COVID-19 wave, or *fall surge*, that began in late October 2020, the first of a series of three infection waves following the Thanksgiving, Christmas, and New Year holidays, respectively. At the beginning of this period, the City instituted a curfew for all nonessential businesses and Chicagoans were again asked to avoid social gatherings of more than six people and end all social gatherings by 10pm.

The fourth period began around January 16, 2021 with declining case rates. This decline was likely due to the approval and rollout of three highly effective COVID-19 vaccines and the implementation of vaccination programs such as *Protect Chicago Plus* (PCP), a citywide equity plan to improve vaccine access and distribution within communities that had experienced the greatest COVID-19 burden according to the Chicago COVID-19 Vulnerability Index (City of Chicago, 2020). This decline was followed by a relatively moderate and brief *spring surge* in mid-April.

The final period, or late *spring decline*, began May 1, 2021 when case rates tailed off as COVID-19 vaccines were administered to a growing number of eligible populations.

Citywide variations in COVID-19 burden

Similar to other socially- and politically polarized US cities, it was feared from the outset that Chicago's communities of color would bear a disproportionate health and economic burden of the pandemic (Kim and Bostwick, 2020). When the City began to publicly disseminate its daily COVID-19 counts by race and ethnicity, these fears were largely borne out. Between March 6 and April 6 2020, the first month of the initial surge, 226 (47%) of all COVID-19 reported cases were Black (non-Latinx), despite this group comprising less than 30% of the city's total population (ACS, 2020).[2] A comparison of incidence proportions for that month suggests that the city's Black population was 4.6 times as likely to die from a COVID-19 related illness as their White counterparts.

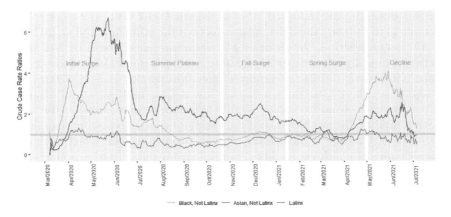

Figure 10.2 Seven-day moving average COVID-19 crude case rate ratios by race, ethnicity (White, not Latinx as comparison group), 3/1/2020 to 7/6/2021.

Notes: Values > 1 indicate greater rates of infection among the specified race, ethnic group relative to similar rates for the White, Not Latinx population. Values < 1 indicate greater rates of infection among the White, Not Latinx populations relative to the specified race, ethnic group. The gray horizontal line represents parity with the White, Not Latinx crude case rates. Data sources: Figures 10.1 and 10.2 are adapted from the City of Chicago's Daily COVID-19 Cases, Deaths, and Hospitalizations (2021); US Census Bureau ACS 5-Year Estimates 2015–2019.

Over time, however, relative rates of infection shifted between demographic groups, likely due to the interplay of socio-cultural, economic, and environmental factors combined with City, State, and federal policy responses to the disease. Figure 10.2 plots rate ratios by race/ethnicity based on 7-day average COVID-19 infection rates using crude case rates for the White population as the comparison group (e.g., the crude case rate ratio is equal to the crude case rate of the selected racial/ethnic group divided by a similar rate calculated for Chicago's White population). Rate ratios exceeding 1 (above the dark gray line) represent days when the crude case rate for the specified racial/ethnic group exceeded that for the White population. It is clear from the figure that Black and Latinx populations experienced greater relative risk of COVID-19 infection compared to the White population throughout most of the pandemic. Our calculations using data downloaded from the City's open data portal suggest that for 271 (55.1%) of the 492 days reviewed, the Black population experienced greater case rates than the city's White population. Even greater disparities existed between Latinx and White populations, with Latinx case rates exceeding that of Whites for 445 (90.4%) of days in the period reviewed. Save for two brief periods in the initial and spring surges (totaling 31 days), the city's White population had average infection rates below that of other racial/ethnic groups.

COVID-19 mortality and hospitalization rates for the city's Black and Latinx populations were also considerably higher than rates for the city's White population throughout most periods reviewed (Table 10.2). The inequitable barriers to accessing testing and care faced by Black and Latinx Chicagoans suggest that the true disparity is likely even greater.

Neighborhood-level variations in COVID-19 burden

These patterns of inequity are even more pronounced at the neighborhood level, where the burden of COVID-19 was consistently higher in predominantly Black and Latinx communities on the city's south and west sides. Figures 10.3a–e show statistically significant high- and low-case rate clusters throughout the city by zip code.[3] Areas shaded in red represent clusters of higher case rates (relative to the mean) and areas in blue represent clusters of lower COVID-19 case rates. For instance, during the initial surge, seven of the city's 58 zip codes on the west side, comprised 13,758 (28.9%) of the city's total COVID-19 cases. Pandemic disease hot spots shifted between the south, southwest, and west sides over the 70-week duration, save for the *spring surge* period when zip codes in the northwest and near west sides reported relatively higher case rates. Figure 10.3f shows the majority racial/ethnic group for each zip code.

DATA TO ACTION

Chicago's COVID-19 response efforts, like those of all cities and states, remain a work in progress. However, from the outset, the City's public health community made a concerted effort to ensure that as the city responded to immediate needs, consideration was given to deep-rooted contextual factors that drive COVID-19 inequities. As resources to support the COVID-19 response were allocated via Federal, State, and local governments, and supplemented by philanthropy, the City of Chicago has been intentional about facilitating collaboration across health systems, academic institutions, public health professionals, community-based organizations, and others to ensure that data is accurately interpreted, that it is disseminated at various levels to those making decisions, and that response is driven by diverse perspectives and wisdom. A key tenant to Chicago's comparative success versus some other urban areas has been its active pursuit of community insights to guide decision making and the inclusion of community leaders and organizations as co-developers of response efforts.

Racial Equity Rapid Response Team (RERRT)

The City of Chicago responded to the first wave of data by establishing the Racial Equity Rapid Response Team (RERRT). Discussing the initial data

Table 10.2 City of Chicago COVID-19 outcomes by period and race, ethnic group, 3/1/20 to 7/6/21

	Period					
	Initial Surge	Summer Plateau	Fall/ Winter Surge	Spring Surge	Decline	Cumulative
Date range	3/1/20 to 6/1/20	6/2/20 to 10/21/20	10/22/20 to 1/15/21	1/16/21 to 4/30/21	5/1/21 to 7/6/21	3/1/20 to 7/6/21
Number of days	93	142	86	105	66	492
Cases	47,586	47,487	130,449	50,207	9,317	285,046
Deaths	2,271	789	1,527	745	286	5,618
Hospitalizations	9,834	4,123	8,660	4,558	1,384	28,559
Cases, Unknown Race	18.3%	15.9%	24.4%	19.2%	18.6%	20.8%
Deaths, Unknown Race	0.1%	0.3%	0.1%	0.7%	0.0%	0.2%
Hospitalizations, Unknown Race	2.4%	4.9%	5.4%	4.5%	4.6%	4.1%
Case Rate (per 100K)						
Black, Not Latinx	1,532.2	1,054.6	2,519.5	1,487.8	475.5	7,069.5
Asian, Not Latinx	590.5	539.6	1,975.5	1,041.3	131.0	4,277.8
White, Not Latinx	631.2	1,130.5	2,900.4	1,314.1	144.4	6,120.5
Latinx	2,362.5	2,426.3	5,550.8	1,636.6	264.7	12,240.9
Total	1,766.4	1,762.7	4,842.3	1,863.7	345.8	10,580.9
Death Rate (per 100K)						
Black, Not Latinx	132.7	35.8	63.8	37.1	19.6	289.0
Asian, Not Latinx	56.8	11.9	44.9	21.1	4.9	139.6
White, Not Latinx	47.8	18.4	44.8	20.3	5.4	136.7
Latinx	89.1	41.5	69.2	29.2	9.9	239.0
Total	84.3	29.3	56.7	27.7	10.6	208.5
Hospitalization Rate (per 100K)						
Black, Not Latinx	578.4	206.1	432.9	288.3	108.4	1,029.4
Asian, Not Latinx	152.6	41.7	155.9	61.2	14.6	425.9
White, Not Latinx	161.5	89.9	194.9	92.2	20.0	558.6
Latinx	377.2	167.6	314.4	127.8	32.1	1,019.1
Total	365.0	153.0	321.5	169.2	51.4	1,060.1

Data sources: Adapted from the City of Chicago's Daily COVID-19 Cases, Deaths, and Hospitalizations (2021); US Census Bureau ACS 5-Year Estimates 2015–2019.

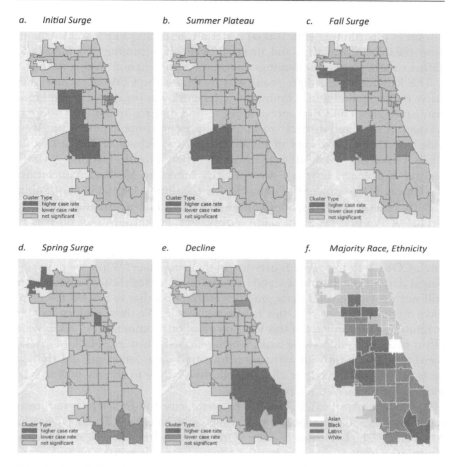

Figure 10.3 (a–f) City of Chicago COVID-19 case rate clusters by zip code and period, 3/1/20 to 7/6/21.

Data sources: Adapted from the City of Chicago's Daily COVID-19 Cases, Deaths, and Hospitalizations (2021); US Census Bureau ACS 5-Year Estimates 2015-2019; TIGER/Line cartographic boundary zip code tabulation area (ZCTA) shapefile (2019).

at a press conference, Mayor Lightfoot stated: "these numbers take your breath away… this is a call-to-action moment for all of us… It is unacceptable, no one should think that this is OK."[4] Moreover, she noted: "When we talk about equity and inclusion, they're not just nice notions… they are an imperative that we must embrace as a city." The RERRT was established in April 2020, with a framework of data-driven, collaborative, and community-driven mitigation of COVID-19 morbidity and mortality. It sought to bring together communities and form coalitions by convening community leaders from the south, west, and southwest sides; to identify needs and advocate for resources (distributing educational materials, tests, and PPE); and to champion reliable information and promote wellbeing (running town halls to gather insights from communities and sharing information with residents).

The RERRT's immediate focus was to flatten the COVID-19 mortality curve in Black and Latinx communities. Its work was organized around four core strategies: education, prevention, testing and treatment, and support services. A data and metrics working group, comprising experts from West Side United, the University of Illinois at Chicago School of Public Health, Rush University Medical Center, Sinai Urban Health Institute (SUHI), DePaul University, Loyola University, the American Medical Association, the Chicago Department of Public Health, the Illinois Department of Public Health, Enlace, NowPow, South Shore Works, and more provided support.

One of the first tasks the data and metrics workgroup took on was to address missing race/ethnicity data for COVID-19 tests. Mayor Lightfoot also underscored that race/ethnicity data was missing in almost half of the city's COVID-19 test records early on in the pandemic: "While we have sufficient data to say that these trends are alarming… Healthcare providers are still not providing total demographic information that is needed for us to have a complete picture… this is not negotiable. We must understand the magnitude of the impact of this virus on all of our communities." A citywide effort needed to address the issue, which reflected a historical lack of investment in public health infrastructure, fractured data collection and sharing systems, and underneath it all, our collective failure to convey why it is so vital to collect race/ethnicity data.

As early as April 2020, missing race/ethnicity for COVID-19 tests was recognized as a national problem. Writing in the *New York Times*, Dr. Aletha Maybank, Chief Health Equity Officer with the American Medical Association noted "this data is central to understanding injustice and ensuring the optimal health of people, but it is gravely missing in this crisis… this is a recipe for undercounting, keeping structural harms and disease burden invisible."[5] Without sufficient race/ethnicity data, we would not have a full accounting of the pandemic, its public health implications, or its economic effects. The RERRT proved to be an effective network from which to develop, validate, and disseminate a statistical solution to address the problem of missing race/ethnicity.[6]

Making data accessible and usable

Through this effort, novel collaborations emerged to address complicated problems related to COVID-19 data. For example, much of the infection data that the City received from the State's database tended to be missing race/ethnicity. Using the data outlined previously, infections reported with unknown patient race/ethnicity make up 20.8% of all cases (Table 10.2). Death and hospitalization records have far fewer missing race/ethnicity data because this information is required to be collected and reported by hospitals and police departments or – in the case of deaths – next-of-kin upon making final funeral home arrangements. COVID-19 infection data, however, are reported by a wide range of providers and, many times, inconsistently. To better monitor case rates across racial/ethnic groups, the City of Chicago worked with faculty, students, and staff in DePaul University's College for Computing and Digital Media – members of the RERRT data and metrics workgroup – to adapt a method for imputing missing race/ethnicity data using residential location and surname (Grundmeier et al., 2015). The City ultimately used this imputed race/ethnicity information to track infection disparities throughout the pandemic (Cherone, 2021).

Collaborations such as the RERRT operated more efficiently by using online resources made available by the City, which made COVID-19 data not only easier to find but also provided documentation on how and when data were produced and corresponding data dictionaries. In the years leading up to the pandemic, the City had established and cultivated its open data portal, initiated through an executive order signed by former Mayor Rahm Emanuel in late 2012. The portal quickly grew to become among one the country's most comprehensive municipal data gateways. The Lightfoot administration further leveraged this digital infrastructure to share detailed information about the pandemic, supporting resident inquiries as well as a wide range of academic research, professional articles, and other online applications.

The idea to develop DePaul University's COVID-19 Community Health Equity Dashboard, launched in September 2020, was largely conceived through conversations during RERRT's data and metrics workgroups concerning the need for better information to determine the location of mobile COVID-19 testing sites (DePaul University, 2020). The website, similar to the popular Johns Hopkins COVID-19 Dashboard (Johns Hopkins, 2020), uses ESRI's ArcGIS Dashboards platform, with much of the data imported directly from the City of Chicago's portal. Through a series of R code (made publicly available via a corresponding GitHub repository), the City's data were processed, combined with other state and nationwide datasets, and transformed to create custom rates and indices designed to guide the optimal location of testing facilities and to broaden public awareness of inequities beyond what was included in the City's own COVID-19 dashboard (Smith, 2021). The DePaul dashboard provides interactive charts and maps showing the progression of COVID-19 cases, deaths, and vaccinations including daily, cumulative, and 7-day moving averages, as well as community-level information on health trends, vulnerabilities, and inequities.

Progressive collaboration

As time has gone on, RERRT's efforts have increased awareness of the type of data available, and communities have been increasingly proactive in seeking out local-level data and using it to drive their response. As one example, North Lawndale Community Coordinating Council (NLCCC), a group of local stakeholders guiding comprehensive planning and implementation in North Lawndale, a predominantly Black (non-Latinx) community area on Chicago's historically disinvested west side, assembled a COVID-19 Response Team early in the pandemic. NLCCC's COVID-19 Response Team asked SUHI to provide data updates at bi-weekly meetings on the six zip codes that comprise its priority areas. SUHI presented on test rates, case rates, positivity rates, and vaccination rates, among others, on a local level, and also kept the group apprised of citywide trends by race/ethnicity. As NLCCC held community forums, SUHI set the foundation for conversation by giving data presentations. NLCCC and its community partners used the data in a multitude of ways, from supporting the need for shelter-in-place support programs, to generating messaging that appealed to different audiences, to increasing vaccine access via convenient pop-up clinics and in-home options, to supporting parents/caregivers of children in the e-learning environment. An important secondary effect of Chicago's data-driven and community-grounded response was the acknowledgment of epidemiologic data's importance to achieving racial/ethnic equity beyond the public health community as well as improved data literacy beyond traditional data users.

CDPH's aim to proactively center racial/ethnic and geographic equity helped establish data systems and methods of interpreting data that prioritized communities for outreach and vaccination based on COVID-19 vulnerability. Researchers have contended that understanding contextual vulnerability provides opportunities to understand and design responses, and to inform preparedness and response strategies for times of crisis. These initiatives have resulted in a higher vaccination rate overall in Chicago and among Latinx and Black (non-Latinx) residents than most other large US cities (data is from March – we will update this before finalizing the chapter, including latest reference). CDPH embraced the Public Health 3.0 model[7], recognizing that protecting the public's health transcends the boundaries of what governmental agencies can do and requires a coordinated effort that engages multiple sectors (e.g., hospitals/health systems, schools, community-based organizations, social service agencies, academic partners, faith-based organizations). The City developed a COVID-19 burden index to inform decisions in the latter stages of the pandemic. In February 2021, CDPH used the COVID-19 Community Vulnerability Index (CCVI) to identify 15 highly impacted communities for concentrated efforts toward expanded vaccine access. The initiative, Protect Chicago Plus, partnered with community stakeholders to ensure limited resources were expended in ways that remove barriers and increase vaccination rates. As time went on, Protect Chicago Plus pivoted to focus on communities with the highest CCVI and lower vaccination rates, and the data continues to guide the response. The effort has increased the proportion of Latinx and Black (non-Latinx) Chicagoans who have received at least one vaccination dose from <10% when the initiative started to 49% and 40%, respectively (as of July 21, 2021).

Over the past 16 months, there has been more intentional collaboration across diverse stakeholders than ever before. These collaborations stemmed from a shared recognition of deep racial and ethnic inequities within the data and have translated to direct response. Some of these partnerships were initiated through governmental agencies such as the Chicago COVID-19 Response Corp (CCRC), which began as the City's community-based contact tracing initiative. The City of Chicago contracted Chicago Cook Workforce Partnership to lead the CCRC in collaboration with University of Illinois at Chicago School of Public Health, NORC at the University of Chicago, Malcolm X College (a City College of Chicago), and SUHI. This team was responsible for identifying 31 community-based organizations that then hired over 600 community residents to serve as contact tracers, contact tracing supervisors, resource coordinators, and resource coordinator supervisors. As time went on and the need for contact tracing was less pressing, the team transitioned to support other aspects of the response from vaccine uptake to messaging to resource coordination. From the beginning, the team was attentive to concurrent social factors that had contributed to COVID-19 inequities, including access to education and stable, good jobs. For example, the team ensured that the 600 community residents in the CCRC received training that would develop skills applicable to future careers once the need for pandemic response waned, including laying a foundation of community health worker (CHW) core skills.

Several other important partnerships were initiated by non-governmental stakeholders, such as the Chicagoland Vaccine Partnership (CVP), which was first initiated in Summer 2020 by health systems serving Chicago's west side communities/suburbs as a mechanism to address low anticipated vaccine confidence. In Fall 2020, Michael Reese Health Trust, a local philanthropic organization, joined the effort, and stakeholders – including the Chicago Department of Public Health and Cook County Department of Public Health, community-based organizations, federally qualified health centers, and others – began coordinating resources and sharing best practices for the anticipated COVID-19 vaccine rollout. Partners in Health was engaged in January 2021 to project manage the initiative, providing structure to convene over 100 organizations weekly to co-learn, share best practices, and coordinate efforts toward equitable vaccine uptake.

LESSONS LEARNED

Several important lessons were learned through Chicago's COVID-19 response that will inform future efforts to address public health emergencies and more endemic public health challenges. First, the importance of getting accessible data to community stakeholders, from residents to organizations to health providers, in real time cannot be overstated. It is also vital that data is shared in digestible ways that mobilize people and organizations to informed action. The pandemic demonstrated a longer term need to build capacity and data literacy across sectors, empowering all Chicagoans to access and interpret public health data and use it to guide decision making and action. While Chicago was fortunate to have a data-sharing portal (https://chicagohealthatlas.org/) prior to the pandemic, partners engaged through the COVID-19 response aim to implement innovative models that translate typically underused epidemiologic data to formats for community members, organizers, and organizations that will help them make strategic decisions going forward. One potential approach being considered is a Community Scientist training center.

As we build broader public and community capacity to access and interpret data, we as data analysts, public health professionals, and scientists need to think critically about how data can be used to tell stories that meaningfully capture underlying health inequities. Data can be used to paint the most complete picture only if we center equity from the moment we conceive of our data collection and analysis methodology. Data further needs to be contextualized with community insights to better distinguish race from racism and to lay bare how data analysis decisions can inadvertently hide inequities (e.g., not disaggregating between subgroups within Latinx or Asian racial/ethnic groups). We need to improve the ways data can be used to uncover and explain injustices. Of particular note, as Chicago's COVID-19 experience underscores, we can begin by stressing the importance of collecting accurate and complete racial/ethnic data. With COVID-19, the City emphasized that all testing and vaccination sites collect race/ethnicity; however, collection of this information should not stop there if we hope to understand and address health inequities beyond COVID-19. While DePaul's work with the City to impute missing race/ethnicity data was a necessary step to improving Chicago's COVID-19 response, it also had its shortcomings and is not a long-term solution. The best data is data directly collected from individuals and accurately recorded. An achievable next step would be to ensure adequate sample size within our commonly used public health datasets to disaggregate by race/ethnicity, by ethnic subpopulations (e.g., within Latino, within Asian), and by special populations such as those with disabilities or LGBTQ+ populations. Finally, there is a continued need for enhanced awareness among data analysts on how to analyze data so that we are moving beyond race as a risk factor to racism as a root cause of inequity.

Another important lesson from Chicago's COVID-19 response is that data itself is power, and therefore it needs to be intentionally shared with community partners. The more directly accessible we can make data to communities, the more we level the playing field toward shared power and decision making. The data and response initiatives highlighted throughout our chapter including the RERRT, Protect Chicago Plus, Chicago COVID-19 Response Corp, Chicagoland Vaccine Partnership, and countless others by community organizations, organizers, and health systems, demonstrate the potential that data can afford if coupled with the insights, lived experiences, and deep knowledge of community members and community-serving organizations. While the data can point us in directions, it is the contextualization provided by these real world experts that allowed the City, organizations, and individuals to implement programs and initiatives that resonated with those they sought to help.

Finally, reflecting on the beginning of this chapter, the racial/ethnic and geographic inequities seen in COVID-19 cases, hospitalizations, and deaths, and the associated economic fallout, were predictable and fell along longstanding, historic lines of injustice. Many individuals and organizations mentioned throughout were acutely aware of these historic injustices before COVID-19 spread throughout our city. Many were also on the path of enhanced collaboration to address their root causes before the pandemic. It was these early-stage efforts that allowed the City to mobilize a full-scale collaborative response to COVID-19. The mobilization transcended silos that – for various reasons – were insurmountable before COVID-19 and demonstrates what can be achieved through intentional and targeted collective effort. We have seen firsthand that no single data analyst, public health professional, physician, organization, foundation, government official, or community member has the complete answer; but, together, we come a lot closer a lot faster. There were undoubted challenges to collaboration at this scale, from onerous months-long development of data sharing agreements, to determining a data infrastructure, to balancing the real and competing priorities of different collaborative members. However, we learned that collaboration is feasible and it can move us toward health equity. The collaborative infrastructure established during the COVID-19 pandemic cannot stop there – it is critical for addressing other endemic and longstanding health inequities throughout our city.

LOOKING FORWARD

As the COVID pandemic slowly comes to a close, the multi-sector capacity built across Chicago is seen by many as a catalyst for longer term change in the way we do public health. Most importantly, the COVID-19 pandemic, coupled with the city's reckoning with longstanding systematic racism, has led to public commitments by local institutions to work alongside communities to dismantle racist systems and to internally dismantle practices that perpetuate inequitable health outcomes. In June 2020, 36 hospitals and health centers signed an open letter to the Chicago community explicitly naming racism as a public health crisis and collectively committing to work to improve health equity by focusing on over-burdened and under-resourced communities most affected by inequities.[8] Specific commitments include examining institutional policies through a health equity lens, improving access to primary and specialty care, continuing focus on reducing the burden of chronic disease on communities, supporting investments "that create innovative solutions to achieve enduring improvements in access, quality and health outcomes for our communities," committing to hire locally and to diversify leadership, providing anti-racism and implicit bias training to healthcare workers, and advocating for a greater emphasis on social needs. As we continue to work through COVID-19, it is imperative to build upon the accelerated progress toward addressing racism and health inequities. Many institutions have these intentions, but it will be important that they be held accountable to their commitments. Data is a critical element in creating transparent accountability.

One mechanism that will undoubtedly aim to hold institutions accountable is the expansion of government- and community-based efforts through Protect Chicago Plus into six officially designated Health Equity Zones across Chicago. Based on a successful model used elsewhere, the central aim of the Zones is to encourage community-driven response to health needs, to pursue multi-sector and community collaboration to rapidly achieve health improvement, and to use ongoing data collection to inform activities and response. Each regional zone is managed by a local community organization, with additional community organizational leads throughout the neighborhoods located in each zone. All leads are compensated for their efforts to ensure that community voice, collaboration, and data are used to move the needle forward on health equity. The City – who oversees the Zones –and its technical partners aim to provide technical assistance and capacity building across the regional and community leads to expand the use of data to inform response. While the efforts are starting with vaccine rollout, the zones are about a longer term response to health inequity, centering approaches in addressing the root causes and systematic racism that perpetuate inequities. In particular, the Zones aim to also address epidemics of gun violence, opioids, diabetes, maternal morbidity and mortality, infant mortality, and so forth.

The mobilization of these efforts in the past year and these ongoing efforts demonstrate our continued work as a city toward a public health 3.0 that is broader than the public health or healthcare system. In many ways, in Chicago, we have embraced the public health 3.0 model in our pandemic response and are building systems of accountability to ensure that these efforts do not cease with the pandemic, but rather continue to mobilize our city, partners, and communities toward sustainable and longstanding health equity.

NOTES

1 https://features.propublica.org/chicago-first-deaths/covid-coronavirus-took-black-lives-first/
2 The City of Chicago and Cook County Medical Examiner's office use racial classifications based on US Census Bureau categories. "Latino" or Latinx is defined as an ethnicity and therefore individuals identified within this category may be

of any racial group. For the remainder of this document, the categories Black, White, and Asian do not include those who also identify as Latino. The American Community Survey 5-year 2015–2019 estimates report the total resident population for the City of Chicago to be 2,693,959 with the following race, ethnic composition (arranged in descending order by share of population): White (33.5%); Latinx (28.8%); Black (28.5%); Asian (6.9%), and Other (2.3%).

3 Figures 10.3a-e show the extent to which zip codes throughout the City of Chicago form statistically significant clusters of COVID-19 case rates by period. Local Moran's I (or local indicators of spatial association, LISA) scores (modeled using "queen" contiguity) were used to identify the clusters (Anselin, 1995).

4 https://abcnews.go.com/Politics/coronavirus-disproportionately-killing-black-community-experts/story?id=70011986 and https://www.washingtonpost.com/nation/2020/04/07/chicago-racial-disparity-coronavirus/

5 https://www.nytimes.com/2020/04/07/opinion/coronavirus-blacks.html

6 Two presentations at the 2020 Health Equity and Social Justice conference: Predicting Missing Race/Ethnicity for Chicagoans in COVID-19: Applying BISG Imputation Methods to Better Understand Racial Disparities – Margarita Reina (Epidemiologist, Chicago Department of Public Health) and (2) Using Bayesian Improved Surname Geocoding Method to Impute the Missing Race/Ethnicity in the Chicago Department of Public Health COVID-19 Surveillance Dataset – Hao Wu **need full author list for both** https://www.youtube.com/watch?v=4_1iFXq75kg

7 Public Health 3.0 shifts the role of governmental public health from having primary responsibility to implement all things public health, to a strategic role whose responsibility is to engage multiple sectors and community partners toward collective impact. https://www.cdc.gov/pcd/issues/2017/17_0017.htm

8 https://cookcountyhealth.org/wp-content/uploads/Racial_Equity_Rapid_Response_Provider_Letter.pdf

REFERENCES

ACS. 2020. "American Community Survey, 2015–2019 5-Year Estimates." *US Census Bureau*. http://census.gov

Anselin, Luc. 1995. "Local Indicators of Spatial Association—LISA." *Geographical Analysis* 27 (2): 93–115.

Bai, Jushan, and Pierre Perron. 2003. "Computation and Analysis of Multiple Structural Change Models." *Journal of Applied Econometrics* 18 (1): 1–22. doi. 10.1002/jae.659.

Benjamins, M. R., Silva, A., Saiyed, N. S., and De Maio, F. G. 2021. "Comparison of All-Cause Mortality Rates and Inequities Between Black and White Populations Across the 30 Most Populous US Cities." *JAMA Network Open* 4 (1): e2032086. doi: 10.1001/jamanetworkopen.2020.32086

Bushnell, Chas J. 1901. "Some Social Aspects of the Chicago Stock Yards. Chapter II. The Stock Yard Community at Chicago." *The American Journal of Sociology* 7 (3): 289–330. doi: 10.1086/211064.

Cherone, Heather. 2021. "67% of Chicagoans Vaccinated are White, Asian: City Data." *WTTW News*. https://news.wttw.com/2021/01/25/67-chicagoans-vaccinated-are-white-asian-city-data.

City of Chicago. 2020. "Chicago COVID-19 Community Vulnerability Index (CCVI) | City of Chicago | Data Portal." https://data.cityofchicago.org/Health-Human-Services/Chicago-COVID-19-Community-Vulnerability-Index-CCV/xhc6-88s9.

Cook County Medical Examiner. 2021. "Medical Examiner Case Archive – COVID-19 Related Deaths." *Cook County*. https://datacatalog.cookcountyil.gov/Public-Safety/Medical-Examiner-Case-Archive-COVID-19-Related-Dea/3trz-enys.

De Maio, Fernando, Raj C. Shah, John Mazzeo, and David A. Ansell, University of Chicago Press, March 29, 2019.

DePaul University. 2020. "Chicago COVID-19 Community Health Equity Dashboard." https://depaul-edu.maps.arcgis.com/apps/MapSeries/index.html?appid=e472138e11264c709f78b77377495021.

Eldeib, D. et al. 2020. COVID-19 Took Black Lives First. It Didn't Have To. – In Chicago, 70 of the city's 100 first recorded victims of COVID-19 were black. Their lives were rich, and their deaths cannot be dismissed as inevitable. Immediate factors could — and should — have been addressed. ProPublica (USA). http://uic.edu. Accessed 8 May, 2022.

Faris, R. E. L., and Dunham, H. W. 1939. *Mental disorders in urban areas: An ecological study of schizophrenia and other psychoses*. University Chicago Press.

Ghinai, Isaac, Tristan D. McPherson, Jennifer C. Hunter, Hannah L. Kirking, Demian Christiansen, Kiran Joshi, Rachel Rubin, et al. 2020. "First Known Person-to-Person Transmission of Severe Acute Respiratory Syndrome Coronavirus 2 (SARS-CoV-2) in the USA." *The Lancet* 395 (10230): 1137–1144. doi: 10.1016/S0140-6736(20)30607-3.

Grundmeier, R. W. et al. 2015. "Imputing Missing Race/Ethnicity in Pediatric Electronic Health Records: Reducing Bias with Use of U.S. Census Location and Surname Data." *Health Services Research* 50 (4): 946–960. doi: 10.1111/1475-6773.12295

Huang, H. 2021. A Spatial Analysis of Obesity: Interaction of Urban Food Environments and Racial Segregation in Chicago. *Journal of Urban Health* 98 (5): 676–686. doi: 10.1007/s11524-021-00553-y

Johns Hopkins. 2020. "COVID-19 Map." *Johns Hopkins Coronavirus Resource Center*. https://coronavirus.jhu.edu/map.html.

Kim, Sage J., and Wendy Bostwick. 2020. "Social Vulnerability and Racial Inequality in COVID-19 Deaths in Chicago." *Health Education & Behavior* 47 (4): 509–513. doi: 10.1177/1090198120929677.

National League of Cities. 2021. "National League of Cities (NLC) COVID-19: Local Action Tracker." *National League of Cities*. https://www.nlc.org/resource/covid-19-local-action-tracker/.

Sampson, R. 2012. "Moving and the Neighborhood Glass Ceiling." *Science* 337 (6101): 1464–1465. https://www.science.org/doi/full/10.1126/science.1227881

Scott Smith, C.. 2021. *GitHub repository*. https://github.com/justenvirons/covid-dashboard

Stier, Andrew J., Marc G. Berman, and Luís M. A. Bettencourt. 2021. "Early Pandemic COVID-19 Case Growth Rates Increase with City Size." *Npj Urban Sustainability* 1 (1): 1–6. doi: 10.1038/s42949-021-00030-0

Chapter 11

Tennessee case study

Cori Cohen Grant
University of Tennessee Health Science Center
Memphis, TN

David Schwartz
University of Tennessee Health Science Center
Memphis, TN

Arash Shaban-Nejado
University of Tennessee Health Science Center
Memphis, TN

CONTENTS

Introduction 161
Shelby county (demographics, poverty, chronic disease) 163
    Poverty 163
    Chronic disease 165
    COVID-19 165
COVID-19 task force 167
Establishing community-based COVID-19 testing 168
Creating an Urban Population Health Observatory (UPHO) for
    Western Tennessee to more equitably manage the COVID-19
    emergency and ongoing public health priorities 169
Digital interventions as cost-effective and scalable means for
    healthcare planning and delivery 170
Social Determinants of Health (SDoH) indicators 171
Bringing it all together: Deploying an integrated COVID-19
    UPHO knowledgebase in Western Tennessee to promote
    an equitable future 171
References 172

INTRODUCTION

American life expectancy has abruptly declined by more than one year in the COVID-19 era [1] Different racial and ethnic groups have not experienced this equally. Life expectancy of White males decreased by about 10 months in the first half of 2020. Over the same period, life expectancy for Black males fell by three years. Before COVID, life expectancy of Black males was four years shorter than that of White males. Six months into the pandemic, this disparity had widened to six years.

The baseline prevalence of health comorbidities, a consequence of environmental, social, and healthcare access hardships experienced by disadvantaged populations, has contributed significantly to COVID-19's inequitable impact. As a result of these pre-existing health disparities, vulnerable populations have suffered higher infection, hospitalization, and death rates from COVID-19 than non-Hispanic Whites.

The U.S. Centers for Disease Control and Prevention (CDC) has reported that COVID-19 deaths among Hispanic or Latino, non-Hispanic Black, and American Indian/Alaskan Native (AI/AN) groups exceeds their numerical representation within the total U.S. population. A study published in June 2020 found that Blacks accounted for 34% of the total national COVID-19 mortality, despite representing only 13% of the population. In New York, Black individuals make up 22% of the population but suffered 28% of COVID-19 deaths [2]. Hispanic individuals constitute 29% of the population but suffered 34% of COVID deaths. Another study analyzed disparities in COVID-19 cases (defined by the authors as >5% actual difference between proportion of cases and proportion of the population for underrepresented racial and ethnic groups) in 205 COVID-19 "hotspot" counties across 33 states [3]. For those counties that reported demographic totals, nearly all (96.2%) noted disproportionately high case rates in minority populations. Latino communities have been particularly hard hit in locations with a higher population prevalence of heart disease and dense residential occupancy [4].

Preexisting lack of health and social resources have made ongoing vaccination efforts more challenging in disadvantaged, minority–majority neighborhoods [5, 6]. Remarkably, no more than half of U.S. states explicitly took race, ethnicity, or social disadvantage into account in their vaccination planning. A survey of 47 publicly available state plans by the Kaiser Family Foundation just prior to vaccine approval revealed that only 25 states explicitly acknowledged health equity issues as part of their vaccine distribution planning [7]. Not surprisingly, vaccination rates in U.S. minority groups have lagged significantly since the introduction of effective immunization programs. The first published report of national, county-level vaccination rates by the Washington Post in March 2021 confirmed majority Black (15.3%) and majority Hispanic (16%) counties to have lower vaccination rates than White majority counties (18.6%) [8].

Our local experience in Memphis, TN mirrors this storyline and lends urgency to the situation. Baseline vaccine hesitancy in African Americans was high. A community survey of 400 Memphians in November 2020 mirrored national trends, confirming that 45% of surveyed Black individuals would refuse a free vaccine [9]. Unfortunately, these attitudes may have heightened the vulnerability of minority populations to COVID-19 transmission. According to publicly available Shelby County Health Department data, over 56% of COVID-19 cases in the county containing Memphis have been diagnosed in African Americans (baseline 48.5% of general population) [10]. Over 11% of cases have been found in Hispanic populations (baseline 5.6% of general population). By late April 2021, Memphis reached a tipping point whereby disproportionate vaccination in White neighborhoods began driving concentration of remaining COVID-19 transmission toward minority communities. The pandemic had split in two, with demographics defining their boundaries. By the end of April, public reporting showed that approximately 30% of the county had received at least one vaccination dose. African Americans (36%) and Hispanics (4%) were disproportionately underrepresented in this population [11]. Most strikingly, 76% of COVID-19 cases surveyed by the county in April self-reported as African American. Over 30% were employed in manufacturing or warehousing industries and 54% were between the ages of 18–44. By June 2021, geospatial mapping of case distribution confirmed that zip codes with the highest median income and proportion of White residents continued to have the highest vaccination and lowest case rates (Figure 11.3) [12]. An inverted distribution of low vaccination and elevated case rates was seen in low-income, minority–majority zip codes.

Taken together, without data-driven vaccination outreach, COVID-19 threatens to linger indefinitely in minority communities, fueled by focal transmission among younger people working in industrial jobs with limited health benefits and protections. The impact could be magnified by emerging COVID-19 variants with higher transmissibility, virulence, and reinfection rates. This risks reemergence of spread across the entire region. Downstream chronic morbidities stemming from COVID-19 (i.e., "long COVID") may eventually become segregated and endemic, with older generations suffering accelerated mortality and younger generations shouldering avoidable chronic debility. The healthcare system, particularly safety net resources, would be forced to shoulder this burden indefinitely.

SHELBY COUNTY (DEMOGRAPHICS, POVERTY, CHRONIC DISEASE)

The population of Shelby County, Tennessee was 9,36,374 in 2019 [13]. Shelby County includes the city of Memphis and several other suburban metropolitan areas (Table 11.1).

Poverty

The Poverty Rate in Memphis and Shelby County Compared to National Rates.

In general, poverty rates for the City of Memphis continue to be higher than poverty rates in Shelby County for every category. Both are higher than poverty rates in Tennessee, with the notable exception of non-Hispanic Whites, for which poverty rates are higher in Tennessee than in Memphis [14].

Table 11.1 Demographics of Memphis, Memphis MSA, Shelby County, Tennessee, and the United States

2019 Demographics	Total Population	% White	% Black	Hispanic	Asian
United States	324,697,795	72.5	12.7	18	5.5
Tennessee	6,709,356	77.6	16.8	5.4	1.8
Shelby County	936,374	39.1	53.7	6.4	2.6
Memphis city, Tennessee	651,932	29.2	64.1	7.2	1.7
Memphis, TN-MS-AR Metro	1,339,623	46.3	47.1	5.6	2.1

Source: U.S. Census Bureau, American Community Survey, 2019 [13].

Table 11.2 Poverty rates in Memphis, Memphis MSA, Shelby County, Tennessee, and the United States, 2019

Geographic area	Overall	Under 18	18–64	65+	Non-Hispanic White	Non-Hispanic Black	Hispanic/ Latino
United States	12.3	16.8	11.5	9.4	9.0	21.2	17.2
Tennessee	13.9	19.7	12.9	9.7	11.2	21.5	23.6
Shelby County	16.8	25.9	14.3	11.8	6.8	23.0	24.5
Memphis city, Tennessee	21.7	35.0	18.3	14.1	9.3	26.1	29.2
Memphis, TN-MS-AR Metro	16.5	25.5	13.9	11.8	6.9	22.6	21.9

Source: U.S. Census Bureau, American Community Survey, 2019 [14].

Memphis is one of the poorest major metropolitan cities in the United States [14], and the racial disparities in poverty are glaring. Memphis has an overall poverty rate of nearly 22%. The rate of poverty for non-Hispanic Whites is 9%, which is markedly lower than Blacks at 26% and Hispanics/ Latinos at 29%. Child poverty is 35%, compared to 14% for people over age 65, which is the lowest of any age group (Table 11.2). Forty percent have public health insurance coverage and 13% under 65 have no coverage at all [14]. Our previous research [15–19] revealed associations between social and environmental determinants of health with several adverse health outcomes in the population living in Memphis.

In the Memphis Metropolitan Statistical Area (MSA), which includes parts of Tennessee, Arkansas, and Mississippi, we see a similar pattern. All three states rank in the top 10 in the United States for the percent of people below poverty level in the past 12 months. Mississippi ranks #1, Arkansas #5, and Tennessee #9 [20]. The overall poverty in the Memphis MSA is 16%, child poverty is 25%, poverty for people over age 65 is 12%. Black

Table 11.3 Cumulative cases, deaths, and vaccinations for COVID-19

Geographic Area	Cumulative Cases*	Rate per 1,00,000*	Cumulative Deaths*	Deaths per 1,00,000*	Number Fully Vaccinated*	% Fully Vaccinated**
Tennessee	1,013,943	14,847	13,304	195	2,823,857	41%
Memphis, TN-MS-AR CBSA	180,556	13,414	2,680	199	523,540	39%
Shelby County	120,884	12,899	1,847	197	377,785	40%

* As of August 27, 2021,[26]
** Fully vaccinated as a percent of the total population [27].

Table 11.4 Case and death rates for COVID-19 by race and ethnicity

Geographic Area	Overall	Cases (White)	Cases (Black)	Cases (Hispanic)	Overall	Deaths (White)	Deaths (Black)	Deaths (Hispanic)
Tennessee*	13,084		10,537	15,221				
Shelby County*		6,444	9,494	12,380	185.2	159.4	201.5	93.4
National**						124.00	178	154.0

* As of July 29, 2021 [26].
** As of March 7, 2021; Rate per 1,00,000 [27].

poverty is 23%, non-Hispanic White poverty is 7%, and Hispanic or Latino poverty is 22%. The childhood poverty rate (under age 18) [14] in the Memphis MSA is the second-highest in the United States for MSAs with more than a million people. The rate for African American children is more than three times that for White children.

Chronic disease

The population in Shelby County suffers greatly from numerous health problems including a high prevalence of heart disease (177/1,00,000) obesity (33%), smoking (38%), and diabetes (33%). Mortality rates from diabetes are 16% for Whites and 44% Blacks [21]. Due to the high prevalence of these risk factors, Shelby County is said to lie within the U.S. "stroke belt"[22, 23], "diabetes belt" [24], and "Tobacco Nation"[25].

COVID-19

In August 2021, there were 1,20,884 cumulative cases and 1,847 deaths from COVID-19 in Shelby County. Sixty percent (n = 1,108) of the deaths were among Blacks and 35% (n = 646) among Whites [26] (Tables 11.3 and 11.4, Figure 11.1).

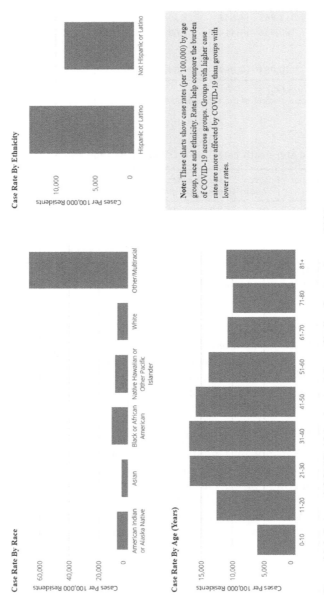

Figure 11.1 Rates of COVID-19 by Age and Race, Shelby County, August 2021.

Source: Dashboards Shelby County [28].

COVID-19 TASK FORCE

In March of 2020, The University of Tennessee Health Science Center in Memphis prepared a COVID-19 Road Map that called for the formation of regional task force. Later that month, at the direction of the Memphis and Shelby County mayors, the Shelby County COVID-19 Task Force (Task Force) was created. Led by the City of Memphis Chief Operating Officer (COO) and Shelby County Chief Administrative Officer (CAO), brought together elected officials from each of the municipalities in Shelby County, and officials from surrounding counties in Tennessee, Arkansas, and Mississippi, as well as representatives from the Shelby County Health Department, school districts, and several nonprofit agencies that provide social services to the most vulnerable populations. This effort included the City of Memphis Office of Emergency Management and Shelby County Office of Preparedness teams together with key healthcare partners including infectious disease specialists, all area hospitals, leadership within the University of Tennessee Health Science Center (UTHSC) and from Federally Qualified Health Centers (FQHCs).

The Task Force was designed to ensure a coordinated and comprehensive response to the coronavirus pandemic for Shelby and surrounding counties in Tennessee, Arkansas, and Mississippi. The early formation of the Task Force created the infrastructure to assess and address the needs of residents of Shelby County. To accomplish this, the group needed data that would allow them to identify vulnerable communities and allocate more resources accordingly.

Preexisting lack of timely access to an integrated consistent health and non-health (e.g. socioeconomic and environmental determinants) data sources made COVID-19 efforts, from testing and contact tracing to vaccinations, and intervention/policy implementation in Memphis and Shelby County challenging. This was not unique – remarkably, no more than half of U.S. states explicitly took race, ethnicity, or social vulnerability into account in their COVID-19 planning. For example, a survey of 47 publicly available state plans by the Kaiser Family Foundation just prior to vaccine approval revealed that only 25 states explicitly acknowledged health equity issues as part of their vaccine distribution planning. Not surprisingly, vaccination rates in U.S. minority groups have lagged significantly since the introduction of the vaccine. The first published report of national, county-level vaccination rates by the Washington Post in March 2021 confirmed majority Black (15.3%) and majority Hispanic (16%) counties to have lower vaccination rates than White majority counties (18.6%).

The activities of the task force were targeted and conducted at the census tract level with a focus on activities and resources in the areas that correspond to the highest levels of social and community vulnerability. To do this the Task Force used mapping to determine where to set up testing and immunization sites and provide enhanced education in the community [29] (Figure 11.2).

Lowest rates of vaccination in zip codes 38127, 38106, 38126, 38114, 38118, 38115, 38141 (Figure 11.3).

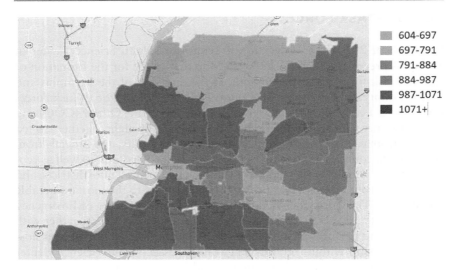

604-697
697-791
791-884
884-987
987-1071
1071+

Figure 11.2 COVID-19 cases per 1,00,000 population, August 11–25, 2021.

Source:https://insight.livestories.com/s/v2/1-4-geographic-data/6bb3072d-e622-4b84-9555-7b0ef390b354, [30].

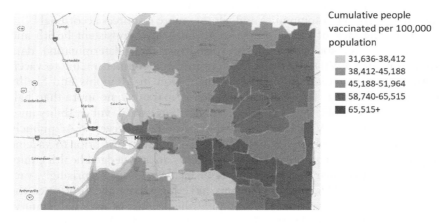

Cumulative people
vaccinated per 100,000
population

31,636-38,412
38,412-45,188
45,188-51,964
58,740-65,515
65,515+

Figure 11.3 Rate of people vaccinated per 1,00,000 population.

Source: https://insight.livestories.com/s/v2/1-4-geographic-data/6bb3072d-e622-4b84-9555-7b0ef390b354, [30].

ESTABLISHING COMMUNITY-BASED COVID-19 TESTING

In March 2020, following guidance from the American Association of Medical Colleges, junior and senior year students at the UTHSC College of Medicine were removed from the clinic due to COVID-19. Leaders at the College identified an opportunity to create a large-scale, community drive-through COVID-19 testing site and solicited student participation. Student leaders were tasked with organizing the site with clinical administrators, representatives from the Memphis Fire and Police Departments, and faculty members. Additional medical student volunteers underwent training in proper personal protective techniques, specimen collection/handling, and electronic health record (EHR)-based patient registration the following day, allowing the testing site to open within 72 hours of initial planning.

First responders from the Memphis community were prioritized for testing while workflow and procedures were fine-tuned. Medical students served as the primary workforce for both the drive-through testing site and a scheduling call center, under direct supervision from faculty and house staff. In late March 2020, the site was open to the public. It was operated by students and supervisors until late May 2020, when the site shifted to professional staffing. Leaders of the UTHSC testing program helped to establish a Safety Net COVID-19 Committee for the City of Memphis, which remains active and is composed of leaders from community providers, including Federally Qualified Health Centers, participating in city-funded COVID-19 testing for underserved neighborhoods. The Safety Net Task Force helped to identify a second UTHSC site which then opened in North Memphis to boost testing in underserved neighborhoods. This coverage quickly expanded to a total of four sites that operated throughout the summer. In conjunction with the City of Memphis, our operations have since been consolidated at a larger facility in East Memphis working in tandem with smaller clinical facilities across the metropolitan region. In all, over 30,000 unique individuals had been tested at UTHSC-run sites as of mid-December 2020.

As noted above, all UTHSC testing sites have required patients to use an automated smartphone-based chatbot application to self-register and report demographic information, COVID-19 exposure history, type of occupation (first responder, healthcare provider, frontline worker, other), as well as medical history highlights and risk factors for COVID-19 complications (diabetes, hypertension, etc.). The chatbot was designed by a third-party vendor (CareCognetics, Las Vegas, NV) in tandem with the UTHSC clinical leadership team to interface with its native EHR system (Nextgen Healthcare, Irvine, CA). This patient self-service registration platform permitted a near-universal collection of key clinical and demographic characteristics, matched to COVID-19 test results for each individual. To permit downstream analysis of anonymized population-level data, the collection process was formally approved by the UTHSC Investigational Review Board.

CREATING AN URBAN POPULATION HEALTH OBSERVATORY (UPHO) FOR WESTERN TENNESSEE TO MORE EQUITABLY MANAGE THE COVID-19 EMERGENCY AND ONGOING PUBLIC HEALTH PRIORITIES

Prior to COVID-19, Memphis had no large-scale population health data warehousing infrastructure. We have leveraged the urgency of the pandemic to establish an Urban Population Health Observatory to rectify this short-fall so that we are prepared to identify and serve marginalized groups more effectively in our community during the ongoing public health emergency and beyond.

Memphis Pandemic Health Informatics System (MEMPHI-SYS) Regional COVID-19 Data Registry is a large-scale data repository created in UTHSC, in collaboration with the City of Memphis, which captures data from community drive-through COVID-19 testing sites across Memphis, TN. MEMPHI-SYS has been used in coordination with private clinical partners to distribute testing across the metropolitan region and to now coordinate large-scale public vaccination. Over 80,000 unique individuals have been tested at UTHSC-run sites as of March 1, 2021. The registry population represents approximately 10–15% of total testing performed in Shelby County. Our testing has been unique from its inception since we have required all test subjects to use an automated smartphone-based chatbot application to collect general demographic information, COVID-19 exposure history, type of occupation (first responder, healthcare provider, front-line worker, or none of the above), and medical history highlights and risk factors for COVID-19 complications (diabetes, hypertension, etc.). This self-service interface permitted a near-universal collection of key clinical and demographic correlates alongside COVID-19 testing results. This data will be leveraged to further strengthen the on-the-ground relevance of the UPHO to the pandemic in Memphis.

DIGITAL INTERVENTIONS AS COST-EFFECTIVE AND SCALABLE MEANS FOR HEALTHCARE PLANNING AND DELIVERY

Precision medicine is [31] "an emerging approach for disease treatment and prevention that takes into account individual variability in genes, environment, and lifestyle." Similarly, precision population health targets public health challenges (e.g., disease prevention, health disparities, etc.) in a population by using omics, social, cultural, behavioral, and environmental data to account for differences between populations in the development and use of health interventions [32, 33]. The targeted use of digital technologies can engage specific populations to improve their health awareness and adoption of healthy behaviors. An efficient Urban Population Health Observatory (UPHO) [34] can help overcome some of the barriers to real-time disease surveillance and intervention planning currently posed by limitations of existing healthcare systems, especially in resource-scarce environments. An integrated UPHO platform can be used to maintain a historical digital representation of populations' health state from diagnosis to monitoring and interventions by integrating local knowledge about their EHR data with global trusted knowledge to produce intelligent, personalized recommendations to improve their health state.

The platform has utilized several components generated through our previous developments, including the Population Health Record (PopHR) [35] that facilitates the integration of various group-level and individual-level data, SIEMA [36] for maintaining interoperability between various data sources, POLE.VAULT for automated health intervention evaluation [37, 38], the Personal Health Library (PHL) [39, 40], and SPACES [41], an intelligent recommender system based on Explainable Artificial Intelligence to facilitate targeted surveillance and resource allocation. While the initial development [31] of the UPHO provides promising results, improving this platform and application package requires employing a wide spectrum of innovative technologies to expand the breadth and depth of the platform and to improve users' experience by providing them with user-friendly digital interventions.

SOCIAL DETERMINANTS OF HEALTH (SDOH) INDICATORS

In collaboration with a private sector partner, we created an integrated Neighborhood Quality data repository consisting of highly granular social, environmental, and behavioral datasets, which is instrumental in understanding the pathways of how SDoH contribute to individual and public health. We did this by applying knowledge modeling tools for integrating SDoH using epidemiological techniques, along with methodologies from data and network sciences.

To enable Memphis Urban Health Surveillance, an integrated dataset consisting of the Memphis Neighborhood Quality data, the U.S. census data on the neighborhood racial composition, poverty level, chronic condition data from the Center for Disease Control & Prevention (CDC) 500 Cities have been aligned and curated.

BRINGING IT ALL TOGETHER: DEPLOYING AN INTEGRATED COVID-19 UPHO KNOWLEDGEBASE IN WESTERN TENNESSEE TO PROMOTE AN EQUITABLE FUTURE

Our UPHO will provide a single secure access point to a metropolitan-wide health database to empower informed health policy decisions via integrated access to large, previously uncoordinated streams of complex data. As urban populations such as Memphis struggle with the pandemic's intensification of longstanding health inequalities, local policymakers and public health agencies must urgently enhance their health surveillance systems to meaningfully support healthy populations at 21st century expectations. Creation of truly "smart cities" will require "harnessing technology and data analytics to ease key challenges of urban life" [3]. The Memphis UPHO will provide ongoing collection, integration, analysis, and dissemination of all data and knowledge relevant to COVID-19, and encode this knowledge in a formal machine-readable format. The UPHO platform promises impact to all Memphians through validation of a novel XAI platform leveraging a unique focus on maintaining healthcare quality in historically vulnerable populations before and after large-scale public health events, such as COVID-19.

Although Memphis and Western Tennessee continue to be severely impacted by newer, more virulent strains of COVID-19, we envision a legacy of nimble, more equitable large-scale public health responses to the unpredictable new emergencies and old stubborn inequities we face presently and in the future. We cannot be satisfied with cataloging the health inequities laid bare by COVID-19, we must have the battlefield data to start eliminating them.

REFERENCES

[1] Santhanam Laura. (2021, Feb 18). *COVID-19 Has Already Cut U.S. Life Expectancy By a Year. For Black Americans, It's Worse.* PBS.org. https://www.pbs.org/newshour/health/covid-19-has-already-cut-u-s-life-expectancy-by-a-year-for-black-americans-its-worse.

[2] Mein SA (2020). COVID-19 and Health Disparities: The Reality of "the Great Equalizer". *Journal of General Internal Medicine*, 35, 2439–2440.

[3] Moore JT, et al. (2020). Disparities in Incidence of COVID-19 Among Underrepresented Racial/Ethnic Groups in Counties Identified as Hotspots During June 5–18, 2020–22 states, February–June 2020. *Morbidity and Mortality Weekly Report*, 69(33), 1122.

[4] Rodriguez-Diaz CE, Guilamo-Ramos V, Mena L, Hall E, Honermann B, Crowley JS, & Millett GA (2020). Risk for COVID-19 Infection and Death Among Latinos in the United States: Examining Heterogeneity in Transmission Dynamics. *Annals of Epidemiology*, 52, 46–53.

[5] Neergaard L and Fingerhut H. (2020, December 9). AP-NORC Poll: Only Half in US Want Shots as Vaccine Nears. *AP News*. https://apnews.com/article/ap-norc-poll-us-half-want-vaccine-shots-4d98dbfc0a64d60d52ac84c3065dac55

[6] Jean-Jacques M, & Bauchner H (2021). Vaccine Distribution—Equity Left Behind?. *JAMA*, 325(9), 829–830.

[7] Kaiser Family Foundation (2020, Nov 18). *States Are Getting Ready to Distribute COVID-19 Vaccines. What Do Their Plans Tell Us So Far?* https://www.kff.org/coronavirus-covid-19/issue-brief/states-are-getting-ready-to-distribute-covid-19-vaccines-what-do-their-plans-tell-us-so-far/

[8] Johnson A (2021, February 13). Lack of Health Services and Transportation Impede Access to Vaccine in Communities of Color. *The Washington Post*. https://www.washingtonpost.com/health/2021/02/13/covid-racial-ethnic-disparities/

[9] COVID-19 Update (11–16). (2021, November 16). Covid 19.memphistn.gov.https://covid19.memphistn.gov/2020/11/

[10] Case Demographic Data. (n.d.) Shelby County Health Department. https://insight.livestories.com/s/v2/1-3-case-demographics/19e3182b-e67e-4d93-b5d2-07c249328d6e. Accessed 30 April 2021.

[11] Vaccine Data. (n.d.) Shelby County Health Department. https://insight.livestories.com/s/v2/1-6-1-shelby-county-vaccine-dashboard/336442d5-36c8-4a10-8e46-130c32a8c3e7. Accessed April 30, 2021.

[12] Shelby County Health Department, (2021, June 22) https://insight.livestories.com/s/v2/1-4geographic-data/6bb3072d-e622-4b84-9555-7b0ef390b354.

[13] U.S. Census Bureau, (n.d.) "ACS Demographic and Housing Estimates 2019," *2014-2019 American Community Survey 5-Year Estimates (DP05)*, https://www.census.gov/acs/www/data/data-tables-and-tools/data-profiles/, accessed August 10, 2021.

[14] U.S. Census Bureau, (n.d.) "Poverty Status in the Past 12 Months, 2019," *2014–2019 American Community Survey 5-Year Estimates (S1701)*, https://www.census.gov/acs/www/data/data-tables-and-tools/data-profiles/, accessed August 10, 2021.

[15] Shin EK, Shaban-Nejad A. (2018). Urban Data Integration for Population Health Surveillance: Urban Decay and Pediatric Asthma Prevalence in Memphis, Tennessee. *IEEE Access* 6: 46281–46289. doi: 10.1109/ACCESS.2018.2866069.

[16] Shin EK, Mahajan R, Akbilgic O, Shaban-Nejad A. (2018 Oct 2). Sociomarkers and Biomarkers: Predictive Modeling in Identifying Pediatric Asthma Patients at Risk of Hospital Revisits. *NPJ Digit Med.*, 1:50. doi: 10.1038/s41746-018-0056-y. PMID: 31304329.

[17] Shin EK, Kwon Y, Shaban-Nejad A. (2019 Aug 1). Geo-Clustered Chronic Affinity: Pathways From Socio-Economic Disadvantages to Health Disparities. *JAMIA Open*, 2(3): 317–322. doi: 10.1093/jamiaopen/ooz029. PMID: 31984364.

[18] Shin EK, LeWinn K, Bush N, Tylavsky FA, Davis RL, Shaban-Nejad A. (2019 Jan 4). Association of Maternal Social Relationships With Cognitive Development in Early Childhood. *JAMA Netw. Open*, 2(1): e186963. doi: 10.1001/jamanetworkopen.2018.6963. PMID: 30646208.

[19] Akbilgic O, Shin EK, Shaban-Nejad A. (2021 Mar 12). A Data Science Approach to Analyze the Association of Socioeconomic and Environmental Conditions With Disparities in Pediatric Surgery. *Front Pediatr.*, 9: 620848. doi: 10.3389/fped.2021.620848. PMID: 33777865.

[20] The Poorest States in America. (n.d.) https://www.safety.com/the-poorest-states-in-america/, accessed August 15, 2021.

[21] Memphis & Shelby County Health Brief. (2018). https://bettertennessee.com/memphis-shelby-county-health-brief/#demographics], accessed August 15, 2021.

[22] Alberts MJ. (1996). The Stroke Belt Consortium. *J Stroke Cerebrovasc Dis.* 6(1):54–58.

[23] Liao Y, Greenlund KJ, Croft JB, Keenan NL, Giles WH. (2009). Factors Explaining Excess Stroke Prevalence in the US Stroke Belt. *Stroke*, 40(10): 3336–3341.

[24] Centers for Disease Control and Prevention. (n.d.) *CDC Identifies Diabetes Belt.* Centers for Disease Control and Prevention. Atalanta GA. https://www.cdc.gov/diabetes/pdfs/data/diabetesbelt.pdf. Accessed August 15, 2021.

[25] Truth Initiative. *Tobacco Nation: An ongoing crisis.* (2019). https://truthinitiative.org/tobacconation. Accessed August 15, 2021.

[26] COVID-19 Community Profile Report. (2021, August 27). https://healthdata.
gov/Health/COVID-19-Community-Profile-Report/gqxm-d9w9, accessed
August 30, 2021.

[27] The COVID Racial Data Tracker. (n.d.) https://covidtracking.com/race, accessed
August 20, 2021.

[28] Dashboards Shelby County. (n.d.) https://covid19.tn.gov/data/dashboards/?
County=Shelby, accessed August 25, 2021.

[29] Joint Task Force. (n.d.) https://covid19.memphistn.gov/resources/joint-task-
force/, accessed August 15, 2021.

[30] https://insight.livestories.com/s/v2/1-4-geographic-data/6bb3072d-e622-
4b84-9555-7b0ef390b354; accessed Aug 25, 2021.

[31] The Precision Medicine Initiative. (2021, August) https://obamawhitehouse.
archives.gov/precision-medicine

[32] Shaban-Nejad A, Michalowski M. (2020).From Precision Medicine
to Precision Health: A Full Angle from Diagnosis to Treatment and
Prevention. In: Shaban-Nejad A, Michalowski M (eds) *Precision Health and
Medicine. Studies in Computational Intelligence*, vol 843. Springer, Cham.
doi.10.1007/978-3-030-24409-5_1

[33] Shaban-Nejad A, Michalowski M, Peek N, Brownstein JS, Buckeridge DL.
(2020, Mar).Seven Pillars of Precision Digital Health and Medicine. *Artif Intell
Med.* 103: 101793. PMID: 32143798.

[34] Brakefield WS, Ammar N, Olusanya OA, Shaban-Nejad A. (2021 Jun 16).
An Urban Population Health Observatory System to Support COVID-19
Pandemic Preparedness, Response, and Management: Design and Development
Study. *JMIR Public Health Surveill.* 7(6): e28269. doi: 10.2196/28269. PMID:
34081605.

[35] Shaban-Nejad A, Lavigne M, Okhmatovskaia A, Buckeridge DL. (2017 Jan).
PopHR: A Knowledge-Based Platform to Support Integration, Analysis, and
Visualization of Population Health Data. *Ann N Y Acad Sci.* 1387(1): 44–53.
doi: 10.1111/nyas.13271. Epub 2016 Oct 17. PMID: 27750378.

[36] Al Manir MS, Brenas JH, Baker CJ, Shaban-Nejad A. (2018 Jun 15). A
Surveillance Infrastructure for Malaria Analytics: Provisioning Data Access
and Preservation of Interoperability. *JMIR Public Health Surveill.* 4(2):
e10218. doi: 10.2196/10218. PMID: 29907554.

[37] Shaban-Nejad A, Okhmatovskaia A, Shin EK, Davis RL, Franklin BE,
Buckeridge DL. (2017). A Semantic Framework for Logical Cross-Validation,
Evaluation and Impact Analyses of Population Health Interventions. *Stud
Health Technol Inform.* 235: 481–485. PMID: 28423839.

[38] Brenas JH, and Shaban-Nejad A. (2020) Health Intervention Evaluation Using
Semantic Explainability and Causal Reasoning. *IEEE Access* 8: 9942–9952.
doi:10.1109/ACCESS.2020.2964802.

[39] Ammar N, Bailey JE, Davis RL, Shaban-Nejad A (2021) Implementation of a
Personal Health Library (PHL) to Support Chronic Disease Self-Management.
In: Shaban-Nejad A, Michalowski M, Buckeridge DL (eds) *Explainable AI
in Healthcare and Medicine. Studies in Computational Intelligence*, vol 914.
Springer, Cham. https://doi.org/10.1007/978-3-030-53352-6_20

[40] Ammar N, Bailey JE, Davis RL, Shaban-Nejad A. (2021). Using a Personal Health Library–Enabled mHealth Recommender System for Self-Management of Diabetes Among Underserved Populations: Use Case for Knowledge Graphs and Linked Data. *JMIR Form Res* 5(3): e24738. doi: 10.2196/24738; PMID: 33724197.

[41] Ammar N, Shaban-Nejad A. (2020 Nov 4). Explainable Artificial Intelligence Recommendation System by Leveraging the Semantics of Adverse Childhood Experiences: Proof-of-Concept Prototype Development. *JMIR Med Inform.* 8(11): e18752. doi: 10.2196/18752. PMID: 33146623.

Chapter 12

Regional modeling

Madeleine McDowell
Sg2/Vizient
Carbondale, CO, USA

Meghan Robb
Vizient
Annapolis, MD, USA

Jim Jacobsohn
SG2
Chicago, IL, USA

CONTENTS

Early case-based hospitalization and critical care data 179
Sample COVID-19 data published online from Italy's National
    Health System 180
Using known data from Italian experience to estimate infected
    population COVID-19 hospitalization rates 182
Sg2 COVID-19 surge demand model evolves to dynamic
    SIR modeling 183
Impact of social distancing measures in Italy 184
Comparing frequently cited models for early US COVID-19 surge 184
Sg2's tracking of state-mandated stay-at-home orders by date of
    implementation for local transmissibility mitigation inputs 186

Understanding the impact of change. That's been our tagline for 20 years. Sg2's cutting-edge expertise and analytics provide health industry leaders the tools to confidently formulate the strategy needed to succeed today while positioning for tomorrow. Knowing how to navigate changing demand, technology adoption, care delivery redesign and enterprise growth strategy has been our lifeblood. But COVID-19 brought about change at a pace not seen before and introduced an unprecedented level of unpredictability. This upending of the system forced us to revisit our strengths, leverage our skills in new ways to meet new needs, learn and adapt at record speed and co-create in novel ways for the greater good.

    Every analytic model we create begins with a healthcare business question communicated to us by our clients. Sg2's first major step into the analytic

DOI: 10.1201/9781003204138-15

space came as a result of clients needing to understand changes in inpatient demand resulting from the evolving healthcare ecosystem. Years later we responded to health systems' increasingly complex questions around care continuum optimization and growth, which required more sophisticated tools and predictive modeling. Decades of modeling healthcare demand did prepare us in some unique ways for responding to US health system needs in the early pandemic, but in many ways, we were forced to rapidly evolve our tools, data and talent.

Sg2 analytics primarily inform strategic planning questions, often with a 3-, 5- or even 10-year horizon. That longer-term planning horizon became far less relevant in early 2020 as COVID-19 first began to spread across the United States and healthcare systems became overwhelmed with patients infected with a disease that was incredibly difficult to treat and extremely resource intensive. Our clients suddenly had a desperate need to predict demand for hospital beds, ICU beds and ventilators in the coming days weeks and months. For many, the need to survive the operational crises of the minute or hour was becoming the overwhelming focus. We asked ourselves – Could Sg2 step in to provide help in managing for the pandemic's immediate future? How could we best aid our member clients on the front lines of battle with this new disease, so that they in turn could be better prepared to care for the communities they served in the trying months ahead? (Figure 12.1)

Our goal was to evolve our demand forecasting methodologies and bed need modeling expertise to provide our health system members with a reliable and defensible means of planning for, and proactively adjusting to, the constant moving target of COVID. We set off on a race against time to adapt our modeling capabilities to include scenarios of COVID-19 infection spread and then translated this disease-driven demand immediately into projected, daily, bed and ventilator needs. We built in a means of direct and rolling comparison to real-world experience via actual capacity data and average daily census benchmarks. And we continually evolved our modeling as both the disease, and our understanding of it, progressed.

But how did we evolve? What did that journey look like? In retrospect, some of our analytic development process seemed to follow what we considered to

> " We're sort of planning for what's going on right now, and we're trying to make up for lost time, but I'm not sure we're planning for a month from now, or even two weeks from now. "
>
> –Christopher M. Tedeschi, MD
> Emergency physician and assistant professor, Columbia University Medical Center

Figure 12.1 The need for disaster planning.

Source: J. Goldstein and B. Rosenthal. New York Times: Coronavirus in N.Y.: Will a Surge in Patients Overwhelm Hospitals? March 14, 2020.

be the obvious next steps forward. Some of it was the result of trial and error, and lots of collaborative creativity. And some of it, admittedly, did seem like fortunate luck.

To tell the story, we should start at the beginning. By late January and into February 2020, many within Sg2 had begun to track international news of COVID. Data was scarce and conjecture on the future seemed to be everywhere. As time went on, the tragic reporting from Europe – and in particular, Italy – heightened our realization of the importance of bed and ventilator demand forecasting, an area of healthcare analytics we knew well. We also observed that hospital admissions had become the one true litmus of disease spread, as COVID-19 seemed to carry a high asymptomatic case rate and testing access was limited to international travel contacts and hospitalized patients. Basing our early analytical work on bed demand mechanics and known hospitalization rates (vs case rates) helped us start with a solid modeling foundation.

Getting from that solid modeling foundation to a functional, useful and defensible analytic was most certainly more difficult than we ever expected.

We gathered what data was available and assessed how we could use it to move our modeling forward. We were astounded to see, in both popular press and professional circles, many COVID-19 positive case-rate based hospitalization data being used interchangeably with population-based hospitalization rates for COVID-19. More than once we scratched our heads at the misinformation circulating and gaining weight in pandemic predictions. The pressures of the crisis and swirl of a seemingly perpetual feed of new and incomplete data had clouded the critical lens of some and had damaged the common-sense filter of others.

We knew that age-adjusted, population-based hospitalization, ICU and ventilator rates for COVID-19 were critical to our modeling success. Unfortunately, because the pandemic was so new and evolving so quickly, these data did not yet exist. We did have, thanks to early reporting from China and Europe, age-adjusted, case-based hospitalization and critical care data.

EARLY CASE-BASED HOSPITALIZATION AND CRITICAL CARE DATA

Even advantaged with early information coming from international hot zones, we were still lacking in population-based hospitalization and critical care rates. Again, we searched for what was known in a vast sea of unknowns. And again, thankfully, an ever-more connected world was allowing us unprecedented access to near-real time data from the front lines of the pandemic in Italy.

By mid-February and throughout March 2020, near-daily COVID-19 case positives, non-ICU and ICU hospital census volumes were being

Age Group (years)	% Symptomatic cases requiring hospitalization	% hospitalized cases requiring critical care
0 to 9	0.1%	5.0%
10 to 19	0.3%	5.0%
20 to 29	1.2%	5.0%
30 to 39	3.2%	5.0%
40 to 49	4.9%	6.3%
50 to 59	10.2%	12.2%
60 to 69	16.6%	27.4%
70 to 79	24.3%	43.2%
80+	27.3%	70.9%

Figure 12.2 Case distribution by age cohort.

Source: Ferguson NM et al. Impact of non-pharmaceutical interventions (NPIs) to reduce COVID-19 mortality and healthcare demand. Imperial College London. March 16, 2020.

reported online by Italy's National Health System (Servizio Sanitario Nazionale) (Figure 12.2). These data gave us the slope of the curve of transmission and hospital census volume trajectories before Italy enacted social distancing policies, which became a critical piece of the puzzle in calculating true, population-based hospitalization rates for the early phase of the COVID-19 pandemic. Thank goodness for transparent, international health data reporting – and web-enabled language translators!

SAMPLE COVID-19 DATA PUBLISHED ONLINE FROM ITALY'S NATIONAL HEALTH SYSTEM

Patterns that emerged from early data out of Wuhan and Lombardy were the first indicators of how this virus would likely behave going forward in the United States (Figure 12.3 and Figure 12.4). Many epidemiologists were looking at past epidemics using SARS CoV-1 or Influenza or even Ebola to model out early predictions. Having actual international transmission data on SARS CoV-2 was the key to making accurate future predictions for the present crisis. Leveraging these data, plus other emerging information – including early SARS-Cov-2 estimates from China on average pre-infectious time period and infectious period – our analytic toolkit evolved to include infectious disease modeling staples such as susceptible-infected-recovered (SIR) modeling.

What we learned from this early international data, we applied to early modeling projections for the United States. By incorporating international infection and hospitalization data, SIR curves as guidance, and triangulating data sources to help back into reasonable assumptions when direct data was not available, we were able to glean what the actual, population-based

Regione	POSITIVI AL nCoV				DIMESSI GUARITI	DECEDUTI	CASI TOTALI	TAMPONI
	Hospitalized with Symptoms	Intensive Care	Home Isolation	Total Currently Positive				
Lombardia	698	167	461	1326	139	55	1520	9577
Emilia Romagna	187	24	187	398	4	18	420	2012
Veneto	49	19	229	297	7	3	307	10176
Piemonte	13	3	40	56			56	458
Marche	27	13	19	59		2	61	200
Campania	11		19	30			30	405
Liguria	12	2	5	19	4	1	24	121
Toscana	10		8	18	1		19	697
Lazio	10		1	11	3		14	877
Friuli V.G.	1		12	13			13	354
Sicilia	2		3	5	2		7	307
Puglia	2		4	6			6	298
Abruzzo	5		1	6			6	52
Trento	1		3	4			4	122
Molise	3			3			3	13
Umbria	1	1	6	8			8	45
Bolzano	1			1			1	20
Calabria			1	1			1	39
Sardegna	1			1			1	29
Basilicata			1	1			1	42
Valle d'Aosta				0			0	12
TOTALE	1034	229	1000	2263	180	79	2502	25856

Figure 12.3 Distribution of cases and care location by region.

Source: Servizio Sanitario Nazionale via https://www.salute.gov.it/

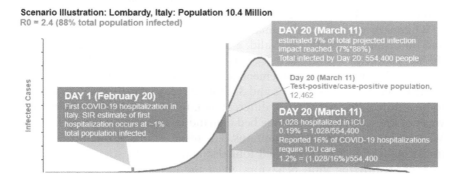

Figure 12.4 Wave modeling approach.

Note: Assumes constant RO of 2.4; pre-infection days = 5; infectious data = 10; 1 day time-step.
Source: Grasselli G et al. Critical care utilization for the COVID-19 outbreak in Lombardy, Italy: early experience and forecast during an emergency response. JAMA Network. March 13, 2020.

hospital rate range was most likely to be. It was discovered to be much lower than what others were predicting, because the number of infected was much higher than reported case positives. Many early models applied the percent hospitalized, as defined as the number hospitalized over reported case positive numbers, to overall populations to estimate hospitalizations, drastically inflating projected bed demand. This distinction, and our drive for observable and defensible data points relevant to the current situation, proved vital to the accuracy of our projections in the early stages of our modeling.

USING KNOWN DATA FROM ITALIAN EXPERIENCE
TO ESTIMATE INFECTED POPULATION COVID-19
HOSPITALIZATION RATES

Emerging data points and expanding modeling techniques helped us pin-point appropriate hospitalization and ICU admission rates. But the utility – and challenges – of incorporating SIR modeling into our traditional resource demand forecasting work was far from over. As mentioned earlier, our approach to COVID-19 demand modeling was always to lean in first on what we knew best, forecasting. Sg2 began forecasting annual year-over-year 10-year inpatient bed demand in 2001. Along our 20-year journey, we adopted many new facets to our analytic approach: expanding from IP fore-casting to all sites of care, refining our approaches to length of stay impacts, migrating to a cross-continuum disease-based forecasting approach, and "hyperlocalizing" aspects of modeling to capture local market conditions impacting healthcare demand. And while Sg2's forecasting had always incor-porated epidemiologic inputs; the refined resolution of SIR infectious disease modeling had never been integrated before. SIR detail allowed for projected outputs at a level of refined time resolution necessary for pandemic planning, but it also introduced many new and different questions about the known and unknown data inputs critical to modeling COVID-19 bed demand.

While early international estimates of the average pre-infectious time period and infectious period proved valid, a crucial SIR modeling input, known as the Reproduction Number, or R_0, was elusive for COVID-19. By the end of February 2020, there was agreement across the international community that the R0 likely ranged between 2 and 3. From there, scenario modeling was key to be able to transparently test different assumptions when the answer to R_0 was not known. What would the bed demand be if the $R = 2$ versus $R = 2.5$? We tested many possible assumptions. The result of this testing produced an initial model which incorporated four distinct, static, R_0 scenarios, intended to project differing viral behaviors given the impact of varying pandemic response: scenario (1) uncontained COVID-19 spread, as observed in the early pandemic in Wuhan, China (R2.40), scenario (2) mildly abated COVID-19 spread, influenced by large event cancellations (R2.00), scenario (3) mod-erately abated COVID-19 spread, influenced by the addition of voluntary social distancing and mask wearing, and scenario (R1.53) (4) a reference pro-jection modeled after benchmarked data for the typical seasonal flu (R1.30).

Almost as soon as it was released, we realized the dynamic nature of cir-cumstances surrounding the pandemic drove the need to evolve our initial model approach from a static view of disease impact progression, to a more dynamic capture of changing circumstances continually affecting projected COVID-19 resourcing. We were quick to appreciate the importance of determining localized impact of COVID response not just because observed data from China and Italy clearly showed high regional variation, but

because model customization for market dynamics was core to our traditional demand forecasting. An important feature of our 10-year demand
forecast was that the national forecast could be "hyperlocalized" or custom-
ized to a market for more accurate growth projections. Much in the same
way, we knew that COVID-19 would not spread uniformly across a country
or region but instead hot spots would develop based initially on international travel patterns and population density and as the pandemic evolved,
by climate, level of indoor activity and human behavior – namely adherence
to social distancing and mask wearing. The static R0 SIR modeling embedded in our COVID-19 surge model quickly advanced into a self-selected
initial, reproductive rate, augmented by a series of disease mitigation inputs
designed to continuously act upon transmission strength (R_0), and resulting
in locally nuanced projections of disease and hospital burden. This shift to
more dynamic COVID surge model allowed for market-relevant accelera-
tion or deceleration in COVID demand – this fundamental shift was the
start in modeling the "blunting of the curve."

SG2 COVID-19 SURGE DEMAND MODEL EVOLVES TO DYNAMIC SIR MODELING

But just how were we able to make this modeling leap? Again, using data
from Italy, we mapped the timing of their lockdown in-step with the observed
decline in cases (12 days) and then the corresponding, but delayed, decline
in hospitalizations (Figure 12.5 and Figure 12.6). These observed statistics
became critical reference data, used to train and inform our go-forward,
dynamic modeling approach. This advance in our surge modeling allowed us
to incorporate the impact of the implementation and timing of social distancing on health system demand and became critical to our ability to project, with
accuracy, a local community's ability to "blunt" the curve of COVID-19 surge.

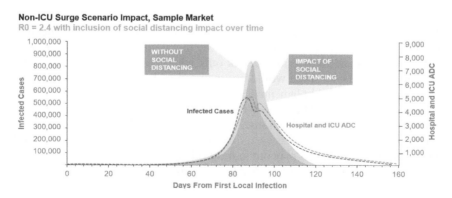

Figure 12.5 Surge impact modeling approach.

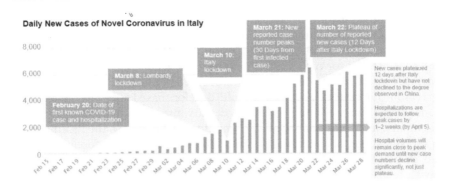

Figure 12.6 Incidence modeling using key dates.

Source: Worldometer. Coronovirus. Accessed March 2020; Remuzzi A and Remuzzi G. COVID-19 and Italy: what next? Lancet. March 13, 2020.

IMPACT OF SOCIAL DISTANCING MEASURES IN ITALY

Our work led us to study market variation and the key drivers in utilization trend differences by market population, local case mix and disease burden, market supply and business affiliations differences, state healthcare policy and level of risk payment contracting. Lessons learned from the valuable data and patterning from early international data helped us understand how to think about dynamic modeling in COVID-19. And, because we had access to that data in near-real time, we could test assumptions quickly and fine tune our own modeling. Testing our assumptions on the data from Italy allowed us to predict the story in New York City with incredible accuracy – we were off to the races.

COMPARING FREQUENTLY CITED MODELS FOR EARLY US COVID-19 SURGE

It turned out, as we learned in the US experience, the timing of implementing social distancing mandates in relation to the first community-spread hospitalizations was critical in determining not only when peak hospitalizations from the initial COVID-19 surge would occur but also the magnitude of the peak itself. Had New York implemented SD mandates just 4 days earlier, the model projected a significant blunting of the curve that would have avoided a significant number of hospitalizations. A few days made a large difference in the magnitude of blunting the curve, as would be expected for non-linear trend lines. This trend did in fact play out in most other cities across the United States, where social distancing mandates occurred in time to prevent COVID-19 surges of the magnitude observed in Wuhan, Lombardy, New York City and early hot spots. The difference being days, not weeks in the timing of mitigation efforts.

While near-real time reference data was critical to internal model builds, we needed to balance this advancing model sophistication with connections to actual environmental and pandemic response reference points, to ensure that even the most novice hospital analyst could still understand how to, and gain value from, running the Sg2 model (Figure 12.7). For the increasing complexity of imputing local disease mitigation approaches, we built into the model more simplistic reference notes tracking things like the timing and expanse of state stay-at-home orders, so that necessary and relevant localized inputs could be as accurate as possible (Figure 12.8).

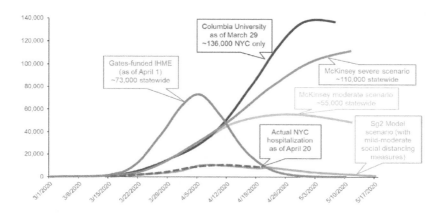

Figure 12.7 Variation in modeling approaches. IHME = Institute for Health Metrics and Evaluation.

Sources: COVID-19 Surge Demand Calculator, Sg2, 2020; NYC Health. COVID-19: Data; New York State. Pressroom: Official News from the Office of the Governor. All websites accessed April 2020.

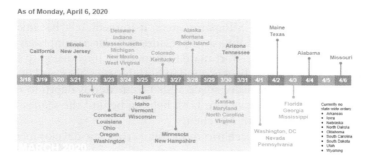

Figure 12.8 Stay at home dates. Note: The Governor of Pennsylvania began ordering stay-at-home orders for some counties on March 23, before implementing a state-wide order effective April 1.

Sources: KFF, State Data and Policy Actions to Address Coronavirus. April 3, 2020; Kates J. et al. Stay-at-Home Orders to Fight COVID-19 in the United States: The Risks of a Scattershot Approach. KFF. April 5, 2020; state government websites; Accessed April 2020.

SG2'S TRACKING OF STATE-MANDATED STAY-AT-HOME ORDERS BY DATE OF IMPLEMENTATION FOR LOCAL TRANSMISSIBILITY MITIGATION INPUTS

To date, the discussion of our COVID-19 model evolution and success has been contingent upon critical data availability and expanded analytic integration. However, none of the work we accomplished would have been possible had we not leveraged the expertise of a diverse set of people in model construction. This proved critical to the success of the project. Some of it was deliberate, but due to this being a race against time, some of it was quite honestly luck and happenstance. The three core developers had not worked as a team before. They came from three different areas of the company with different backgrounds and skillsets, that in retrospect allowed for an effective combination of complementary talents and capabilities. In addition, each had in common a history tackling unchartered territories and were comfortable in investigating the unknown and areas not within their direct expertise. Being new to the field of epidemiology was of course challenging but there was the benefit of bringing a fresh perspective that enabled us to question existing assumptions made by other modelers and experts in the field, as well as apply modeling methodologies not used in epidemiology that had born out in other work we had done. None of this was intentional at the onset though, as the urgency of developing this tool required expediency over process and planning. In fact, the emergency at hand allowed for taking risks and breaking down silos that enabled nimble innovation, something that was similarly observed as a by-product of the pandemic across healthcare. An important question is, under normal circumstances, would we have brought together as effective a team? Would the heavy burden of planning and traditional silos have prevented this accelerated innovation?

It became evident early on that there was a gap in expertise in the field of epidemiology. Recognizing what you don't know and solving for that is as important as leveraging what you know. Once we had developed a basic beta model, incorporating SIR parameters, it immediately became evident that we needed an epidemiologist to pressure test our assumptions and ask the hard questions. We were fortunate enough to be introduced to David W Hutton, PhD. Dr. Hutton's background in both health policy and mathematical modeling in the healthcare space added tremendous depth to our team and we were grateful to have him both helping behind the scenes and also on a series of webinars with our clients.

Triangulating data and scenario modeling across our development group became the foundation for pressure testing our model. Every day our team asked ourselves dozens of questions and questioned our assumptions. Was the R0 for SARS-CoV-2 like SARS CoV-1 or other Coronaviruses of Influenza? What was the doubling time of COVID-19 hospitalizations in Lombardy Italy? If NYC behaved like Lombardy, what would the ICU bed demand be on any given day after the first known hospitalization due to community spread?

As always, our clients provided us with feedback and direction that allowed us to pressure test early versions of the model but pushed us to iterate on our analytic approach. Almost as soon as our first, four-scenario, static model was release, we received impassioned pleas to quickly solve for a more dynamic view that allowed for multiple scenarios that evolved over time. We tried our best to scale our resources and in addition to the direct model, live, online Office Hour sessions, methodology documents, training videos and FAQ files helped socialize our work. But we also rolled up our sleeves and held hundreds of calls with individual clients at the market level, to help understand, and model to the best of our ability, the dynamic nature of COVID-19.

Sg2 and its parent company, Vizient, are both member organizations. We spend our time and resources dedicated to meet member need. Demonstrating value to our members is absolutely core to all that we do. And yet, our discussion on how to and whom to release our COVID-19 Surge Model was a fast one. While our clients would receive the model first, shortly afterward it would be made publicly available to all at no cost.

Predicting the impact of an evolving pandemic meshed with highly variable human behavior and local politics made our task nearly impossible. In the end, we did not produce a predictive model, but rather a scenario

CHICAGO, IL (V6.1)

The Sg2 model was able to accurately model the actual ADC peak magnitude and timing that Chicago experienced, as well as the ongoing trajectory of virus within the region.

ADC Surge Scenario Impact for COVID-19

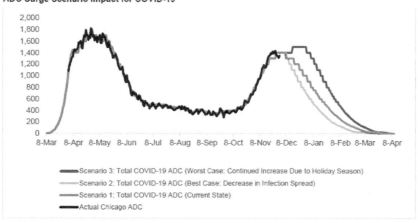

Source: City of Chicago. COVID-19 hospital capacity metrics. Chicago Data Portal. Accessed December 2020.

Starting R_0: 2.2 (See Appendix Table 2 for guidance regarding starting reproductive rates.)

• Accuracy of the model:
  – Peak timing and magnitude were predicted with accuracy.
  – Average of 5% variance between actual Chicago ADC and Sg2 projected total COVID-19 ADC

Figure 12.9 Hospital Average Daily Census (ADC) modeling in Chicago, Illinois.

DALLAS, TX (V6.1)

The Sg2 model accurately modeled both the initial ADC peak magnitude and timing that Dallas experienced and the resurgence that occurred with reopening the economy.

ADC Surge Scenario Impact for COVID-19

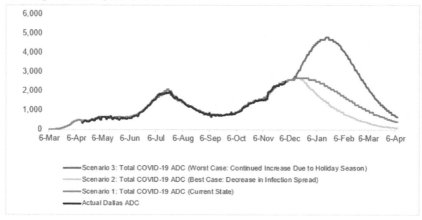

Note: Actual Dallas ADC from July 23, 2020, to July 28, 2020, may be incomplete due to transition in the reporting process.
Source: Texas Health and Human Services. COVID-19 hospitalizations by trauma service area. Accessed December 2020.

Starting R_0: 1.8

• Accuracy of the model:
  – Peak timing and magnitude were predicted with accuracy.
  – Average of 6% variance between actual Dallas ADC and Sg2 projected total COVID-19 ADC

Figure 12.10 Hospital Average Daily Census (ADC) modeling in Dallas, Texas.

planning tool based on international and national disease experience that also allowed for manipulability in critical variables, giving users more control in localizing the impact of change (Figure 12.9 and Figure 12.10).

The tool uses accessible data inputs, such as bed capacity and population demographics, and allows scenario modeling around true "unknowns" – the speed and magnitude of the infection in a given market, and the hospitalization rate and average length of stay (ALOS) under evolving practice patterns. Ultimately, its true utility was not in demonstrating novel analytic approaches but in distilling highly practical outputs for critical pandemic planning. The tool allowed health systems to compare projected demand over existing capacity based on occupancy rates, and to see week-over-week and day-over-day prospective patterns in ADC, plus how many days or weeks away from peak surge they were likely to be.

The statistician, George Box, is attributed with saying, "All models are wrong, but some are useful." Our hospitals and health systems needed the best possible information to inform decisions around bed demand,

MILWAUKEE, WI (V6.1)

The Sg2 model continues to accurately match and follow the COVID-19 hospitalization data reported by Milwaukee.

ADC Surge Scenario Impact for COVID-19

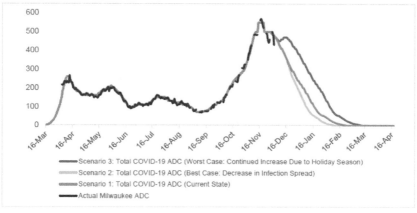

Source: County of Milwaukee. Milwaukee County COVID-19 Dashboard. Accessed December 2020.

Starting R_0: 1.9

- Accuracy of the model:
  - Peak timing and trajectory of virus spread were predicted with accuracy.
  - Average of 5% variance between actual Milwaukee ADC and Sg2 projected total COVID-19 ADC

Figure 12.11 Hospital Average Daily Census (ADC) modeling in Milwaukee, Wisconsin.

PPE, staffing, equipment and how to handle the rest of their business including elective procedures during a period of unprecedented uncertainty. While we strived for accuracy, we demanded, at the very least, the model be useful/reliable in its outputs to directly support critical decision making by hospitals. Frequent validation testing of our model was performed using publicly available or member hospital census data, in near real time, to ensure the model was meeting these objectives (Figure 12.11 and Figure 12.12).

While the validation of model projections against actual pandemic experience across all markets Sg2 followed closely provided gratification, true member impact provided the most important evidence of a job well done. Nowhere was this more apparent than in the close working relationship that Sg2 had with UTSA and their regional COVID-19 response planning hub, who leveraged Sg2's modeling and expertise extensively throughout the early pandemic, and even invited Sg2 to present at the UTSA Infectious Disease Symposium, held in August 2020. Direct member-created data

NEW YORK CITY, NY (V6.1)

The Sg2 calculator modeled the timing of the peak ADC in New York City as well as ongoing COVID-19 ADC trajectory with accuracy.

ADC Surge Scenario Impact for COVID-19

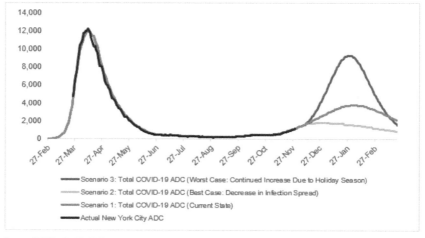

Scenario 3: Total COVID-19 ADC (Worst Case: Continued Increase Due to Holiday Season)
Scenario 2: Total COVID-19 ADC (Best Case: Decrease in Infection Spread)
Scenario 1: Total COVID-19 ADC (Current State)
Actual New York City ADC

Source: NYC Health. COVID-19: data; New York State. Pressroom: Official news from the Office of the Governor. All websites accessed December 2020.

Starting R_0: 2.6

• Accuracy of the model:
  – Peak timing and trajectory of the virus spread were predicted with accuracy.
  – Average of 5% variance between actual New York City ADC and Sg2 projected total COVID-19 ADC

Figure 12.12 Hospital Average Daily Census (ADC) modeling in New York, New York.

comparisons, and comments on the model, follow (Figure 12.13 and Figure 12.14):

> On behalf of The University of Texas Health San Antonio, our city and regional planning teams, I want to thank you again for all of your support and efforts over the past 5 months. This surge demand model, and the work your team has put into the development of it, has allowed us to accurately plan for our COVID-19 response and taking care of the citizens of this community. The precision to which this model has predicted hospitalizations, in a county of 2 million people, is extremely impressive.
>
> I want to personally thank you for the collaboration and time you've provided. It's been a great working relationship, your team is professional and extremely knowledgeable. We appreciate you helping make a difference in San Antonio (where Sg2 is now a household name!).
>
> August 2020

SAN ANTONIO, TX (V6.1)

The Sg2 model accurately fits the actual surge trajectory for San Antonio.

ADC Surge Scenario Impact for COVID-19

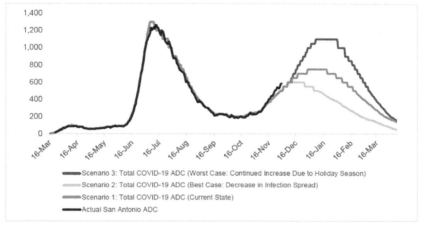

Note: From early November, the Sg2 model slightly underestimates the actual ADC data from San Antonio due to transfers to the local hospitals from outside the service area.
Source: City of San Antonio. COVID-19 trends. Accessed December 2020.

Starting R_0: 1.5

* Accuracy of the model:
    – Peak timing, magnitude and trajectory of COVID-19 census were predicted with accuracy.
    – Average of 6% variance between actual San Antonio ADC and Sg2 projected total COVID-19 ADC

Figure 12.13 Hospital Average Daily Census (ADC) modeling in San Antonio, Texas.

The success of our predictive modeling stemmed from our decision to beta test early and update modeling regularly based on new information, validation testing and user feedback. This directly enabled the model to evolve quickly and adopt new learnings from the scientific community and the unique US experience. In all, we created six versions of the model over the timespan of 10 months. The unprecedented crisis at hand fostered an environment of experimentation and rapid learning, lessons that could be replicated in less turbulent times.

The scale and pace of change introduced by the COVID-19 pandemic were unprecedented and had notable ramifications on the evolution of healthcare planning. The work of strategy leaders and planning teams was now routinely carried out in multiple time frames: connecting to and supporting operations in the here and now while also ensuring the prioritization and execution of longer-term opportunities to differentiate, transform and serve their communities. Along with this, new data analytics and predictive modeling solutions are required to meet these evolving needs. Our

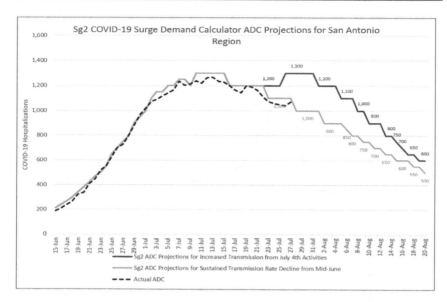

Figure 12.14 Surge demand modeling in San Antonio, Texas.

Source: Graph Provided by UTSA.

exploration into local scenario modeling and near-term forecasting for COVID-19 accelerated our learning curve in new areas of predictive modeling and has provided long-term, enduring approaches for future modeling.

Section 3

Topics

Chapter 13

Healthcare analytics

The effects of the pandemic on behavioral health

Kasey Knopp
University of Maryland School of Medicine
Baltimore, MD, USA

Naakesh (Nick) Dewan
GuideWell-Florida Blue
Jacksonville, FL, USA

CONTENTS

Introduction 195
Telehealth/telepsychiatry/tele-mental health and COVID-19 196
Mental health and COVID-19 197
Economic downturn and mental health 198
Loneliness and isolation and mental health 198
Mental health and substance abuse/substance use disorder 199
Issue to address 212
    One: Use of electronic medical records 212
    Two: Linking data systems 212
    Three: Big data and policy in the era of COVID-19 pandemic 213
    Four: Collecting socio-demographic data 213
Conclusion 214
References 214

INTRODUCTION

The COVID-19 pandemic has ushered in a new wave of analytics. Generally, data analytics are aimed at prediction – anticipating future trends and needs. The unpredictability of COVID-19 has resulted in excess pressure for researchers in health sciences to determine what data is readily available, reliable and appropriate for collection and analysis to identify, understand and predict trends in healthcare during and after COVID-19. To date, evidence points to a "second" pandemic nested within COVID-19: a mental health pandemic. Government organizations and researchers are reporting increasingly negative mental health outcomes with increases in depression and anxiety across age cohorts, resulting in greater need for mental health treatment. This demand, coupled with COVID-19 preventative precautions, led to policy and regulation flexibilities to allow for greater accessibility of services via telepsychiatry and tele-mental health. However, there are noted issues in the application of telepsychiatry as it relates to populations experiencing substance abuse disorder (SUD). Due to the rapidly changing nature of the COVID-19 pandemic, new and constantly changing data from a variety of sources, many of which are not publicly available, make it difficult to capture the full scope of impact of these aspects of healthcare provision through data.

This chapter will focus on the rapid and expansive implementation of telehealth, specifically, telepsychiatry/tele-mental health as it relates to the COVID-19 pandemic as a result of both COVID-19 precautions and increasingly poor mental health outcomes experienced across U.S. populations. Due to the varying levels (e.g. regional, state, national), type (e.g. electronic health records, insurance claims) and accessibility of data, the main goal of this chapter is to provide guidance on best practices of methods recording and analytics when using such varied data as the topic necessitates a fast turn-around.

A brief background of the expansion of telehealth, telepsychiatry/tele-mental health in response to the COVID-19 pandemic will be provided. Then, the chapter will lay out the most recent data on COVID-19's impact on the state of mental health and substance abuse in the U.S. and its intersectionality with emergency department (ED) utilization as a result of opioid overdoses. A systematized review of the literature will be presented with particular focus on the methodologies used with regard to the sample population, outcome measures, and strategies as well as themes. Finally, a detailed list of recommendations in approach to data and methodologies for future COVID-19 studies will be provided as a framework to guide researchers in conducting studies in such situations that require immediate analysis and results when data may not be readily available and is constantly in flux.

TELEHEALTH/TELEPSYCHIATRY/TELE-MENTAL HEALTH AND COVID-19

In March 2020, federal, state and private agencies enacted numerous policy and regulatory changes to expand the use of telehealth to address continuity of care and to practice precautions during the COVID-19 pandemic (Weigel, Ramaswamy, Sobel et al., 2020). Telepsychiatry is the application of telehealth within the specialty of psychiatry. Other associated terms are tele-mental health and tele-psychology, which refers to the administration of therapy or psychological treatment through technological means, such as video conferencing or telephone call (O'Brien & McNicholas, 2020). Prior to the pandemic, forms of telehealth (e.g. telepsychiatry) were limited to a small group of individuals living in designated rural settings, as long as the visit took place in a licensed medical facility (Showalter, 2020; Weigel et al., 2020). In addition, any telehealth visit could only occur with previously established providers, of which, a license to practice had to be valid in the state in which they were located at the time of services, as well as being licensed in the state in which the patient received care (Showalter, 2020; Weigel et al., 2020). Other important change affecting uptake up telehealth included cost sharing benefits, which allowed providers to reduce or waive all cost sharing for telehealth visits, as well as the inclusion of telephone calls as opposed to application or video-based platforms (Showalter, 2020). While there is no guarantee these emergency flexibilities to policies and regulations will outlast COVID-19, they made a clear and substantial impact on telepsychiatry utilization.

Pre COVID-19 research determined that services received via telepsychiatry were comparable to those received in-person as it relates to reliability and treatment outcomes (Hubley et al., 2016). However, utilization of telehealth to provide care services for mental health and/or substance use disorders (SUD) was uncommon, accounting for roughly 1% of visits between 2010–2017 (Huskamp et al., 2018; Patel et al., 2020). During COVID-19, the odds of completing a telepsychiatry visit were three times higher than completing an in-person visit and was associated with higher rate of visit completion. By comparison, by October 2020, 41% of mental health/SUD visits occurred virtually (Mehrotra et al., 2021). An ebb and flow of telehealth visits across all healthcare domains followed patterns of sudden spikes and/or decline from March 2020–October 2020; no matter, mental health services received via telehealth remained steady across this time period compared to other specialties (Mehrotra et al., 2021).

MENTAL HEALTH AND COVID-19

Beyond (physical) morbidity and mortality rates, the COVID-19 pandemic infiltrated nearly every aspect of peoples' lives. Rapid and dramatic changes in employment, personal relationships, finances, schooling and housing have all negatively affected mental health outcomes. Precautions at federal, state and regional levels were implemented by public and private entities in an attempt to "stop the spread". Unfortunately, these precautions resulted in a number of policies that encouraged and/or enforced social distancing and, in many instances, social isolation. Early on, the state of people's mental well-being amidst such changes was the central concern of clinicians and care providers. In the onslaught of stress, loneliness, fear and depression has caused a second health crisis amidst the pandemic: a behavioral health crisis.

Reports from the Center for Disease Control (CDC) National Health Interview Survey (NHIS) found that one in ten adults experienced symptoms of anxiety or depression between January-June 2019 (Falk et al., 2021) compared to four in ten adults surveyed in January 2021 in the CDC's Household Pulse Survey (CDC, 2021); this statistic is similar to that at the beginning of the pandemic. A significant amount of research prior to the pandemic identifies a number of pandemic-related experiences as being correlated with poor mental health outcomes.

ECONOMIC DOWNTURN AND MENTAL HEALTH

Like other countries, the U.S. experienced a sudden economic downturn at the onset of COVID-19 with unemployment rates more than tripling between February and May 2020: from 6.2 million to 20.5 million respectively- or-from 3.8% to 13% (Kochnar, 2020). Increased unemployment and nationwide stay at home orders lead to an unexpected economic recession, which has been correlated to having poor mental health outcomes such as increased depression, anxiety, substance abuse, and suicide rates (Frasquilho, Matos, Salonna et al., 2016). While the CDC's recent data from the Household Pulse Survey shows that unemployment rates are dropping, easing strain on households, these rates remain low as many are struggling to catch up with rent while experiencing difficulties obtaining enough food (Center on Budget and Policy Priorities [CBPP], 2021). Furthermore, as is the nature of any health crisis, nobody can estimate when it will end.

LONELINESS AND ISOLATION AND MENTAL HEALTH

Before COVID-19, research found that loneliness and social isolation were prevalent across age groups in the U.S. (Leigh-Hunt, Bagguley, Bash et al., 2017). This attributed to poor mental health outcomes, such as increased symptoms of depression and anxiety (Lee et al., 2020), increased suicide risk (Calati et al., 2019) and a growth in high risk behaviors, such as substance abuse (Hosseinbor, Ardekani, Bakhschani et al., 2014). Roughly 28% of American live alone (U.S. Bureau of Census, 2019), and even among those who do not, feelings of loneliness and social isolation occurred across age groups (Clair, Gordon, Kroon et al., 2021). A study by Clair et al. (2021) indicates that these feelings are exacerbated by lack of socialization outside of the household across households of all sizes, but are especially prevalent in younger adults in their 20s (Clair et al., 2021).

A survey of psychologists conducted in the first six months of the pandemic by the American Psychological Association (APA) reported that psychologists found their patients experienced a 74% and 60% increase in patients with anxiety and depression disorders compared to before the pandemic (American Psychological Association [APA], 2020).

MENTAL HEALTH AND SUBSTANCE ABUSE/SUBSTANCE USE DISORDER

Previous research has reported strong correlations with SUD and presence of substance use among individuals with anxiety symptoms or disorders (Conway, Compton, Stinson et al., 2006; Brady, Haynes, Hartwell et al., 2013; Magidson, Liu, Lejuez et al., 2012; Lai et al., 2015). Individuals with some form of SUD are more than twice as likely to have anxiety disorder or symptoms (Lai et al., 2015). Similarly strong associations are found among individuals with depression, of whom, are 1.3 to 2.6 times more likely to experience SUD (CDC, 2010). A web-based survey distributed by the CDC during June 24–30, 2020 found that 40% of adults were experiencing adverse mental or behavioral health conditions, including symptoms of anxiety or depressive disorder (30.9%) and those with trauma-stress-related disorder (TSRD) (26.3%) and those who started or increased substance use to cope with stress related to COVID-19 (13.3%) (Czeisler et al., 2020). A Kaiser Family Foundation (KFF) tracking poll from July 2020 also found that increases in substance abuse or alcohol consumption had increased by 12% due to worry and/or stress related to coronavirus (Panchal et al., 2021). Substance abuse rates were especially high among young adults (18–24), who were more 25% more likely to report substance abuse (Panchal et al., 2021).

Given the relationships between the COVID-19 pandemic, its negative impact on mental health, and the need for and expansion of telehealth resulting from these moving pieces, it is important to review the evidence-based information available on these topics. The main aim of the following section is to provide a systematized review of the available literature which looks at a number of domains: telehealth/telepsychiatry and COVID-19; perceptions of telehealth/telepsychiatry changes during COVID-19; changes in mental health during COVID-19; and the impact of COVID-19 on substance abuse and ED utilization. The primary goal in presenting this systematized review is to provide examples of studies using Big Data to find trends in the ways COVID-19 impacts the aforementioned domains. Secondary is to highlight the aligned trends found across the literature despite utilizing different forms of data. The final goal is to address the intricacies and obstacles in working with Big Data during a time of constant, rapid changes while providing insight on how to address them in future research.

Author	Year	Duration	Type of Study	Sample Size	Setting
Avalone et al.	2021	Pre-COVID 19: October 8-November 8, 2019 COVID-19: Aril 8-May 8,2020	Quantitative	COVID-19 Period: N = 37,809 Pre COVID-19 period: N = 40318	U.S. (NYC Health + Hospitals)
Bojdani et al.	2020	March 2020– May 2020	Scoping Review/ Quantitative (Survey)/ Qualitative (informal discussions)	13 samples	U.S.
Ettman et al.	2020	March 31– April 13, 2020 Pre- COVID-19 2017–2018	Quantitative (Survey/ Longitudinal Survey)	April 15–20,2020 N=1,441 "pre" COVID 2017–2018 N=5,065	U.S.

Outcome Measures	Study Characteristics	Results
Visit completion rates (telepsychiatry vs. in-person) (primary) Visit cancelations/no show (secondary)	Use of EMR[1] data The majority of participants in both groups were female Mean age for pre and during COVID-19 were 49.5 ± 16.0 and 49.28 ± 15.9 respectively. Across all race categories except those who identify as White (-29.8%), the distribution of (all) visits increased across races, the highest increase experienced among "Others" (+19%) In both time frames, the majority of participants were enrolled in Medicaid or Medicare.	During the pandemic, the odds of completing a telepsychiatry visit were >6 times the odds of completing a face-to-face visit During the pre-COVID-19 period, the odds of completing a telepsychiatry visit were 3 times the odds of completing a face-to-face visit.
Articles including terms "COVID-19" and "psychiatric care"; resulted in 37 articles, only 13 were relevant Must be literature that focuses on first-hand experiences of the impact of COVID-19 on the psychiatric care provided to patients Survey of psychiatric physicians, themes found from informal discussions with fellow psychiatric physicians Provision of "how to" process what is occurring during the COVID-19 pandemic	Scoping review of literature on "COVID-19" and "psychiatric care" in the U.S. No data on participant characteristics for survey or informal interviews provided.	Main themes of concerns of psychiatric physicians: (1) personal prevention (i.e. PPE availability/guidance); (2) Personal treatment (if infected- what treatment options are available?; (3) Effects on others (i.e. family, roommates, family planning); (4) Economic stress (i.e. disruption in income, job loss, quitting to avoid potential infection); (5) ethical considerations for self (i.e. maintaining Hippocratic oath); (6) Ethical considerations towards others (i.e. informed consent, telepsychiatry); (7) training considerations (i.e. learning opportunities, graduation competencies)
Depression symptoms defined using the Patient Health Questionnaire Categories of depression symptoms: non (0–4), mild (5–9), moderate (10–14), moderately severed (15–19) and severe (≥20); 13 stressors related to traumatic events were utilized	COVID-19 period participants derived from the Life Stressors Impact on Mental Health and Well-being study (AmeriSpeak panel). Pre-COVID-19 estimates were derived from the National Health and Nutrition Examination Survey (NHANES) conducted from 2017–2018. In both the pre and during COVID-19 periods, Women were most likely to experience symptoms of depression. Across both time periods individuals with less education, with a low household income were more likely to experience depressive symptoms.	In the U.S., prevalence of depression symptoms was over 3 times higher during the COVID-19 pandemic than before (2017–2018). Those individuals with fewer economic resources and greater exposure to stressors, such as job loss, reported higher burden of depression symptoms. Prevalence of depression symptoms was higher in every category during COVID-19 than before COVID-19.

(Continued)

Author	Year	Duration	Type of Study	Sample Size	Setting
Fischer et al.	2021	May 1–6, 2020	Quantitative (Longitudinal Survey)	N=2,052	U.S. (American Life Panel)
Gentry et al.	2021	March 2020– June 2020	Quantitative (Survey)	N=112	U.S.
Guinart et al.	2020	April 2020– June 2020	Quantitative (Survey)	N=3,070	U.S. (CT, FL, ME, MI, NH, NY, OR, RI, SC, TX, UT)

Outcome Measures	Study Characteristics	Results
Receipt of treatment for chronic physical or behavioral health condition when the pandemic began OR consideration of seeking care for a new or recurring condition during the pandemic For each condition, telehealth (video of phone) due to pandemic If treating physician was their own doctor, or, a different doctor	The majority of the sample was female (51.9%) The sample was nearly equally divided across age groups (20-39, 40-59, 60+) The majority were White (63.9%) Over 90% were insured Nearly half (48%) used telehealth, mostly for behavioral health conditions.	The majority of participants were continuing to seek treatment with their own physicians whether prior or new condition. The largest amount of reports of seeing another doctor occurred with a new condition. Between mid-March and early May, over 40% of participants with a physical health condition utilized telehealth. Between mid March and early May, over 50% of participants with behavior health conditions utilized telehealth.
Likert scale survey of clinicians (psychiatrists, psychologists, trainees, advanced practice providers and licensed mental health counselors) with implementation experience of video telehealth visits between March-June2020. Following measures of attitudes of appropriateness/suitability, and feasibility of telehealth as a way to deliver mental health services during COVID-19:Rate telehealth implementation of measures:Acceptability of Intervention (AIM), Feasibility of Intervention (FIM) and Intervention Appropriateness Measure (IAM) Relay respondents' view of patients' attitudes towards tele-mental-health (TMH) Respondent views of technology, IT support, and training pertaining to TMH Respondents' attitudes about future use of telehealth	Most respondents were faculty psychiatrists (33%), between the age of 30-30[sic][2] (33.3%), female (59.8%) and in practice 0–5 years (30.4%) During the pre-COVID-19 timeframe, most practitioners had 0-5 telehealth visits (82.6%) compared to 20+ telehealth visits (55.9%) after COVID-19	Video telehealth was rated highly in terms of acceptability, appropriateness and feasibility (83-97%) Participants felt their patients were highly satisfied with video visits (79.5%), and that they seemed as comfortable in video visits as they did in-person among established and new patients. More than half (59%) agreed that video was more efficient than in-person visits. Overall quality of technical support and training for telehealth was high. Nearly half (49.1%) of participants felt they would prefer to continue the use of video telehealth for a significant part of their practice once COVID-19 is over; ideally, the majority (42%) would refer their practice to be 50% telehealth and 50% in-person.
11 question survey delivered electronically to patients receiving telepsychiatry care at 18 participating centers across 11 U.S. states Questions were answered via Likert scale and focused on: (1) age, (2) length of service, (3) experience with telepsychiatry and (4) satisfaction with telepsychiatry	Most participants were 45-55-64 (23.7%) and were receiving psychiatric care at their institution between 1-5 years (44.6%) Telephone was used for most telepsychiatry appointments (63.7%) followed by video (23.4%) and a combination of telephone and video (12.9%). The majority of respondents preferred telephone over video (64.1% and 35.9% respectively).	Most patients' experiences utilizing telepsychiatry was "excellent" or "good" (82.2%). Patients agreed or strongly agreed that telepsychiatry sessions (video or phone) were as helpful as in-person treatment. The most frequently identified advantages of telepsychiatry were lack of commute (46.1%), flexibility in scheduling (45.5%). Disadvantages commonly identified were missing the clinic/hospital (30.7%) and feeling less connected to their service provider (24.6%). Once the pandemic is over, the majority (64.2%) would consider using remote, telepsychiatry, for future treatment sessions.

(Continued)

Author	Year	Duration	Type of Study	Sample Size	Setting
Hall et al.	2021	Pre-COVID-19 period: October 20, 2019–March7, 2020 COVID-19 period: March 8, 2020-July 25, 2020	Quantitative	Pre-period: N=96,824 COVID-19 period:N=80,581	U.S. (7 Chicago EDs)
Herring et al.	2021	Pre-COVID-19 period: May 2019–March 2020 COVID-19 period: April 2020	Quantitative	Pre-COVID-19: ≈ 8,685 COVID-19 period: ≈ 675	U.S. (CA)

Outcome Measures	Study Characteristics	Results
Opioid and alcohol related ED visits identified using Agency for Healthcare Research Quality Clinical Classifications Software Refined (AHRQ-CCSR) Evaluate weekly trends of ED visits for opioid and alcohol related disorders over the 40-week study period	The pre-COVID-19 and COVID-19 periods experienced similar mean weekly visits at 4,841 and 4,029 respectively. The median age in the pre-pandemic period was 42, while it was 46 in the pandemic period. The majority of visits were experienced by females-over 50% in each period. During both periods, the majority of ED visits related to opioid or alcohol occurred among White individuals (69.1% and 68.6% respectively).Most visits were ranked "Level 3" (urgent) in the Emergency Severity Index in both pre and pandemic periods.	In aggregate, there were more weekly alcohol-related visits than opioid related visits per 1,000 ED visits. There was an immediate and significant negative effect on alcohol related ED visits when the pandemic starts, followed by an immediate increase beginning in June, 2020. The weekly rates of ED visits for opioid-related diagnoses were not significantly altered once the pandemic period began.
Identify the change in activity of hospital and emergency department (ED)[3] initiated buprenorphine for opioid use disorder (OUD_ during California's COVID-19 state of emergency. Looking at California Bridge Program (CA Bridge) hospitals cross the state: 70 hospitals in all, some in rural areas and other in urban areas. Total number of patients identified with OUD Number of patients who accepted a referral Number of patients who received a buprenorphine prescription Number of patients who were administered buprenorphine within the hospital Number of patients who attended at least one follow-up visits (outside institution) for addiction treatment within 30 days	In total, 52 CA Bridge hospitals report medications for opioid use disorder (MOUD) related monthly activity in pre-COVID-19 and COVID-19 period data. 25% are from a hospital with a teaching program and 23% are located in rural settings.	In the pre-period, there was a linear increase in the number of patients who met each of the five main CA Bridge outcomes: 66 patients with identified OUD, 41 patients who accepted a referral, 34 patients were prescribed buprenorphine and 29 patients attended a follow-up visit for addiction treatment within 30-days. Compared to pre-pandemic time period, the overall observed number of patients and patients per outcome in April 2020 was lower than expected: a 37% decrease in patients identified with OUD, 48% decrease in those prescribed buprenorphine, 53% decrease in patients who were administered buprenorphine and a 33% decrease in the number of patients who attended at least one follow up visit for addiction treatment. Overall, the proportion of individuals administered buprenorphine in the hospital in April was the lowest observed over the entire 12-month period

(Continued)

Author	Year	Duration	Type of Study	Sample Size	Setting
Holland et al.	2021	December 30, 2018– October 10, 2020	Quantitative	N=187,508,065	U.S. (48 states + D.C) (National Syndromatic Surveillance Program)
Koonin et al.	2020	Pre COVID-19 period: January– March 2019 COVID-19 period: January– March 2020	Quantitative	Pre COVID-19 period: N=1,084,000 COVID-19 period: N=1,629,000	U.S.
Pierce & Stevermer	2020	Pre-COVID-19 periods: March 17– April 16, 2019 COVID-19 period: March 17-April 16, 2020	Quantitative	Pre-COVID-19 period: N=10,953 COVID-19 period: N=7,742	U.S. (University of Missouri Health System, MU Health)

Outcome Measures	Study Characteristics	Results
Examine the changes in U.S.> emergency department (ED) visits for Mental health conditions (MHC), Suicide Attempts (SA), all drug overdoses (OD), Intimate partner violence (IPV), opioid ODs, suspected child abuse and neglect (SCAN)	Women accounted for 53.6% of ED visits (results stratified by sex). The greatest mean number of ED visits occurred in individuals ≥10 years of age and those ≥18 years of age.	Overall total ED visit volume decreased after COVID-19 "stop the spread" measures were implemented in the U.S. beginning on March 16, 2020. Weekly ED visit counts for all outcome measures decreased between March 8 and 28, 2020. Overall ED visit rates increased during the week of March 22–28, 2020. Comparing the period of March 15-Octoer 10, 2020 to the same time period in 2019, there were increases in outcomes during the COVID-19 period: SAs, ODs and opioid ODs were significantly higher. Comparatively, there were significantly lower rates of IPV Ed visits and SCAN ED visits.
Trends of frequency of use of telehealth services during the early months of the pandemic as compared with encounters during the same weeks in 2019 Whether the reason for visit was for COVID-19 related encounters as defined by: COVID-19 like symptoms, Coronavirus related ICD-10 code items, or Coronavirus-related text string.	The majority of telehealth encounters in both time periods happened among adults aged 18-49 (66% in 2019 and 69% in 2020). Female patients were the highest utilizers of telehealth in both time periods, accounting for 63% in each.	Overall, there were 50% more encounters during the pandemic period than the pre-pandemic period. During week 13 in 2020, telehealth visits increased by 154% compared to the same time period in 2019. Overall, number of ED visits in the last 3 weeks of March 2020 decreased exponentially compared to the same time period in 2019 (no data provided). Between January-March 2020, more than 90% of telehealth patients sought care for conditions other than COVID-19, but the COVID-19 related encounters more than tripled in the last three weeks of March.
Comparing those family medicine encounters during the initial month of COVID-19 to the same time period in 2019. Outcomes to compare were within groups: COVID-19 period telehealth vs. face-to face visits; demographics of those using full audio–video vs audio-only. Demographics collected were: rurality, payer status, age, race, ethnicity, and sex. Demographic of patients were compared to those in the non-pandemic year.	Compared to pre-pandemic, the distribution of encounters of any type increased among women (+2.2%), individuals identifying as Black (+1.1%) and Hispanic (0.5%) The distribution of telehealth visits increased with age. Those with Medicare, Medicaid or self-pay were most likely to use telehealth. Having a full audio–video encounter was least likely among adults 45+, Blacks, those living in rural areas. and patients with Medicare and Medicaid	During the first 30 days of the pandemic, 51% of encounters occurred face-to-face encounters and 41% vi telehealth. Among telehealth encounters, most (37.9%) were full audio–video encounters and 11.2% were audio-only. Overall, fewer encounters occurred in the 2020 study period compared to the 2019 period (-29.3%).

(*Continued*)

Author	Year	Duration	Type of Study	Sample Size	Setting
Rodda, West & LeSaint	2020	January 1–April 18, 2020	Quantitative	N=459	U.S. (San Francisco)
Shreffler et al.	2021	Period 1: March 6, 2019-June 25, 2019 Period 2: COVID-19 March 6-June 26, 2020 Period 3: 16 weeks prior to COVID-29: November 15, 2019-March 5, 2020	Quantitative	Period 1: N=259 Period 2: N=340 Period 3: N=274	U.S. (KY-University of Louisville Level 1 Trauma Center)

Outcome Measures	Study Characteristics	Results
Prevalence and characteristics of individuals in San Francisco whose use of opioids resulted in an emergency department (ED) visit AND accidental death during the time of social distancing in the COVID-19 pandemic. Deaths were all accidental and were measured as: fentanyl, norfentanyl, 6-monoacetylmorphine (heroin), morphine, and/or codeine.	Men accounted for the majority of ED presentations and deaths (81% and 82% respectively). The majority of ED presentations occurred in the 25-34 age group, while the highest mortality rate occurred in the 35-44 age group. The median age for accidental death was 45.	During the study, 365 ED patients were seen with the final diagnosis of "overdose"; only 189 patients were seen for opioid-related overdose. Most ODs were caused by non-specified opioids (81%) followed by fentanyl (16%) and heroin (1%). Once the shelter in place was enacted (April 18, 2020), ED saw 2.5 patients per day with opioid overdose compared to 1.4 prior to that period. Within the first 109 days of 2020 (prior to shelter in place), 121 opioid-related accidental overdoses were identified by the Chief Medical Examiner; 75% were fentanyl, 11% heroin, and 11% fentanyl and heroin.
Outcome measures include emergency department (ED) diagnoses and county overdose deaths for the same time period	The median age across all three time frames for ED overdose was 35. Among those who experienced an OD overdose, men were the majority across all time frames: 61.8%, 67.9% and 68.5% Across all time periods, most ED overdose diagnoses occurred among individuals identified as White: 77.2%, 72.6% and 70.3% respectively. Similar patterns were found among county OD deaths, with the exception of median age by time period, which were 40.5, 41, and 54 respectively. Among both ED overdose diagnoses and county overdose deaths, daily and weekly counts increased steadily across all time periods.	ED volume decreased between Period 3 and Period 2, but overdose diagnoses increased. A pattern of increased deaths occurred after the state of California's declaration of emergency.

(Continued)

Author	Year	Duration	Type of Study	Sample Size	Setting
Slavova et al.	2020	Pre-COVID-19 period: January 14–March 5, 2020 COVID-19 period: March 6-April26, 2020	Quantitative	Pre-COVID-19 period: N=1,133 COVID-19 period: N=1,323	U.S. (KY-Kentucky State Ambulance Reporting System)
Soares et al.	2021	January 1, 2018–December 31, 2020 broken into 3 periods; Period 1: 2018 Period 2: 2019 Period 3: 2020	Quantitative	Period 1: N=1,215,250 Period 2: N=1,283,303 Period 3: N=1,074,936	U.S. (25 EDs in AL, CO, CT, NC, MA, RI)
Yu, Casalino & Pincus	2021	January–June 2020 broken down by month	Quantitative	January: N=115,765 February: N=223,200 March: N=2,227,081 April: N=2,973,141 May: N=2,686,330 June: N= 1,383,537	U.S. (FAIR Health)

[1] Electronic Medical Records=EMR.
[2] Frye et al. (2021) table stated 30-30, but likely meant 30–39.
[3] Methods stated "primarily from EDs but can include inpatient units" (pp. 1).

Outcome Measures	Study Characteristics	Results
Evaluation of change in daily number of Kentucky emergency medical service (EMS) runs for opioid overdose calls. Opioid Overdose Runs (OOR) were described algorithm (Lasher et al., 2019) Outcome measures included types of EMS runs as identified by: (1) EMS opioid OD runs with transportation to ED, (2) EMS opioid OD runs with refused transportation, (3) EMS runs for suspected opioid OD with death at scene, (4) All other EMS runs (excluding opioid OD) with transportation to ED, (5) all other EMS runs (excluding opioid OD) with refused transportation to ED.	No participant-specific data was collected (e.g. sociodemographic, medical history, prior use of EMS, etc.)	An increase of EMS OOR during the COVID-19 period compared to the previous year; increased 17%. There was a 71% increase in OOR-refusal. Overall, a 50% increase in suspected OOD with death at the scene. A decline of 22% occurred in the total number of EMS transport runs excluding OOR-Transport and <1% change in EMS refusal runs excluding OOR refusal. A daily drop in EMS transport runs excluding OOR-transport was noted after the COVID-19 declaration, from 1074 to 836. However, EMS OOR transport increased post-COVID-19 declaration. After March 18, 2020, EMS OOR-transport sustained an average rate of increase of one opioid OD per week.
Primary outcome measure was weekly counts of ED visits with 1 or more ICD-10 diagnoses code associated with an opioid OD (T40.0* to T40.4* and T40.6*)	The only sociodemographic information collected on patients was age (18+) any information collected was hospital system based (e.g.: academic hospital, county, urbanicity, state EMS refusal law) Across all periods, the majority of hospital systems were non-academic systems in urban/suburban areas in which the state did not have an EMS refusal law. OD rates increased in both urban and suburban areas (29%) and rural areas (20.9%).	Opioid OD ED visits increased substantially in 66% of healthcare systems in 2020 compared to 2018 and 2019: in all, sites experienced a 10.6% increase in OD visits compared with the average of 2018 and 2019 despite a decrease of 14% in all-cause ED visits. OD visit rates per 100 all-cause ED visits increased by 0.32 (28.5%) from 0.25 OD visit per 100 all-cause adult EE visits in 2018 and 2019.
Using FAIR Health data (commercial insurance), calculated telehealth use rates as a percentage of all mental health services by condition category utilizing in-patient and outpatient claims. As a comparison for telehealth utilization, data will be collected on individuals who have used telehealth for acute respiratory disease and infection care services during this time period.	Participant characteristics were broken down in age, gender, and location (rural, urban). Across all time periods, women were the highest utilizers. Over all time periods, telehealth utilization rates among those ≥65 to 70.1% for those ages 25-34. From April to June 2020, differences in telehealth rates between rural and urban areas from by 12.1%; decreasing utilization among rural patients.	After shelter in place orders relaxed, telehealth visits continued to account for roughly two-thirds of mental health services. Comparatively, telehealth rates for acute respiratory disease and infection care services dropped by 16.2% from April to June 2020

ISSUE TO ADDRESS

Discussions about the application of Big Data to healthcare have been happening for decades as technology has improved and infiltrated most healthcare systems. Applications of such data are being used across a variety of research and quality improvement (QI) domains, such as: improved staffing, electronic medical records (EMR), improving patient care/treatment (predictive analytics), and reducing healthcare costs. Despite the widespread collection of data, there are a number of obstacles which make it difficult to use in healthcare research, as is identified in the studies above. Below are four key recommendations to consider when applying Big Data to studies focused on COVID-19 and telehealth/telepsychiatry/tele-mental health.

One: Use of electronic medical records

These systems were originally created specifically for clinical settings for billing/claims purposes settings (DeAlmeida, Paone & Kellum, 2014). In addition, EMR systems do not have interoperability across all settings of care, leading to a lack of ability to follow patients in data sets for needed lengths of time, and/or missing important data points, such as healthcare utilization (Reisman, 2017). Comparatively, the incorporation of data from a Practice Management Software (PMS) allows for more rich data points: tracking patient schedules, medical billing and claims management and socio-demographic information. Compared to EMR, using this software has potential to view and understand how these various aspects impact patient care and outcomes, as well as potential barriers to seeking care- especially when utilizing telehealth models.

Two: Linking data systems

While transactional databases are useful in managing healthcare in terms of time-sensitive processing of financial and clinical function, it is difficult to use in large scale analytics. As it is often difficult to link variables from a variety of data sets due to the lack of one-to-one relationship between variables, it is key to look at other, freely available, widely representative data. The majority of the studies identified utilized some form of EMR (Avalone et al., 2021; Hall et al., 2021; Herring et al., 2021, etc.), two utilized at least one national survey (Ettman et al., 2020; Fischer et al., 2021). While each have their share of shortcomings (e.g. missing data points and data errors in EMR, attrition of participants in surveys), linking the two has the potential to impact the quantity and quality of empirical research. Survey data is widely available compared to EMR, which often requires a large pay out, data use agreements, etc. Linking these two sets of data can result in complimentary analyses and, in times such as COVID-19 when data is constantly changing, the use of survey data can help evaluate whether outcomes in a new area of research follow the themes of related longitudinal data points. For example, the CDC initiated the Household Pulse Survey on April 23, 2020, with new phases/waves being released every 90 days in order to capture the constantly changing social and economic impacts COVID-19 is having on households across the country (CDC, 2021). This provides for an up-to-date comparison of themes in exploratory research using other data points, such as EMR.

Three: Big data and policy in the era of COVID-19 pandemic

The data points which are available now, may not be available in a month or a year. The continuously changing policies and regulations affecting accessibility of mental health services do not ensure that the same groups can be followed, nor, the same data points collected. Of the studies mentioned above, only one (Koonin et al., 2020) was acknowledged when policies affecting accessibility to telehealth were implemented (Koonin et al., 2020, pp. 1596). As previously addressed, these policies, specifically the CMS telehealth waivers, provided more access to telehealth/telepsychiatry than was previously available. At the very least, this should be acknowledged, especially if a pre-post analysis is conducted. At best, separate analyses should be conducted within the study to examine the impact of the policy. This will result in a stronger study, and, help provide a case to policymakers when it comes time to decide to make these policy changes permanent.

Four: Collecting socio-demographic data

As mentioned in recommendation one, a shortcoming of EMR is the lack of availability of rich socio-demographic data. This point also ties in with recommendation three: consider policy changes. Avalone et al. (2021) and Pierce & Stevermer (2020) noted that the majority of uptake of telepsychiatry and/or tele-mental health visits occurred in the Medicare and Medicaid populations; a population previously having limited to no access per CMS coverage guidelines. This was a result of new telehealth waivers/expansions that went into effect March 6, 2020. In addition, Pierce & Stevermer (2020) note that the EMR data indicates an increase in telehealth visits among minorities and individuals in rural areas; groups in which recent reports have found continued and exacerbated disparities in care during COVID-19 (Velasquez & Mehrotra, 2020; Weber et al., 2020). Such data would also help to verify clinicians' first-hand experiences in coverage gaps for at-risk groups. This is especially important as these policy and regulatory expansions are temporary. This may be related to a second set of temporary policies implemented by the Federal Communications Commission (FCC) to address accessibility and infrastructure issues affecting these populations (FCC, 2020; FCC 2021).

CONCLUSION

Clinicians, researchers and policymakers alike should prioritize the importance of data analytics in the midst of a pandemic. The COVID-19 pandemic has created an elevated interest in mental health and telehealth use. COVID-19-related traumatic stress, even for those who were not hospitalized or those with mild clinical symptoms, is expected to have long-lasting impacts across all age cohorts for years to come. This necessitates the prioritization of neuropsychotic registries which will provide long-term follow up and monitoring of neuropsychiatric sequela of individuals who experienced moderate to severe COVID-19 infections. As the pandemic continues, it is equally important to address the chronic, unresolved, grief and bereavement which will further strain the workforce treating these individuals. As the state of mental health declines and telehealth utilization continues to rise, these topics require constant vigilance for data analytics. COVID-19 highlighted the chronic health inequities and necessity to prioritize monitoring those inequities in the years ahead. Addressing these issues in an expedient manner has resulted in rapid alterations to policies and regulations in order to provide greater accessibility and affordability of care related to the poor mental health outcomes created by the pandemic. It is of the utmost importance to understand the intersection of COVID-19, mental health outcomes and telehealth during a time of such immediate change, especially in the emerging value-based environment for behavioral health.

REFERENCES

American Psychological Association (APA). (2020, November). *Patients with depression and anxiety sure as psychologists respond to the coronavirus pandemic*. https://www.apa.org/news/press/releases/2020/11/telehealth-survey-summary.pdf

Avalone, L., Barron, C., King, C. et al. (2021). Rapid telepsychiatry implementation during COVID-19: Increased attendance at the largest health system in the United States. *Psychiatric Services*, 72 (6): 708–711. doi:10.1176/appi.ps.202000574

Bojdani, E., Rajagopalan, A., Chen, A. et al. (2020). COVID-19 pandemic: Impact on psychiatric care in the United States. *Psychiatry Research*, 289. doi.10.1016/j.psychres.2020.113069

Brady, K.T., Haynes, L.F., Hartwell, K.J. et al. (2013). Substance use disorders and anxiety: A treatment challenge for social workers. *Social Work in Public Health*, 28(3–4): 407–423. doi:10.1080/19371918.2013.774675.

Calati, R., Ferrari, C., Brittner, M., Oasi, O. (2019). Suicidal thoughts and behaviors and social isolation: A narrative review of the literature. *Journal of Affective Disorders*, 245: 653–667. doi:10.1016/j.jad.2018.11.022

Center on Budget and Policy Priorities (CBPP). (2021, August 9). *Tracking the COVID-19 recession's effects on food, housing and employment hardships*. https://www.cbpp.org/sites/default/files/8-13-20pov.pdf

Centers for Disease Control and Prevention (CDC). (2010). Current depression among adults—United States, 2006 and 2008. *Morbidity and Mortality Weekly Report*, 59: 1229–1235.

Centers for Disease Control and Prevention (CDC). (2021). *Household Pulse Survey*. https://www.census.gov/programs-surveys/household-pulse-survey/data.html

Clair, R., Gordon, M., Kroon, M. et al. (2021). The effects of social isolation on well-being and life satisfaction during pandemic. *Humanities and Social Sciences Communications*, 8(28). doi:10.1057/s41599-021-00710-3

Conway, K.P., Compton, W., Stinson, F.S. et al. (2006). Lifetime comorbidity of DSM-IV mood and anxiety disorders and specific drug use disorders: Results from the National epidemiologic survey on alcohol and related conditions. *Journal of Clinical Psychiatry*, 67(2):247–257. doi:10.4088/jcp.v67n0211

Czeisler, M.É., Lane, R.I., Petrosky, E., Wiley, J.F., Christensen, A., Njai, R., Weaver, M.D., Robbins, R., Facer-Childs, E.R., Barger, L.K., Czeisler, C.A., Howard, M.E., Rajaratnam, S. (2020). Mental health, substance use, and suicidal ideation during the COVID-19 pandemic – United States, June 24–30, 2020. *MMWR. Morbidity and Mortality Weekly Report*, 69(32): 1049–1057. doi:10.15585/mmwr.mm6932a1

DeAlmeida, D., Paone, S., Kellum, J. (2014). Experiences with linking data systems for analyzing large data. In K. Marconi & H. Lehman (Eds.), *Big Data and Health Analytics*. (pp. 45–56). CRC Press

Ettman, C., Abdalla, S., Cohen, G. et al. (2020). Prevalence of depression symptoms in U.S. adults before and during the COVID-19 pandemic. *JAMA Network Open*, 3(9). doi:10.1001/jamanetworkopen.2020.19686

Falk, G., Romero, D., Carter, J. et al. (2021, June 15). Unemployment rates during the COVID-19 pandemic. *Centers for Disease Control and Prevention (CDC)*. https://fas.org/sgp/crs/misc/R46554.pdf

Federal Communications Commission (FCC). (2020). Lifeline Support for Affordable Communications. FCC.gov. Available from: https://www.fcc.gov/sites/default/files/lifeline_support_for_affordable_communications.pdf

Federal Communications Commission (FCC). (2021). Emergency Broadband Benefit. FCC.gov. Available from: https://www.fcc.gov/broadbandbenefit

Fischer, S., Uscher-Pines, L., Roth, E. et al. (2021). The transition to telehealth during the first months of the COVID-19 pandemic: Evidence from a national sample of patients. *Journal of General Internal Medicine*, 36(3):849–851. doi:10.1007/s11606-020-06358-0

Frasquilho, D., Matos, M., Salonna, F. et al. (2016). Mental health outcomes in times of economic recession: A systematic literature review. *BMC Public Health*, 16 (115). doi.10.118/s12889-016-2720-y

Gentry, M., McKean, A., Breitinger, M. et al. (2021). Clinician satisfaction with rapid adoption and implementation of telehealth services during the COVID-19 pandemic. *Telemedicine Journal and E-Health*. doi:10.1089/tmj.2020.0575

Green, K.M., Zebrak, K.A., Fothergill, K.E. et al. (2012). Childhood and adolescent risk factors for comorbid depression and substance use disorders in adulthood. *Addictive Behaviors*, 37: 1240–1247. doi:10.1016/j.addbeh.2012.06.008

Guinart, D., Marcy, P., Hauser, M. et al. (2020). Patient attitudes towards telepsychiatry during the COVID-19 pandemic: A nationwide, multisite survey. *JMIR Mental Health*, 7(12). doi:10.2196/24761

Hall, G., Cruz, D., Lank, P. et al. (2021). Opioid-related emergency department visits during COVID-19 in a large health system. *Journal of Addiction Medicine*, 15(4): 345–348. doi:10.1097/ADM.0000000000000850

Herring, A., Kalmin, M., Speener, M., Goodman-Meza, D. et al. (2021). Sharp decline in hospital and emergency department initiated buprenorphine for opioid use disorder during COVID-19 state of emergency in California. *Journal of Substance Abuse Treatment*, 123. doi:10.1016/j.jsat.2020.108260

Holland, K., Jones, C., Vivolo-Kantor, A., Idaikkadar, N. et al. (2021). Mental health, overdose, and violence outcomes and the COVID-19 pandemic. *JAMA Psychiatry*, 78(4): 372–378. doi:10.1001/jamapsychiatry.2020.4402

Hosseinbor, M., Ardekani, Y., Bakhschani, S. et al. (2014). Emotional and social loneliness in individuals with and without substance dependence disorder. *International Journal of High Risk Behavior and Addiction*, 3(3). doi:10.5812/ijhrba.22688

Hubley, S., Lynch, S., Schneck, C. et al. (2016). Review of key telepsychiatry outcomes. *World Journal of Psychiatry*, 6(2): 269–282. doi:10.5498/wjp.v6.i2.269

Huskamp, H., Busch, A., Souza, J., Uscher-Pines, L. et al. (2018). How is telemedicine being used in opioid and other substance use disorder treatment? *Health Affairs*, 37(2): 1940–1947. doi:10.1377/hlthaf.2018.05134

Kochnar, R. (2020, June 11). Unemployment rose higher in three months of COVID-19 than it did in two years of the Great Recession. *Pew Research Center*. https://www.pewresearch.org/fact-tank/2020/06/11/unemployment-rose-higher-in-three-months-of-covid-19-than-it-did-in-two-years-of-the-great-recession/

Koonin, L.M., Hoots, B., Tsang, C.A., Leroy, Z., Farris, K., Jolly, T., Antall, P., McCabe, B., Zelis, C., Tong, I., Harris, A.M. (2020). Trends in the use of telehealth during the emergence of the COVID-19 pandemic – United States, January-March 2020. *MMWR. Morbidity and Mortality Weekly Report*, 69(43): 1595–1599. doi:10.15585/mmwr.mm6943a3

Lai, H., Cleary, M., Sitharthan T. et al. (2015). Prevalence of comorbid substance use, anxiety and mood disorders in epidemiological surveys, 1990–2014: A systematic review and meta-analysis. *Drug and Alcohol Dependency*, 154: 1–13. doi:10.1016/j.drugalcdep.2015.05.031

Lasher, L., Rhodes, J., Viner-Brown, S. (2019). Identification and description of non-fatal opioid overdoses using Rhode Island EMS data, 2016–2018. *Rhode Island Medical Journal*, 102(12): 41–45. Available from: http://rimed.org/rimedicaljournal-2019-03.asp

Lee, E., Dep, C., Palmer, B., Glorioso, D. et al. (2020). High prevalence and adverse health effects of loneliness in community-dwelling adults across the lifespan: Role of wisdom as a protective factor. *International Pscyhogeriatric Association*, 31(10): 1447–1462. doi:10.1017/S1041610218002120

Leigh-Hunt, N., Bagguley, D., Bash, K. (2017). An overview of systematic reviews on the public health consequences of social isolation and loneliness. *Public Health*, 152: 157–171. doi:10.1016/j.puhe.2017.07.035

Magidson, J.F., Liu, S.M., Lejuez, C.W. et al. (2012). Comparison of the course of substance use disorders among individuals with and without generalized anxiety disorder in a nationally representative sample. *Journal of Psychiatric Research*, 46(5): 659–666. doi:10.1016/j.jpsychires.2012.02.011.

Mehrotra, A., Chernew, M., Linetsky, D. et al. (2021, February 21). The impact of COVID-19 on outpatient visits in 2020: visits remained stable, despite a late surge in cases. *The Commonwealth Fund*. https://www.commonwealthfund.org/publications/2021/feb/impact-covid-19-outpatient-visits-2020-visits-stable-despite-late-surge

O'Brien, M., McNicholas, F. (2020). The use of telepsychiatry during COVID-19 and beyond. *Irish Journal of Psychological Medicine*, 37(4): 250–255. doi:10.1017/ipm.2020.54

Panchal, N., Cox, C., Garfield, R. (2021, February 10). *The Implications of COVID-19 for Mental Health and Substance Use*. The Kaiser Family Foundation (KFF). https://www.kff.org/coronavirus-covid-19/issue-brief/the-implications-of-covid-19-for-mental-health-and-substance-use/

Patel, S., Huskamp, H., Busch, A. et al. (2020). Telemental health and U.S. rural-urban differences in specialty mental health use, 2010–2017. *American Journal of Public Health*, 110(9): 1308–1314. doi:10.2105/AJPH.2020.3056557

Pierce, R., Stevermer, J. (2020). Disparities in use of telehealth at the onset of the COVID-19 public health emergency. *Journal of Telemedicine and Telecare*. doi: 10.1177/1357633X20963893

Reisman, M. (2017). EHRs: The challenge of making electronic data usable and interoperable. *Pharmacy and Therapeutics*, 42(9):572–575.

Rodda, L., West, K., LeSaint, K. (2020). Opioid overdose-related emergency department visits and accidental deaths during the COVID-19 pandemic. *Journal of Urban Health*, 97:808–813. doi:10.1007/s11524-020-00486-y

Showalter, G. (2020, May 7). Telehealth before and after COVID-19: Telehealth in original Medicare fee for service. *Caravan Health*. https://caravanhealth.com/CaravanHealth/media/Resources-Page/Telehealth_BeforeAfter_COVID19.pdf

Shreffler, J., Shoff, H., Thomas, J. et al. (2021). Brief report: The impact of COVID-19 on emergency department overdose diagnoses and county overdose deaths. *The American Journal on Addictions*, 30: 330–333. doi.10.1111/ajad.13148

Slavova, S., Rock, P., Bush, H. et al. (2020). Signal of increased opioid overdose during COVID-19 from emergency medical services data. *Drug and Alcohol Dependence*, 214. doi:10.1016/j.drugaledep.2020.108176

Soares, W., Melnick, E., Nath, B., D'Onofrio, G. et al. (2021). Emergency department visits for nonfatal opioid overdose during the COVID-19 pandemic across six US health care systems. *Annals of Emergency Medicine*, S0196-0644(21): doi.10.1016/j.annemergmed.2021.03.013

United States Bureau of Census (BOC). (2019, November 21). *One-person households on the rise*. Available at: https://www.census.gov/library/visualizations/2019/comm/one-person-households.html

Velasquez, D., Mehrotra, A. (2020). Ensuring the growth of telehealth during COVID-19 does not exacerbate disparities in care. *Health Affairs Blog*, May 8, 2020. doi:10.1377/hblog20200505.591306

Weber, E., Miller, S., Astha, V. et al. (2020). Characteristics of telehealth users in NYC for COVID-related care during the coronavirus pandemic. *Journal of the American Medical Informatics Association*, 27(12): 1949–1954. doi:10.1093/jamia/ocaa216

Weigel, G., Ramaswamy, A., Sobel, L., Salganicoff, A., Cubanski, J., Freed, M. (2020). Opportunities and barriers for telemedicine in the U.S. during the COVID-19 emergency and beyond. Kaiser Family Foundation (KFF). https://www.kff.org/womens-health-policy/issue-brief/opportunities-and-barriers-for-telemedicine-in-the-u-s-during-the-covid-19-emergency-and-beyond/

Yu, J., Casalino, L., Pincus, H. (2021). Telehealth use for mental health conditions among enrollees in commercial health insurance. *Psychiatric Services*. doi:10.1176/appi.ps.202000778

Chapter 14

Digital transformation in healthcare
How COVID-19 was an agent for rapid change

Bala Hota
Rush University System for Health
Chicago, IL, USA

Tendo Systems
Chicago, IL, USA

Omar Lateef
Rush University Medical Center
Chicago, IL, USA

CONTENTS

Introduction 219
Rush pre-COVID: innovation pilot in telemedicine 221
    Telemedicine pilot for movement disorders 221
        Business model immaturity 222
        Lack of regulatory clarity 222
        Acceptability to a wider population of patients 222
Public health as a laggard in data sharing 222
Rush and COVID-19 224
    Telemedicine growth 225
    Transfers and clinical outcomes 225
Chicago Department of Health (CDPH) and data hub 226
Future directions 230
Acknowledgments 230
References 231

INTRODUCTION

Over 20 years ago, innovation expert Clayton Christensen first predicted the disruption of the healthcare industry through digital transformation [1]. He imagined disruptive innovation, a term he and colleagues coined, redesigning the health industry with a more consumer-focused approach and presented arguments for how technology could improve the patient experience, convenience, and reduce healthcare cost, modeled after other industries that had been affected in a similar fashion by technology. The

DOI: 10.1201/9781003204138-18

US healthcare system could have much to benefit from a transformation through use of technology, as it is well known that while highly advanced, US healthcare is among the most expensive systems in the world, without an associated excellence in overall outcomes.

Yet change in the healthcare industry has been slow. Fragmentation of data, long wait times, and poor communication continue to be noted as gaps in the experience of care. Federal legislation has driven significant change in the industry: meaningful use of legislation has increased the digitization of electronic health records, and the affordable care act and hospital quality measurement programs have created metrics-driven assessments of healthcare performance. But the actual implementation of these programs, and the use of electronic health records themselves, has led to new problems: data silos; burdens due to software use and documentation requirements; physician burnout; and new technology budget costs. The transition to new technology has in most cases led to incremental change and has been overlaid on existing systems, not disrupting the historical approach to clinical care, billing, and documentation.

Several new technologies and approaches have been developed over the last several years that promise more convenient and cost-effective care, but their use has been limited due to multiple barriers. Telemedicine, in which patients can connect with their providers over video or audio formats; "appification" of patient experiences and consumer facing care, in which elements of the traditional patient–provider interaction are abstracted into app-based workflows; ML/AI-based algorithms, in which prior data sets are used to train learning models that guide workflows and automate some elements of care; and sensor-based data collection using internet of things design patterns for home care are all new models of care and interaction with patients that were being developed prior to 2019. Adoption of these tools was slow, however, due to unclear reimbursement models, ambiguous regulatory guidance, a lack of broadly available healthcare data for model training, and skepticism on the part of the healthcare industry for care models outside of clinical offices. Christensen has observed that change has taken longer than he originally forecast, but the industry appears poised for adoption of new technology [2].

COVID-19 served as an accelerator for digital transformation initiatives. First, new models of care in which face-to-face visits were deferred were needed to reduce risk to healthcare workers and patients. While this has been a goal of digital transformation advocates for many years, COVID-19 served as a catalyst to resolve regulatory hurdles, experiment with workflows, and drive adoption. Second, gaps in the data sharing infrastructure were demonstrated. The novel virus and a hunger for information about outcomes by physicians and patients exposed a basic absence of timely data to study and report on clinical data. Finally, the successes and gaps in public health adoption of technology progress, despite inclusion in meaningful use standards, were made strikingly clear and a drive to fix these gaps was started. In this chapter, using the experience of Rush University Medical

Center and its partner, the Chicago Department of Public Health, we will describe how digital innovation and transformation was accelerated by the COVID-19 pandemic, and how we sought to leverage interoperability, data aggregation, and analytics to improve outcomes due to infection with SARS-COV-2 for our community.

RUSH PRE-COVID: INNOVATION PILOT IN TELEMEDICINE

Rush University Medical Center pursued technological innovation prior to the COVID-19 pandemic – and like most medical centers, innovation was most often implemented in pilot programs. Pilot programs enable stakeholders in the organization both to build new technologies and workflows, and/or partner with external programs to promote new technologies and solutions. An example of one of these initiatives at Rush was a nascent telemedicine program which was integrated with the Epic Electronic Health Record using a third-party tool to facilitate video and media content. Adoption was limited, however, with under 100 visits per week and ongoing consensus-driven planning around program design and implementation. This rollout was conducted in a typical setting for healthcare providers using electronic health records: industry-wide usability issues, documentation burden, and burnout. The target population during the pilot was movement disorder patients [3]. The program represents an excellent example of typical innovation programs at health systems, and how during the era prior to COVID-19, change was slow related to adoption of digital technology.

Telemedicine pilot for movement disorders

Conceptualized between 2017 and 2018, the program was imagined as a method to deploy telemedicine for patients in remote settings and to facilitate expansion of access to Rush Medical Center specialists. This program was established to design, implement, and evaluate the use of telemedicine and examine how scaling of use of telemedicine services could occur. A third-party provider of integrated video, Vidyo, was integrated into the Epic electronic record at Rush to enable the technology; staffing of telemedicine services occurred from within the sponsoring department (Neurology); and a focus of the program was on acceptability from patients, limitations of the technology, and clinical services that could be safely offered. Overall, the program was deemed a success, as shown in strongly positive satisfaction scores among both patients and providers. The implementation was considered a pilot, however, and was conducted in a limited number of patients, in a research context through a grant, and without a business plan. At the end of the pilot, discussions of wider scaling of the program identified key issues preventing a broader rollout. The process of building consensus on scaling pilots to larger deployments, thereby truly disrupting current models of care, has been noted to be a cause of delay in innovation [4]. Issues being discussed at Rush were as follows:

Business model immaturity

In the pilot, all telemedicine care was offered for free, through institutional grants for its implementation. Given the national approach to billing for telemedicine services, reimbursement for care in person would exceed that of telemedicine, and the business case for scenarios in which a telemedicine visit would be favorable over an in person visit was not clear. At-risk contract scenarios, like Accountable Care Organizations, Medicare Advantage, or commercial ACOs seemed to potentially weigh in favor of telemedicine economics, but when analyzed in specific business plans the value was not clear.

Lack of regulatory clarity

Internally, issues such as licensure and liability were also considered. Licensure requirements for telemedicine were identified as confusing and unclear. Issues such as in-state licensure requirements, and how to limit appropriateness of patients to the visit were addressed. Liability in the case of adverse events with virtual visits was also considered and the uncertainty of the legal environment was felt to be a barrier to implementation.

Acceptability to a wider population of patients

Though the pilot demonstrated strong acceptance, uncertainty about the generalizability of the response of a larger population was present. Further study was desired to evaluate the ability to scale the platform to broader populations with workflows, physician staffing for the growth and suitable patient populations.

PUBLIC HEALTH AS A LAGGARD IN DATA SHARING

While hospitals focus on workflows as a target of innovation, public health relies on multi-stakeholder, multi-hospital data to drive its innovation in decision making, surveillance, and research. The potential for public health to be an innovator in the data ecosystem is substantial: as a central point for data submission and feedback, a well-functioning public health data infrastructure could be a resource for researchers, reduce administrative burden, and be a tool for the characterization of regional illness and planning of resource use. The onset of the COVID-19 pandemic brought gaps in the penetration of digital transformation and data access in the public health sphere into sharp relief.

Public health has been a part of national planning in interoperability and electronic record use as a part of the meaningful use program. In theory, the standard data formats and exchange methods provided by meaningful use should enable rapid healthcare data exchange in the setting of disruptive healthcare events like a pandemic. In reality, access to data has remained challenging, and even if available, often lacks conformity to regulated standards. The current COVID-19 pandemic has also revealed gaps in data liquidity and the resultant difficulty in gathering information quickly. Since the declaration of a global pandemic on March 11, 2020 [5], health departments, researchers, and clinicians have sought the best evidence to plan regional responses and provide the best clinical care. Disease surveillance is a critical function of public health and provides essential information about disease burden, clinical and epidemiologic parameters of disease, and is an important precursor to effective and timely case and contact tracing. In addition to individual and aggregate level patient data, this pandemic has required careful monitoring of healthcare capacity and utilization to ensure clinical care needs could be met. Though meaningful use has resulted in significant progress in data sharing for public health, significant gaps continue to exist, which may be solved through the FHIR API standards.

Support for the surveillance and epidemiology of disease has been embedded in key national informatics initiatives for nearly two decades. These efforts have included syndromic surveillance [6], electronic laboratory reporting [7], and registry submission [8] in the meaningful use program [9], and the growth of the National Healthcare Safety Network (NHSN) [10]. These technology-enabled programs have created linkages between hospitals, commercial labs, and public health to enable the collection and organization of data through the EHR and order workflows and improve the timeliness and completeness of reporting.

Electronic laboratory reporting (ELR) systems have resulted in improvements in the reporting of data to public health for surveillance: the volume and timeliness have improved 2.3–4.4-fold and 3.8–7.9 days earlier, respectively [11]; ELR also improves the completeness of reporting over what is found through passive surveillance [12, 13].

But ELR data can be incomplete. The completeness of fields reported via ELR within basic HL7 v 2.x messages ranges from 38% (race) to 98% (date of birth) [13]. To improve completeness, groups have proposed (1) increased mandatory fields in ELR HL7 2.x messages [11]; (2) augmenting ELR feeds with data from a health information exchange, which improved completeness for race to 60% [13]; and (3) electronic case report forms which are completed either through automated data capture or manual completion [14]. Significant limitations in case reporting have identified during the COVID-19 pandemic, including limited data on key variables such as age, race/ethnicity, hospitalization, and ICU status [15]. Additionally, co-morbid conditions, a significant predictor of disease outcome, are rarely captured. Improving the completeness of reportable data is necessary for epidemiological studies of risk factors for emerging pathogens like SARS-CoV-2.

To date, electronic reporting from registries and EHRs for public and population health has also not reduced administrative burden. The average cost per physician to complete federally mandated quality reporting has been estimated to be $40,069 per physician per year in the United States [16]. A study of data quality has found electronic reporting via eCQMs has a sensitivity of 46%–98%, specificity from 62% to 97%, and has underestimated the rate of proper care by over half for asthma and vaccine adherence [17]. Reporting programs may also show a lack of alignment, with differences between clinical, payor and public health needs, and compliance risks [18].

RUSH AND COVID-19

As the COVID-19 pandemic emerged on the west and east coasts of the United States, in Chicago leaders at Rush University Medical Center watched and learned about the key issues noted by early sites. In the spring of 2020, published data were lacking on characteristics and outcomes of individuals infected with SARS-CoV-2; the lack of information early in the pandemic led to social media becoming an outsized source of information on outcomes and clinical pathways [19]. The prominence of social media in the response opened the door to the creation of the "infodemic" [20–22].

Early on, leaders recognized the need for real-time data in the decision making process for COVID-19. As detailed in the Rush COVID-19 response playbook [23], following the convening of a command center, dashboards with key metrics were created for the medical center. These dashboards covered national, regional, and local rates of COVID-19; patients tested and positive with infection for SARS-CoV-2; supply chain information related to PPE; bed occupancy and capacity; and outcomes of infection. As the pandemic progressed, forecast models were developed and incorporated into the dashboards for PPE supply needs and bed capacity [24]. Given the rise of telemedicine visits which were used to provide care to COVID-19 and general patients, dashboards on ambulatory care utilization and virtual visits were created. These efforts led to a standardized COVID-19 registry within Rush that was used to aid in rapid data analysis for operations and for research. These foundational data efforts created an ecosystem of benefits, including successful applications for a national COVID-19 registry for the study of post-acute sequelae of COVID-19 (PASC) [25, 26]; a national data sharing network for COVID-19 outcomes (Health Data for Action) [27], as well as numerous peer reviewed publications from Rush.

Telemedicine growth

COVID-19 also created intense demand for new models of care. Given the need to identify methods to reduce face-to-face contact with individuals potentially infected with SARS-CoV-2, regulatory and financial barriers were removed for telemedicine visits with elimination of liability, reduction of technical requirements, and patient acceptance of telemedicine solutions. Rush was able to scale its internally developed telemedicine program rapidly. Within two weeks, Rush was able to address an average of over 1000 visits per week (i.e. 10x growth), with a net promoter score as of 9/21/2021 of 83. While COVID-19 drove rapid adoption of virtual visits to support city-wide triage and scheduling of potential COVID-19 cases, thereby supporting better infection control protocols, Rush transitioned to general ambulatory use of telemedicine by June 2020 and has continued to grow usage over time. Over 20,000 visits have used telemedicine in the last 18 months, with average wait times of under 20 minutes for scheduled or unscheduled visits. COVID-19 has been the catalyst of this transformation, but the clinical system and patients were ready to capitalize on the practice change.

Transfers and clinical outcomes

A part of the Rush strategic plan is to serve as an anchor hospital for its regional populations and hospitals [28]. To achieve that aim, it seeks to provide capacity for transfers and offer care and wellness solutions to reduce health inequities. A thesis as leaders at Rush learned about COVID-19 was that infection and mortality difference noted between race and ethnic groups [29] were manifestations of access to care differences. A specific focus early in the pandemic was access to high intensity, high skill care such as proning for critically ill COVID-19 patients. In addition, the Rush belief in the spring and summer of 2020 was that reaching out to potential high risk populations was an effective strategy to save lives.

Rush made it known in the Chicago region that it was willing to provide expert care for the sickest COVID-19 patients through media communications, promotion of free COVID-19 video visits combined with testing, and direct outreach to essential hospitals serving Chicago neighborhoods with a high proportion of African American and Hispanic residents. As a result, during the initial COVID-19 surge Rush cared for a substantial proportion of Illinois patients with COVID-19: 1032 admissions for COVID-19 disease, representing 8% and 20% of the ICU patients and 4.5% and 23% of the ventilated patients for Illinois and Chicago, respectively. In this high-volume experience, Rush witnessed firsthand the disproportionate impact COVID-19 has had on African American and Hispanic populations. Overall, Hispanic ethnicity accounted for 48%, 48%, and 47% of admissions, ICU stays, and mechanical ventilation episodes, respectively; African American race accounted for 37%, 37%, and 34% of admissions, ICU stays, and mechanical ventilation episodes. Among Hispanic and African American patients at Rush, no mortality difference was noted: inpatient mortality was 11% vs 13% for non-Hispanic and non-African American patients. These outcomes compare favorably to data from other sites [29].

Our well-developed community programs and relationships were crucial for facilitating transfers of critically ill COVID-19 patients. We knew under-resourced community hospitals serving African American and Hispanic neighborhoods could be short on either beds, supplies, or staff. Regardless of knowledge and expertise of their staff, these hospitals could be limited in critical care delivery options, likely resulting in poorer outcomes. Through active outreach to these regional community hospitals, we made our bed capacity and level of care available to their patients. As a result 164, or 16%, of our COVID-19 admissions were transfers; 87% of these transfers were either Latino or African American, and 32% of transfers were Medicaid recipients or uninsured, among the highest in the state [30].

The Rush pandemic playbook set the foundation for the excellent outcomes seen in these populations [23]. Leaders were able to monitor bed capacity through the data and analytics work, and inferred from early data at Rush and from other sites the best guidelines, protocols, and care to yield the best outcomes. Rush could confidently receive transfers and build process to act as a regional resource. The pandemic exposed a need for the regionalization of critical care in times of crisis; critical care access is essential for health equity. Interestingly, Liebman and Patel described COVID-19 referral centers as a potential solution [31]; we believe that academic medical centers should receive those referrals, achieving equitable, high-quality outcomes while continuing other types of care. We observe that our openness to transfers allowed us to have a regional impact: our view was that we had an opportunity and obligation to serve as a resource institution – an oasis for the community.

What we also realized from this experience and past infectious disease crises [32] that regional coordination with local health departments and other medical centers is a critical part of a successful response. Respectful and collaborative interactions with regional partners, linked to a digital and data transformation approach, could be a foundation for a novel method to improve the public health infrastructure and drive better data.

CHICAGO DEPARTMENT OF HEALTH (CDPH) AND DATA HUB

Enabling public health to function as a central node in the data ecosystem is an opportunity for better regional health. More streamlined integration of data from EHRs to public health-based registries offers an opportunity to improve data quality and reduce administrative burden of reporting for the clinical, research, and public health domains. Data flows from healthcare entities could pass to local health departments for registry needs, and then be passed onward; in this way detailed data stays in the location with greatest actionability, in alignment with existing policy, including HHS' recent guidance on ensuring COVID-19 lab results are reported, eventually, to HHS [33]. Public health could, as an aggregator of data, act as an efficient broker of information for stakeholders provided the appropriate security models and API endpoints for data can be supplied. Consumers of data throughout the system could leverage the data curation that occurs through this pipeline for multiple uses, including population health and research. The availability of a common data platform with detailed data could enable reporting to multiple stakeholders to be sourced from public health registries, reducing administrative burden [18].

A recent evaluation of the interoperability of clinical EHR data with registries has found that the registry community "has not benefitted from, is not aligned with, and does not contribute to interoperability efforts" [34], and that fragmentation of data models and data elements was present between certified registries that were surveyed. Manual data collection is the dominant model for data collection for registries, and in only 1 case were fields aligned with the USCDI. For COVID-19, the CDC released a manually collected form for persons under investigation (PUIs) for COVID-19 registry data [35] as the initial primary method of capture of data for PUIs with COVID-19. The administrative burden of manual data collection was a cause of poor data quality in PUI form submissions. Disease surveillance is a critical function of public health and provides essential information about disease burden, clinical and epidemiologic parameters of disease and is an important element to effective and timely case and contact tracing. In addition to individual and aggregate level patient data, this pandemic has required careful monitoring of healthcare capacity and utilization to ensure clinical care needs be met. The barriers to reporting, such as manual data collection and interoperability challenges, have proven to be issues in collection of accurate data.

In Chicago, we struggled with two dimensions of interoperability – first, the ability to exchange "real-time" clinical data for public health, and second, the ability to capture aggregate capacity data for resource planning in an administratively efficient manner. On clinical exchange, despite significant EHR investments among the city's hospitals and health systems, case investigators have had to rely on the phone or fax to understand clinical context. On the absence of transparent, real-time capacity data across the city, public health officials lacked enough information to effectively coordinate care between institutions throughout the city.

As for administrative burden, the inability for electronic health records systems to automate delivery of the important data elements for the CDC PUI form [35] meant that due to the high volume of cases, much of that information never reached public health. By April, 2020, multiple agencies had requested bed and surge capacity information, including NHSN, FEMA, the National Guard, the Illinois Department of Public Health, and the local health department, all with slightly varying definitions. Reporting for these groups tied up over 2 FTEs at our medical center daily just to meet bed capacity reporting requirements, and in total, 108 measures – 58 for bed usage alone – were included in the measures sites were obligated to report, with considerable administrative overhead.

In a partnership between Rush University Medical Center and the Chicago Department of Public Health to leverage existing healthcare IT infrastructure for COVID-19 disease, a platform was developed to address the gaps in interoperability. Our goals were to use regulated interoperability standards already in production to generate regional bed capacity awareness, enhance the capture of epidemiological risk factors and clinical variables among COVID-19 tested patients, and reduce the administrative burden of reporting for stakeholders in a manner that could be replicated by other public health agencies. As an example of clinically relevant fields of interest for reporting, we compared available fields in data feeds to the CDC PUI form. We also evaluated the completeness of various data sources supplied to the platform and the capacity to link these sources.

To solve the issue of interoperability, Chicago took an innovative step through the issuance of a public health order. On April 6, 2020, the CDPH issued public health order 2020-4[36] requiring hospitals in Chicago to share electronic health record data with the public health department for all patients tested for COVID-19. The order outlined a constrained set of data to be submitted for all COVID-19 tested patients. The order mandated the sharing with CDPH of three main data types: (1) Electronic laboratory record (ELR) feeds of SARS-CoV-2 tested individuals, which were an existing state mandate; (2) CCDA records from hospitals for SARS-CoV-2 tested patients; and (3) NHSN capacity module reporting, which was asked to be sent centrally to CDPH. These data were requested to be sent at a minimum once per day, by 10 am. Sites also provided contact information for key Rush University Medical Center personnel who were leading the implementation. ELR feeds were accessed from the Illinois' National Electronic Disease Surveillance System (I-NEDSS) to provide baseline information on lab confirmed cases in the city. To meet public health order 2020–2024, hospitals were provided multiple mechanisms to submit consolidated clinical data architecture (CCDA) records for COVID-19 tested patients.

This order was disseminated through CDPH's clinical health alert network and shared with city hospital leadership on calls. CDPH constituted a governance committee comprising medical directors and informaticists from hospital systems in Chicago. The committee was composed of 12 site CMO, CMIO, or technical leads. These leaders also brought content and guidance back to site participants and sought to bridge varying degrees of internal technical capabilities among systems. The committee met weekly and helped to build trust among participating sites. While the local health department, with its public health orders, was a necessary recipient and user of the data, participants recognized the value of a larger sharing initiative, plus site participation to engage on use cases and mechanisms to leverage the information.

General principles were modeled after rules implemented for use of CMS data [37] and were established among sites through this committee. These were:

- Openness: Promoting and facilitating the open sharing of knowledge about COVID-19 data.
- Communication: Promoting partnerships across the region to eliminate duplication of effort, a source of truth for regional data that may enable reduced administrative burden, and a valuable regional and national resource.
- Accountability: Ensuring compliance with approved data management principles and policies. Understanding the objectives of current and future strategic or programmatic initiatives and how they impact, or are impacted by, existing data management principles and policies as well as current privacy and security protocols.

A cloud hosted and isolated environment was established, with five individual modalities for connectivity; all feeding into a centralized data hub for hundreds of thousands of transactions per week. Over the next 30 days, sites were approached for data sharing; a CDPH data governance committee composed of chief medical officers and chief medical informatics officers from select institutions was created through which issues could be discussed and additional roadmaps could be generated; collaboration with Epic and Cerner EHR developers was established, and mechanisms for enterprise scale sharing was created; and data was sent centrally to the CDPH cloud instance. Following a rapid implementation, a reference implementation of the data hub was created that leverages cloud-based microservices in Amazon Web Services, including Amazon HealthLake and analytics tools [38]. This infrastructure was made available as an open source toolkit to enable broader adoption by health departments and public health stakeholders.

As of 9/15/21, 992,651 unique patient records were stored in the data hub from CCDAs, with an average of an additional 25k patient CCDA records with data recorded weekly. Data from 15 hospitals was present, with 7 additional hospitals ready to submit. 5,953,756 ELR records, with a weekly average of over 200,000, were present, and 4,308,261 immunization records, with a weekly average of over 80,000 new records, were present in the data set. ELR represents a significant proportion of reported cases of SARS CoV-2 infection. ELR alone provided 73.7% of cases, while ELR combined with other modalities accounted for a total of 94% of reported cases.

FUTURE DIRECTIONS

As originally described by Christensen, disruptive innovation occurs when incremental progress occurs in adjacent markets, with cheaper, better, and faster workflows desired by customers. In healthcare, this type of innovation has been difficult to sustain due to a high regulatory barrier, and cultural barriers in healthcare preventing change. COVID-19 caused a rethinking of the role of rapid change in healthcare. Due to the critical need for data, as shown by the Chicago use cases outlined above, multiple rapid, agile, projects were implemented to respond to the pandemic. More importantly, these changes yielded benefits for multiple stakeholders: patients, the health system, and the public health department.

If we are fortunate, these changes will be the catalyst that brings sustained disruptive innovation to the US healthcare system in the coming years. At the time of writing, the United States was seeing a new surge in the delta variant strain of SARS-CoV-2, and new strains worldwide had been identified. These facts alone have justified continued investment in mitigation strategies for COVID-19 and data-driven decision making. But leaders are considering which of the foundational elements put in place in the last two years should persist and drive new workflows and care patterns for the future.

Telemedicine represents a new and dynamic method to provide care for patients. It is now accepted and desired by patients, and well staffed by providers. How this can become a new standard for lower cost, more convenient care, will depend on the permanence of regulatory and billing changes implemented during the pandemic. The value proposition of data interoperability has been clearly demonstrated – from federal agencies to hospital researchers, the hunger for databases and clinical registries for COVID-19 has highlighted why good connections and data infrastructure is critical.

We envision a future in which we build on the tools that have been established to improve the patient's care. We have plans to take our data hub efforts developed in health lake and shine a light on health inequities, barriers to access, and prevention of disease. By scaling the connections between data sets, we can connect the longitudinal health records of the most vulnerable. Much as we did for COVID-19, by enhancing access, we believe we can improve outcomes for a whole host of diseases beyond COVID-19, but into the new normal.

ACKNOWLEDGMENTS

The authors gratefully acknowledge the leadership and contributions of the following individuals: Marisa Truesdell and Amanda Tosto who were responsible for the Rush Telemedicine deployment Meeta Shah who led Telemedicine expansion during COVID-19 Shafiq Rab and Jawad Khan who were critical for the initiation and development of the CDPH data hub.

REFERENCES

[1] Christensen CM, Bohmer RMJ, Kenagy J. Will Disruptive Innovations Cure Health Care? *Harvard Business Review [Internet]*. 2000 Sep [cited 2021 Sep 26]; Available from: https://hbr.org/2000/09/will-disruptive-innovations-cure-health-care

[2] Christensen C, Waldeck A, Fogg R. *How Disruptive Innovation Can Finally Revolutionize Healthcare [Internet]*. 2017. Available from: https://www.christenseninstitute.org/wp-content/uploads/2017/05/How-Disruption-Can-Finally-Revolutionize-Healthcare-final.pdf

[3] Hanson RE, Truesdell M, Stebbins GT, Weathers AL, Goetz CG. Telemedicine vs Office Visits in a Movement Disorders Clinic: Comparative Satisfaction of Physicians and Patients. *Movement Disorders Clinical Practice [Internet]*. 2019 [cited 2021 Sep 26]; 6(1): 65–69. Available from: https://onlinelibrary.wiley.com/doi/abs/10.1002/mdc3.12703

[4] Jain SH. Healthcare Holdups, Death-By-Pilot, And The Scourge Of Incrementalism [Internet]. *Forbes*. 2021 [cited 2021 Sep 26]. Available from: https://www.forbes.com/sites/sachinjain/2021/03/16/healthcare-holdups-death-by-pilot-and-the-scourge-of-incrementalism/

[5] WHO Director-General's opening remarks at the media briefing on COVID-19 - 11 March 2020 [Internet]. [cited 2020 Apr 27]. Available from: https://www.who.int/dg/speeches/detail/who-director-general-s-opening-remarks-at-the-media-briefing-on-covid-19---11-march-2020

[6] Syndromic Surveillance (SS) | Meaningful Use | CDC [Internet]. 2020 [cited 2020 Apr 25]. Available from: https://www.cdc.gov/ehrmeaningfuluse/Syndromic.html

[7] Electronic Laboratory Reporting (ELR) | Meaningful Use | CDC [Internet]. 2020 [cited 2020 Apr 25]. Available from: https://www.cdc.gov/ehrmeaningfuluse/elr.html

[8] Public Health & Promoting Interoperability Programs | Meaningful Use | CDC [Internet]. 2020 [cited 2020 Jun 6]. Available from: https://www.cdc.gov/ehrmeaningfuluse/index.html

[9] Guides | Meaningful Use | CDC [Internet]. 2020 [cited 2020 Apr 25]. Available from: https://www.cdc.gov/ehrmeaningfuluse/guides.html

[10] Arnold KE, Thompson ND. Building Data Quality and Confidence in Data Reported to the National Healthcare Safety Network. *Infection Control & Hospital Epidemiology* [Internet]. 2012 May [cited 2020 May 3]; 33(5): 446–448. Available from: https://www.cambridge.org/core/journals/infection-control-and-hospital-epidemiology/article/building-data-quality-and-confidence-in-data-reported-to-the-national-healthcare-safety-network/DA0B1FE51A558BB4C5A4AB7CD77BE730

[11] Rajeev D, Staes CJ, Evans RS, Mottice S, Rolfs R, Samore MH, et al. Development of an Electronic Public Health Case Report Using HL7 v2.5 to Meet Public Health Needs. *Journal of the American Medical Informatics Association: JAMIA*. 2010; 17(1): 34–41.

[12] Samoff E, Dibiase L, Fangman MT, Fleischauer AT, Waller AE, MacDonald PDM. We Can Have It All: Improved Surveillance Outcomes and Decreased Personnel Costs Associated with Electronic Reportable Disease Surveillance, North Carolina, 2010. *American Journal of Public Health*. 2013 Dec; 103(12): 2292–2297.

[13] Dixon BE, McGowan JJ, Grannis SJ. Electronic Laboratory Data Quality and the Value of a Health Information Exchange to Support Public Health Reporting Processes. *AMIA Annual Symposium proceedings AMIA Symposium*. 2011; 2011: 322–330.

[14] Dixon BE, Taylor DE, Choi M, Riley M, Schneider T, Duke J. Integration of FHIR to Facilitate Electronic Case Reporting: Results From a Pilot Study. *Studies in Health Technology and Informatics*. 2019 Aug; 264: 940–944.

[15] CDCMMWR. Severe Outcomes Among Patients with Coronavirus Disease 2019 (COVID-19) United States, February 12 March 16, 2020. MMWR Morbidity and Mortality Weekly Report [Internet]. 2020 [cited 2020 Jun 5]; 69. Available from: https://www.cdc.gov/mmwr/volumes/69/wr/mm6912e2.htm

[16] Casalino LP, Gans D, Weber R, Cea M, Tuchovsky A, Bishop TF, et al. US Physician Practices Spend More Than $15.4 Billion Annually To Report Quality Measures. *Health Affairs* [Internet]. 2016 Mar [cited 2020 May 29]; 35(3): 401–406. Available from: https://www.healthaffairs.org/doi/full/10.1377/hlthaff.2015.1258

[17] Kern LM, Malhotra S, Barrón Y, Quaresimo J, Dhopeshwarkar R, Pichardo M, et al. Accuracy of Electronically Reported "Meaningful Use" Clinical Quality Measures. Annals of Internal Medicine [Internet]. 2013 Jan [cited 2020 May 29]; 158(2): 77–83. Available from: https://www.acpjournals.org/doi/abs/10.7326/0003-4819-158-2-201301150-00001

[18] Strategy on Reducing Burden Relating to the Use of Health IT and EHRs | HealthIT.Gov [Internet]. [cited 2020 May 29]. Available from: https://www.healthit.gov/topic/usability-and-provider-burden/strategy-reducing-burden-relating-use-health-it-and-ehrs

[19] Rosenberg H, Syed S, Rezaie S. The Twitter pandemic: The Critical Role of Twitter in the Dissemination of Medical Information and Misinformation During the COVID-19 Pandemic. *Canadian Journal of Emergency Medicine* [Internet]. 2020 Jul [cited 2021 Sep 27]; 22(4): 418–421. Available from: https://www.cambridge.org/core/journals/canadian-journal-of-emergency-medicine/article/twitter-pandemic-the-critical-role-of-twitter-in-the-dissemination-of-medical-information-and-misinformation-during-the-covid19-pandemic/9F42C2D9-9CA00FBAE50A66D107322211

[20] Diseases TLI. The COVID-19 Infodemic. The Lancet Infectious Diseases [Internet]. 2020 Aug [cited 2021 Sep 27]; 20(8): 875. Available from: https://www.thelancet.com/journals/laninf/article/PIIS1473-3099(20)30565-X/fulltext

[21] Gruzd A, De Domenico M, Sacco PL, Briand S. Studying the COVID-19 Infodemic at Scale. *Big Data & Society* [Internet]. 2021 Jan [cited 2021 Sep 27]; 8(1): 20539517211021115. Available from: doi.10.1177/20539517211021115

[22] Managing the COVID-19 Infodemic: Promoting Healthy Behaviours and Mitigating the Harm From Misinformation and Disinformation [Internet]. [cited 2021 Sep 27]. Available from: https://www.who.int/news/item/23-09-2020-managing-the-covid-19-infodemic-promoting-healthy-behaviours-and-mitigating-the-harm-from-misinformation-and-disinformation

[23] Rush Covid Response Playbook.Pdf [Internet]. [cited 2021 Sep 27]. Available from: https://www.rush.edu/sites/default/files/2020-09/RushCovidResponse Playbook.pdf

[24] Locey KJ, Webb TA, Khan J, Antony AK, Hota B. An Interactive Tool to Forecast US Hospital Needs in the Coronavirus 2019 Pandemic. *JAMIA Open [Internet]*. 2020 Dec [cited 2021 Sep 27]; 3(4): 506–512. Available from: https://doi.org/10.1093/jamiaopen/ooaa045

[25] Hota B. Innovative Support for Patients With SARS-COV2 Infections (COVID-19) Registry (INSPIRE) [Internet]. clinicaltrials.gov; 2021 Jun [cited 2021 Sep 23]. Report No.: NCT04610515. Available from: https://clinicaltrials.gov/ct2/show/NCT04610515

[26] O'Laughlin KN, Thompson M, Hota B, Gottlieb M, Plumb ID, Chang AM, et al. Study Protocol for the Innovative Support for Patients with SARS-COV-2 Infections Registry (INSPIRE): A Longitudinal Study of the Medium and Long-Term Sequelae of SARS-CoV-2 Infection [Internet]. *Cold Spring Harbor Laboratory Press*; 2021 10(18): 1–37. [cited 2021 Sep 27]. Available from: https://www.medrxiv.org/content/10.1101/2021.08.01.21261397v1

[27] New Initiative Aims to Build a Model Open COVID-19 Patient Data Registry Network | AcademyHealth [Internet]. [cited 2021 Sep 27]. Available from: https://academyhealth.org/blog/2020-04/new-initiative-aims-build-model-open-covid-19-patient-data-registry-network

[28] Ansell DA, Oliver HD, Goodman LJ, Lateef OB, Johnson TJ. Health Equity as a System Strategy: The Rush University Medical Center Framework. *NEJM Catalyst [Internet]*. 2021 [cited 2021 Sep 27]; 2(5): 1–19. Available from: https://catalyst.nejm.org/doi/full/10.1056/CAT.20.0674

[29] Price-Haywood EG, Burton J, Fort D, Seoane L. Hospitalization and Mortality Among Black Patients and White Patients with Covid-19. *New England Journal of Medicine [Internet]*. 2020 Jun [cited 2020 Jul 7]; 382(26): 2534–2543. Available from: https://doi.org/10.1056/NEJMsa2011686

[30] Calgary O. Claims Reimbursement to Health Care Providers and Facilities for Testing and Treatment of the Uninsured | Data | Centers for Disease Control and Prevention [Internet]. [cited 2020 Jul 20]. Available from: https://data.cdc.gov/Administrative/Claims-Reimbursement-to-Health-Care-Providers-and-/rksx-33p3

[31] To Save Staff And Supplies, Designate Specialized COVID-19 Referral Centers | Health Affairs Blog [Internet]. [cited 2021 Sep 27]. Available from: https://www.healthaffairs.org/do/10.1377/hblog20200324.547284/full/

[32] Lateef O, Hota B, Landon E, Kociolek LK, Morita J, Black S, et al. Chicago Ebola Response Network (CERN): A Citywide Cross-hospital Collaborative for Infectious Disease Preparedness. Weinstein RA, editor. *Clinical Infectious Diseases [Internet]*. 2015 Nov [cited 2020 Apr 30]; 61(10): 1554–1557. Available from: https://academic.oup.com/cid/article-lookup/doi/10.1093/cid/civ510

[33] COVID-19 Pandemic Response, Laboratory Data Reporting: CARES Act Section 18115 [Internet]. 2020. Available from: https://www.hhs.gov/sites/default/files/covid-19-laboratory-data-reporting-guidance.pdf

[34] Registry Data Standards [Internet]. DCRI. [cited 2020 Jun 5]. Available from: https://dcri.org/registry-data-standards/

[35] CDC. Coronavirus Disease 2019 (COVID-19) [Internet]. *Centers for Disease Control and Prevention*. 2020 [cited 2020 May 3]. Available from: https://www.cdc.gov/coronavirus/2019-ncov/php/reporting-pui.html

[36] COVID-19 Orders [Internet]. [cited 2020 May 3]. Available from: https://www.chicago.gov/content/city/en/sites/covid-19/home/health-orders.html

[37] CMS Information Systems Security and Privacy Policy [Internet]. 2019. Available from: https://www.cms.gov/Research-Statistics-Data-and-Systems/CMS-Information-Technology/InformationSecurity/Downloads/CMS-IS2P2.pdf

[38] Rush University Medical Center creates COVID-19 analytics hub on AWS [Internet]. *Amazon Web Services*. 2021 [cited 2021 Sep 27]. Available from: https://aws.amazon.com/blogs/publicsector/rush-medical-center-aws-analytics-hub/

Chapter 15

Telehealth

Richard Fine

Zocdoc
New York, NY, USA

CONTENTS

Introduction 235
Telehealth before 236
Telehealth's watershed moment 237
Telehealth's new normal 240
Percentage of in-person appointments from May 2020 to May 2021 241
Conclusion 242
References 242

INTRODUCTION

Telehealth has been "the future of healthcare" for so many years that describing it as such has become an insider joke. The dream has long been on-demand, cheaper, easier-to-access healthcare untethered to geography. The reality is that despite multiple decades of boosterism, subsidies, and mandates, telehealth represented just ~1% of care before COVID-19 turned the world upside-down. Prior to the pandemic, the success and adoption of telehealth was hamstrung by low demand, low supply, and fragmented options.

Then, at the outset of the pandemic and stay-at-home orders in early 2020, the use of telehealth spiked rapidly; doctors quickly pivoted to video calls and virtual diagnoses as patients demanded a way to safely get the care they needed. To give some perspective on the size and speed of the shift to telehealth, according to Medicare claims data, 1.3 million patients received telehealth services in the week ending April 18th, compared to just 11,000 a month earlier, an increase of more than 11,718%. While that growth has almost certainly leveled off since, there is no longer any question that telehealth will make up a much larger share of healthcare visits going forward.

In short, decades of progress happened at warp speed. Finally, telehealth saw its long-hyped, rapid, broad adoption.

Then, as the pandemic evolved, people's booking behavior changed again; they began to resume many of their pre-pandemic activities, including

DOI: 10.1201/9781003204138-19

returning to doctors' offices. After all, we all have bodies and there are some things doctors can only do when a patient is physically in the exam room: it's not possible to feel someone's arm through a screen.

We will look at these changes through the unique data available to Zocdoc – a New York City headquartered marketplace where millions of patients come to find and book care every month across 100+ specialties and 50 states. At Zocdoc in February 2020, less than 1% of appointment bookings were for virtual care. By May 2020, the share of telehealth appointments skyrocketed to between 30% and 40%.

As we look toward the future, our data is showing that – while virtual healthcare appointments will certainly remain part of the mix at a much higher percentage than pre-pandemic – the new format is very different from the model that past telehealth evangelists presented. It will largely be a supplement to, not a substitute for, in-person care. Patients will want the option to decide between in-person and virtual care, and their choices will differ by specialty and need. In many cases, they will want online–offline continuity of care with their neighborhood doctor. It will not be a type of healthcare cafe unbound by geography.

Zocdoc's comprehensive data – national, multi-specialty, across telehealth and in-person care – gives us a bird's eye view of these changes. This appointment booking data tells the story of a profound and rapid change in healthcare behaviors and offers hints for the future.

TELEHEALTH BEFORE

For as long as there has been modern technology, there have been attempts to incorporate it into the practice of medicine. In fact, since Alexander Graham Bell got help with an acid burn by making a call on his phone in the 1880s, the idea of remote communication for medical purposes has captured our collective imagination. However, for more than a century, telehealth's utopia has outpaced its utilization.

There were two key barriers to telehealth's widespread adoption: technology and policy. On the technology front, Zocdoc's founder and CEO, Oliver Kharraz, M.D., discussed the tools he relied on most when he was a practicing physician, in a July 6, 2021 article in Fortune:

> As the CEO of a healthcare technology company, I see many ways that new innovations can help doctors provide better care and create a better experience for patients. But before I became a CEO, I was a physician – one who comes from a 300-year family tradition of providing care. Throughout those three centuries, and despite significant leaps forward in medical innovation, my ancestors and I all relied on the very same primary diagnostic tool: the human body itself. Its unmatched sense of touch, sense of sight, and sense of connection are all more powerful in person.

It is only within the 21st century that technological advancements such as high-speed internet, high definition cameras, remarkable sensors, and more, could even begin to support physicians in providing remote care. As the costs of these tools rapidly decreased, and the quality of these tools rapidly increased, it started to become technologically possible for physicians to evaluate patients virtually.

Although the technology had advanced, the policy barriers were still in place and severely restricted both the telehealth supply and demand. There were manifold state and federal regulations – as well as commercial policies – which deterred patients from seeking virtual care, and deterred providers from offering it. There are two, in particular, which hamstrung telehealth's ability to thrive.

The first is a rule around patient relationships. Before the pandemic, many patients were not allowed to see doctors whom they had not previously seen in-person. This meant that if none of your existing providers offered telehealth (and hardly any did), a patient would have no way of even trying virtual care services.

The second is regarding how providers were paid for virtual care. Many payors, public and private alike, either held back reimbursements for healthcare services delivered virtually, or only offered very low reimbursement rates. In addition to their role as caregivers, doctors are also rational economic actors. Without payment and coverage parity, there was no financial incentive for providers to offer these virtual services, and so telehealth was relegated to a fringe phenomenon … until March of 2020.

TELEHEALTH'S WATERSHED MOMENT

When the COVID-19 pandemic overtook America, it changed the way we work, the way we live, and the way we engage with medical care. The urgency around this public health emergency did what decades of work hadn't done: it forced down the barriers that had long prevented the rapid adoption of telemedicine.

While the pandemic certainly increased demand, policy changes at state and federal levels are what actually enabled its rapid and broad adoption. Policymakers moved quickly to make sure that adoption wasn't hampered by longstanding regulatory hurdles around existing provider relationships, reimbursements, and insurance coverage.

On March 17, 2020, the Centers for Medicare and Medicaid Services released new guidelines that eliminated the 'prior relationship' rule. And quickly thereafter, payors – public and private alike – announced that they would offer payment and coverage parity for most virtual care services.

Once these policies changed, so did the market. Providers finally had the permission – and economic incentive – to welcome new patients to their practices virtually, and patients could have their first encounter with a new provider – covered by their insurance – from the comfort of their homes.

Concurrently, in New York City – where Zocdoc was founded and is headquartered – the COVID-19 pandemic surged. While stay-at-home orders were put in place in NYC and beyond, and the way Americans utilized healthcare changed rapidly, New Yorkers felt the acuteness and severity of the situation immediately and acutely. From the seemingly constant sounds of ambulances heading to hospitals across the city, to the cheers for essential workers at 7:00 each evening, to the frequent updates from public health officials, the city felt the weight of the global health crisis – and so did Zocdoc employees.

But while the pandemic certainly presented unprecedented business challenges to Zocdoc, the leadership team saw the severity of the COVID-19 crisis as a call to action. We moved quickly to a remote workforce, to protect the health and safety of our employees, and shifted all our resources to enabling people to continue seeing providers. In a company-wide email sent on March 4, 2020, Zocdoc's founder and CEO Oliver Kharraz, M.D., wrote:

> This is one of the critical moments where we must live our commitment to our Patients First value ... Continuing product development at Zocdoc as if this event was not happening is a failure to ourselves and our patients. We need to act with urgency to change our roadmap so we can get ahead of the needs of patients and the system.

This rapid change in direction allowed Zocdoc to quickly adapt its platform to support the sea change in needs for patients, providers, and the healthcare system as a whole: in April 2020, Zocdoc quickly introduced the ability for providers to offer bookings for video visits through our marketplace. This helped our nationwide network of providers keep their virtual doors open for business, while allowing patients to continue to access care, safely, from home. Then, in May 2020, we launched Zocdoc Video Service: a free, HIPAA-compliant video solution that any provider could use to facilitate their telehealth visits.

In short order, more than 10,000 providers across more than 100 specialties in 50 states were offering telehealth services through Zocdoc – a network on par with some of the large, legacy telehealth platforms. And virtually overnight, patients adopted this novel offering (Figures 15.1 and 15.2):

This volume of virtual care bookings gave us unmatched insight into users' booking behaviors and choices.

For example, we observed that nine out of ten patients who booked telehealth appointments chose an appointment at a scheduled time with the provider they preferred (just as they do when booking in-person care), versus an "on demand" model where they were randomly assigned doctor who could see them now, after waiting in a digital queue.

We also observed that when given a choice, most patients – about seven in 10 – make an appointment with a nearby doctor when booking a virtual visit. This implies that instinctively know that at some point, they'll want or need to physically be in the same room with their doctor. And they understand that choosing a local provider makes it possible to pick up the conversation in-person right where it left off online.

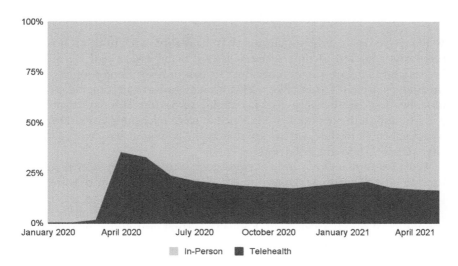

Figure 15.1 Overall percentage of telehealth and in-person appointments from May 2020–May 2021.

(Source: Zocdoc booking data)

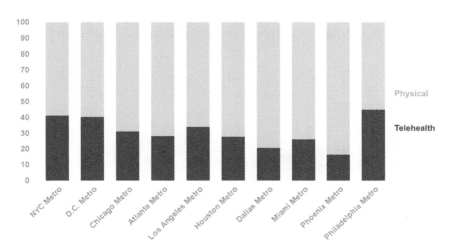

Figure 15.2 Percentage of telehealth bookings by region, April and May 2020.

(Source: Zocdoc booking data)

All of this pointed to the fact that people want an ongoing relationship with their providers, and further data reinforces the importance patients place on continuity of care.

TELEHEALTH'S NEW NORMAL

While we've reached the conclusion that the reality of telehealth is nuanced, there was a period of time when – despite being aware that we all have bodies and there are some things doctors can only examine properly when the body is present – it felt like telehealth was going to become the primary modality for care delivery. In May 2020, across the U.S., an astounding 33% of appointments booked via Zocdoc were telehealth visits! However, with the benefit of time, we can see that as the pandemic has evolved, so too have patients' booking behaviors.

When we took a closer look at trends, we were struck by how much utilization of telehealth services differed by specialty and healthcare need (Figure 15.3).

In particular, when Zocdoc evaluated data for patterns of online–office continuity of care (patients who booked a virtual visit with a new provider and then rebooked an in-person appointment at the same practice), there were three distinct groups of specialties.

The first group, which includes ENTs, podiatrists, OB-GYNs, and orthopedic surgeons, had a high likelihood of in-person rebooking; 50–60% of people who booked a virtual visit with a new provider in these specialties booked a second, in-person appointment, with that same practice.

The second group, which exhibited a medium likelihood of in-person rebooking, includes dermatologists, gastroenterologists, primary care physicians, and the average of all specialties excluding mental health. 20–30% of

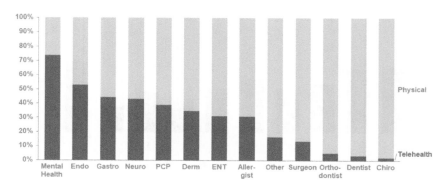

Figure 15.3 Percentage of in-person and telehealth appointments by specialty, May 2020.

(Source: Zocdoc booking data).

people who booked a virtual visit with a new provider in these specialties booked a second, in-person appointment, with that same practice.

Finally, mental health providers had the lowest likelihood of in-person rebooking; the conversational nature of these interactions – and the discretion, ease, and efficiency of talking to a therapist from home – lends itself to telehealth. Just ~5% of people who booked a telehealth appointment with a new mental health provider booked a second, in-person appointment with that same practice. Conversely, More than 95% of people who booked a virtual visit with a mental health provider booked a second, virtual appointment with that same practice.

In short, it's about what works for a particular specialty, not a one-size-fits-all solution. The through line is consistency of care, and a relationship with a particular provider, regardless of the type of appointment.

As of the time of writing this chapter, nearly 200 million Americans have received at least one dose of a COVID-19 vaccine. Many people have resumed their pre-pandemic activities, including returning to doctors' offices. As such, Zocdoc has seen in-person appointments surge and hold steady at around 85% – meaning that roughly 15% of appointments are conducted virtually. Internally, we expect telehealth to settle in between 10 and 20% of all care delivery.

In every specialty outside of mental health, we've seen a widespread return to physical care:

PERCENTAGE OF IN-PERSON APPOINTMENTS FROM MAY 2020 TO MAY 2021

- Primary Care Physician: 58% → 87%
- OB-GYN: 85% → 97%
- Dermatologist: 62% → 91%
- Dentist: 96% → 99%
- Optometrist: 92% → 100%
- Orthopedic Surgeon: 77% → 96%
- Podiatrist: 82% → 96%
- Chiropractor: 98% → 100%
- ENT: 64% → 95%
- Psychiatrist: 25% → 15%
- Ophthalmologist: 89% → 97%
- Gastroenterologist: 60% → 79%
- Urologist: 74% → 94%
- Pediatrician: 75% → 89%
- Allergist: 64% → 91%
- Cardiologist: 75% → 92%
- Neurologist: 52% → 86%
- Psychologist 20% → 13%

CONCLUSION

It's tempting to look at this data and conclude that telehealth is the Segway of medicine – a much-hyped innovation that failed to achieve long-term traction. The reality, however, is more nuanced. In-person appointments are surging, but at the same time, there are a number of areas where telehealth has caught on and is likely to stick.

Qualitatively, we have seen that telehealth is quite useful for certain kinds of consultations or triage. Doctors can do an initial assessment via video, asking questions about patients' symptoms and deciding whether a trip to the office is necessary. These virtual visits might also lead directly to a specialist referral, streamlining the process for both doctors and patients. And, telehealth is undoubtedly useful for patients located in rural areas that are often medically underserved.

There is also the potential to significantly improve the speed of access to healthcare. Right now, it takes an average of three weeks for someone to get an appointment for primary care. In contrast, 70% of in-person appointments booked on Zocdoc take place within three days and telehealth is making this waiting period even shorter.

Further, there are significant financial benefits to access in terms of reducing the cost of treatment. Imagine a world where people didn't have to go to a hospital to get an issue checked out, and instead, they could get medical advice or a prescription after a high-quality telehealth appointment. The opportunity for telehealth to improve the general care experience while reducing costs is huge.

So rather than the Segway, telehealth might be more like the X-ray. When electromagnetic imaging was first invented, the discovery led to a wide variety of uses, from optimizing shoe size in retail stores to recording tongue and teeth movement to studying languages. Eventually, the X-ray's primary value as a tool for specific diagnostic circumstances became apparent.

It is possible to incorporate telehealth into our care delivery system in a way that gives patients choice and power and strengthens the patient–provider relationship.

REFERENCES

Kharraz, O. The Pandemic boosted telehealth – but the future of health care is still in person. *Fortune*. July, 2021. https://fortune.com/2021/07/06/covid-telehealth-virtual-health-care-therapy-in-person-doctor-visits/ Accessed July, 2021.

Chapter 16

The COVID-19 pandemic and development of drugs and vaccinations

Pradeep S. B. Podila

Methodist Le Bonheur Healthcare

Memphis, TN, USA

CONTENTS

COVID-19 pandemic 244
Challenges created by COVID-19 pandemic 244
Preventative measures 245
    Social distancing 245
    Isolation 245
    Quarantine 246
    Contact tracing 246
Drugs and vaccines 246
    The basics 246
    Key similarities between drugs and vaccines 248
    Key differences between drugs and vaccines 248
Herd immunity and its significance 248
Vaccine development process 248
    Traditional vaccine development process 248
COVID-19 vaccine development process 251
Drug development – stages in clinical trials[11] 251
Emergency Use Authorization (EUA)[12] 252
COVID-19 vaccines 253
    Types of vaccines 253
    COVID-19 vaccines approved in the United States 254
        Pfizer/BioNTech/Fosun Pharma[13] 254
        Moderna/National Institutes of Health[13] 254
        Johnson & Johnson[13] 255
Other COVID-19 vaccine projects[12] 255
COVID-19 treatments[12] 256
Conclusion 260
References 261

DOI: 10.1201/9781003204138-20

COVID-19 PANDEMIC

The COVID-19 or coronavirus pandemic is an ongoing pandemic caused by severe acute respiratory syndrome coronavirus 2 (SARS-CoV-2). The disease was first identified in Wuhan, China, sometime around November/December 2019[1]. The initial lockdown efforts in Wuhan and the Hubei province failed and the virus very quickly spread throughout mainland China and around the world. Due to this the World Health Organization (WHO) declared COVID-19 an "outbreak" via Public Health Emergency of International Concern (PHEIC) on January 30, 2020 and "a pandemic" on March 11, 2020[2].

Infectious Disease Terms[3]

ENDEMIC – A disease or condition found among particular people or region.

OUTBREAK – A greater than expected increase in the number of endemic cases. A single case in a new region can be called an outbreak, and when not quickly controlled, an outbreak can become an epidemic.

EPIDEMIC – A disease or condition that impacts a large number of people within a community, population, or region.

PANDEMIC – An epidemic that has spread over multiple countries or continents.

The virus spreads by a human-to-human transmission through direct contact or by droplets. The incubation period (defined as the time from the first entry of the disease agent or virus (exposure) until the disease becomes apparent or symptomatic in the host[4]) is typically around five days but may range anywhere from a day to 14 days; and the propagation period for the infection has been projected to be within 2–14 days (Lei et al. 2020). Countries like the United States, Brazil, India, Russia, and South Africa were mostly infected whereas the other nations were not far behind them. Many variants of the virus have emerged and have quickly become dominant in many countries. The most virulent among them are – Delta, Alpha, and Beta. As of 30 September 2021, more than 233 million cases and 4.77 million deaths have been confirmed, making it one of the deadliest pandemics in history and even surpassed the 1918 Flu pandemic numbers.

CHALLENGES CREATED BY COVID-19 PANDEMIC

The virus is so contagious that it has been spreading every single day and has wreaked havoc on the lives of individuals and has caused a global, social, and economic disruption across various sectors (e.g., financial, healthcare, public health, airline, tourism, education). It changed people's life; people now have to stay indoors by choice or by the order of the government. The COVID-19 pandemic is fast moving, making some existing crisis plans unable to handle it and making businesses suffer greatly causing a significant drop in revenues forcing them to adjust their strategies and the ways in which they operate. Small and micro businesses suffered larger decline than medium and large businesses in business activity. Thus, the impact of the pandemic depends on the nature of the business, size, and complexity; furthermore, the diverse sectors are unevenly affected by COVID-19 pandemic.

The pandemic has stressed the importance of (a) better coordination between healthcare and public health sectors; (b) setting up the necessary public health infrastructure for quickly managing the ground-level efforts; (c) better planning and management of the supply-chain sector to ensure essentials were made available at every nook and corner of the world with a very quick turnaround; and (c) strategizing efforts toward establishing real-time data analytics for situational awareness and better coordination of activities.

PREVENTATIVE MEASURES

While the scientific community around the world is running against time to develop vaccines and drugs to protect the population, the general population would still need to rely on basic preventative measures such as (a) social distancing, (b) isolation, (c) quarantine, and (d) contact tracing as recommended best practices by governments via the public health agencies and healthcare systems to protect themselves from exposure to the virus.

Social distancing

Social distancing, also known as physical distancing is recommended as the best way to curb the spread of COVID-19. This is focused on avoiding non-essential travel and staying at home to reduce the exposure to the virus. Other practices suggested as a part of this are – (1) maintaining at least 6 feet distance with others, (2) avoiding gathering in groups (incl. family or known individuals), and (3) staying out of crowded places[5].

Isolation

Isolation separates sick people with a contagious disease from those who are not sick[6]. This is a great public health practice to protect the public by preventing exposure to people who have or may have a contagious disease. During isolation, it is recommended to (1) stay at home for 14 days after the last contact with a person suspected to be infected by COVID-19, (2) avoid contact during these 14 days with even the individuals within the same household, and (3) monitor for symptoms such as – fever/temperature, chills, body aches, cough, shortness of breath, sore throat, etc.

Quarantine

Quarantine separates and restricts the movement of people who were exposed to a contagious disease to see if they become sick[6]. These are usually those individuals who may have been exposed to the virus and not aware of it, or they may not show any symptoms even after being infected with the virus. During quarantine, it is recommended to (1) monitor for symptoms such as— fever/temperature, chills, body aches, cough, shortness of breath, sore throat, etc. (2) avoid contact with household members and pets, (3) if possible, use separate restrooms, (4) avoid sharing personal items, and (5) wear mask when around people.

Contact tracing

Contact tracing is used to quickly identify individuals who have been exposed to infectious disease (COVID-19, measles, Ebola, TB, and Sexually Transmitted Diseases (STDs)) and alert their contacts of their potential exposure[7]. The goal of contact tracing is to help prevent the further spread of infection, to identify hotspots of infection, and to protect friends, families, and communities from potential infection. The Personal Identifiable Information (PII) of the individuals who test positive (+) are kept confidential as per the guidelines under Health Insurance Portability and Accountability Act (HIPAA). The public health staff works with the individuals who are tested positive to help identify all those who came in contact with them while they were infectious so that the exposed individuals could be alerted via phone and directed to appropriate medical facilities for getting tested. The individuals would be instructed to self-quarantine to prevent the spread of the disease and follow appropriate social distancing practices. The individuals would be asked to check their temperature twice daily and monitor for symptoms and schedule a COVID-19 test before the end of their quarantine period.

DRUGS AND VACCINES

The basics

The following table highlights the key features related to drugs and vaccines[8].

Criteria	Drug	Vaccine
What is it?	A chemical, herbal or biological product used to diagnose, cure, treat or prevent disease. They affect the structure or any function of the body. A molecule that binds and neutralizes virus.	Vaccines are product that stimulates a person's immune system to produce immunity to a specific disease, protecting the person from that disease. A non-infectious virus and/or piece of virus your immune system will recognize.
What is the Goal?	Directly treat some infected with the virus. Drugs treat the infection by preventing spread to other parts of the body or even preventing symptoms while the body clears the infection itself.	Train a healthy immune system to protect from a future infection. The goal is to teach our immune system how to fight the disease causing germs.
Examples	Oseltamivir – prevents production of new influenza A, B particles Raltegravir – prevents integration of HIV genetic material into human chromosomes	Chickenpox vaccine – Live attenuated (weakened form of the germ) Polio vaccine – Inactive (dead form of the germ) Hepatitis B vaccine – Recombinant (specific piece of the germ) Tetanus vaccine – Toxoid (product made by the germ)
How are they administered?	Orally as tablets, capsules, suspensions (Intravenous), dermally, etc.	Usually through needle injections, but can also be administered orally (polio) or nasally.
How quickly does it work?	Immediately	1–2 weeks after vaccination
How long will the protection last?	Weeks to months	Years to lifetime (sometimes need booster doses to retain the effectiveness)
Components	Active ingredient Additives (binders such as starch) Lubricants (Aluminum) Disintegrants Colorants Sweeteners (liquid products) Preservatives (parenteral preparations) Others	Antigen (protein) – active ingredient Suspending fluid (sterile water, saline, or fluids containing protein) Preservatives and stabilizers (albumin, phenols, glycine) Adjuvants or enhancers that help improve vaccine's effectiveness Very small amounts of the culture materials used to grow the virus or bacteria used in the vaccine, such as chicken egg protein

Key similarities between drugs and vaccines

1. Like drugs, vaccines are also medical products
2. Both vaccines and drugs can cause adverse events
3. Both contain multiple ingredients
4. Both have the potential for interaction with disease, drugs, and other vaccines
5. Both have to comply with standards of safety, quality, and "efficacy" (efficacy for drugs and protective efficacy for vaccines)

Key differences between drugs and vaccines

1. Vaccines are almost always biological products, whereas drugs may be chemical or biological.
2. All vaccines require special conditions of storage (maintain the cold chain to keep them for getting damaged) whereas some chemical drugs do not usually require cold storage, but some biological drugs may require cold storage (e.g., insulin).
3. Vaccines are normally given in schedules to the whole population ("herd immunity") and/or age groups whereas drugs are targeted toward individuals.[4]

HERD IMMUNITY AND ITS SIGNIFICANCE

As mentioned in the earlier section, vaccines are usually administered to the whole population and/or targeted groups before they are exposed to the virus or the disease to reduce the spread of the virus or disease. Vaccines train the immune system to recognize and attack a virus, even one it hasn't seen before. The vaccinations which fall into the prevention category help reduce the number of susceptible individuals in the population. This protection is known as herd or community immunity[9]. In other words, herd immunity occurs when a large portion of a community (or herd) becomes immune to a virus or disease, making the spread of the virus or disease from person to person highly unlikely. As a result, the whole community (or herd) becomes protected – not just those who are immune. Figure 16.1 highlights the concept of herd immunity.

VACCINE DEVELOPMENT PROCESS

Traditional vaccine development process

The licensed vaccines that are currently available followed a five-stage linear process[10] (Figure 16.2) because of the involvement of high costs and risk of failure.

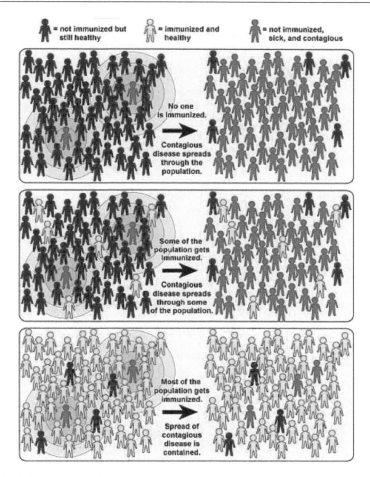

Figure 16.1 Immunity and contagious disease spread.

Stage#1 – Discovery research: Usually takes 2–5 years and involves lab-based research that involves exploring ways to induce an immune response at a molecular level.

Stage#2 – Pre-clinical stage: Takes up to 2 years and involves testing in animals to assess the safety and suitability of potential vaccines for humans.

Stage#3 – Clinical development: The potential vaccines are tested in humans. This has three phases:

- *Phase I – Safety tests:* Takes 2 years and requires 10–50 healthy individuals to participate in trials.
- *Phase II – Understanding the Immune response, safety and dosage:* Takes 2–3 years and requires hundreds of individuals to take part in randomized trials (placebo is administered for control group).

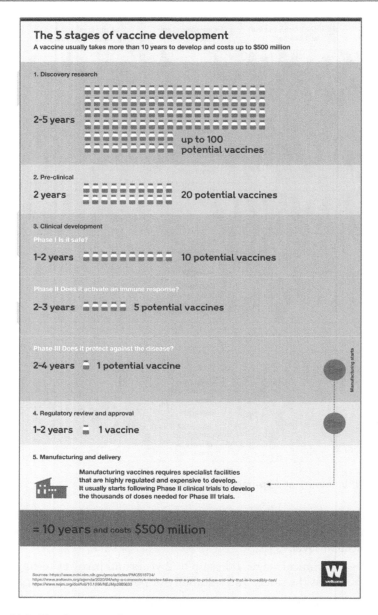

Figure 16.2 The 5 stages of vaccine development.

- *Phase III – Assessing if the vaccine safely protects against the disease:* Takes 5–10 years and requires thousands of people to take part in randomized trials (placebo administered for control group). The immune responses due to the vaccine under test are studied here.

Stage#4 - **Regulatory approval:** Takes about 2 years and involves submitting data and information on the vaccine's safety and efficacy to regulatory authorities for review and approval. Pharma companies continue to monitor effectiveness/safety after it has been licensed.

Stage#5 – **Manufacturing and delivery:** Require specialist facilities that are highly regulated and expensive to set up. This entire process takes about 10 years and $200–$300 million.

COVID-19 VACCINE DEVELOPMENT PROCESS

Given the gravity of the public health emergency generated by COVID-19, the larger scientific and research community had to find ways to speed up the vaccine development process (Figure 16.3) without compromising on testing and safety measures to curtail the spiking cases and mortalities.[10]

- To make the vaccine available faster, different stages of development and production were carried out at the same time. Many production sites were set up to ensure the manufacturing of regular vaccines for MMR and polio, and these are not impacted due to the production of COVID-19 vaccines.
- Vaccine trials were carried out around the world as well as using different innovations and technologies to increase the odds of finding vaccine candidates that are safe and effective for diverse population.

DRUG DEVELOPMENT – STAGES IN CLINICAL TRIALS[11]

Phase-1: The drug is given to a small number of healthy people and people with a disease to look for (a) side effects and (b) figure out the best dose.

Phase-2: The drug is given to higher number of people (usually, several hundred) who have the disease to identify (a) if it works, and (b) if there are any side effects that missed during the phase-1.

Phase-3: This is a large-scale randomized trial where the drug is administered to several hundred and at the same time a similar group of individuals are given a placebo (e.g., sugar pill). This usually goes on more than a few years to better gather evidence about (a) drug's performance and (b) common side effects.

Phase-4: Continuous monitoring of approved drugs is performed to make sure there are no other side effects, i.e., particularly serious or long-term ones.

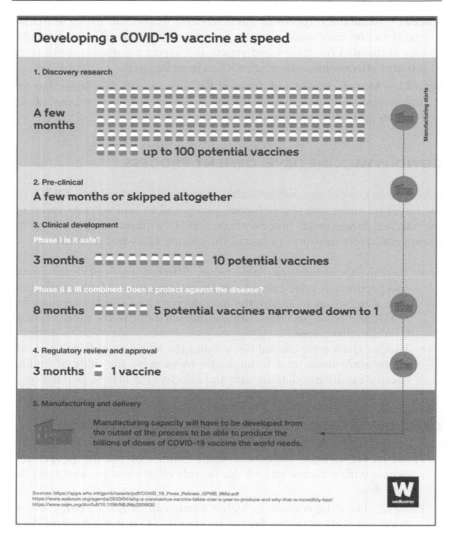

Figure 16.3 Developing a COVID-19 vaccine at speed.

EMERGENCY USE AUTHORIZATION (EUA)[12]

The Emergency Use Authorization (EUA) is a mechanism that allows Food and Drug Administration (FDA) to help strengthen the nation's public health protections against chemical, biological, radiological, and nuclear (CBRN) threats including infectious diseases, by facilitating the availability and use of medical countermeasures (MCMs) needed during public health emergencies. Under section 564 of the Federal Food, Drug, and Cosmetic Act (FD &C Act), when the Secretary of Health and Human Services (HHS) declares that an EUA is appropriate, the FDA may authorize unapproved medical products or unapproved uses of approved medical products to be used in an emergency to diagnose, treat, or prevent serious or life-threatening diseases or conditions caused by CBRN threat agents when certain criteria are met, including there are no adequate, approved, and available alternatives.

COVID-19 VACCINES

The scientific community around the world has started working on a number of vaccine candidates and treatments for COVID-19 as soon as the genetic sequence of the novel coronavirus was shared by the Chinese authorities on January 11, 2020. Several companies are working on antiviral drugs, some of which are already in use against other illnesses to treat people who have COVID-19.

Types of vaccines

There are three main types of COVID-19 vaccines that are authorized and recommended or undergoing large-scale (Phase 3) clinical trials in the United States.[13]

Vaccine type	What does it contain?	How does it work?
mRNA	Material from the virus that causes COVID-19 gives our cells instructions for how to make a harmless protein that is unique to the virus.	After our cells make copies of the protein, they destroy the genetic material from the vaccine. Our bodies recognize that the protein should not be there and build T-lymphocytes and B-lymphocytes that will remember how to fight the virus that causes COVID-19 if we are infected in the future.
Protein Subunit	Harmless pieces (proteins) of the virus that causes COVID-19 instead of the entire germ.	Once vaccinated, our bodies recognize that the protein should not be there and build T-lymphocytes and antibodies that will remember how to fight the virus that causes COVID-19 if we are infected in the future.
Vector	Modified version of a different virus than the one that causes COVID-19. Inside the shell of the modified virus, there is material from the virus that causes COVID-19. This is called a "viral vector."	Once the viral vector is inside our cells, the genetic material gives cells instructions to make a protein that is unique to the virus that causes COVID-19. Using these instructions, our cells make copies of the protein. This prompts our bodies to build T-lymphocytes and B-lymphocytes that will remember how to fight that virus if we are infected in the future.

COVID-19 vaccines approved in the United States

Pfizer/BioNTech/Fosun Pharma[13]

Drugmaker Pfizer teamed up with German biotech company BioNTech, and Chinese drugmaker Fosun Pharma to develop a two-dose mRNA vaccine. It was the first regulatory approval in the United States for a COVID-19 vaccine and the details are provided below:

- **Name:** BNT162b2
- **Brand name:** COMIRNATY
- **Manufacturer:** Pfizer, Inc., and BioNTech
- **Type of Vaccine:** mRNA
- **Number of Shots:** 2 shots, 21 days (3 weeks) apart
  - Moderately to severely immunocompromised people should get an additional shot (3rd dose) at least 28 days after their 2nd shot. Other groups of people are recommended to get a booster shot at least 6 months after getting their 2nd shot.
- **Dose Volume:** 0.3 ml
- **How Given:** Shot in the muscle of the upper arm
- **Full List of Ingredients:**
  - *Active ingredient:* Nucleoside-modified mRNA encoding the viral spike (S) glycoprotein of SARS-CoV-2
  - *Inactive ingredients:* 2[(polyethylene glycol (PEG))-2000]-N, N-ditetradecylacetamide, 1,2-distearoyl-sn-glycero-3-phosphocholine, Cholesterol, (4-hydroxybutyl)azanediyl)bis(hexane-6,1-diyl)bis(2-hexyldecanoate), Sodium chloride, Monobasic potassium phosphate, Potassium chloride, Dibasic sodium phosphate dehydrate, Sucrose

Moderna/National Institutes of Health[13]

The details are provided below:

- **Name:** mRNA-1273
- **Manufacturer:** ModernaTX, Inc.
- **Type of Vaccine:** mRNA
- **Number of Shots:** 2 shots, 28 days (1 month) apart. Some immunocompromised people should get 3 shots
- **Dose Volume:** 0.5 ml
- **How Given:** Shot in the muscle of the upper arm
- **Full List of Ingredients:**
  - *Active ingredient:* Nucleoside-modified mRNA encoding the viral spike (S) glycoprotein of SARS-CoV-2
  - *Inactive ingredients:* PEG2000-DMG: 1,2-dimyristoyl-rac-glycerol, methoxypolyethylene glycol; 1,2-distearoyl-sn-glycero-3-phosphocholine; Cholesterol; SM-102: heptadecan-9-yl

8-((2-hydroxyethyl) (6-oxo-6-(undecyloxy) hexyl) amino) octano-
ate; Tromethamine; Tromethamine hydrochloride; Acetic acid;
Sodium acetate; Sucrose

Johnson & Johnson[13]

The details are provided below:

- **Name:** JNJ-78436735
- **Manufacturer:** Janssen Pharmaceuticals Companies of Johnson &
  Johnson
- **Type of Vaccine:** Viral Vector
- **Number of Shots:** 1 shot
- **Dose Volume:** 0.5 ml
- **How Given:** Shot in the muscle of the upper arm
- **Full List of Ingredients:**
  - *Active ingredient:* Recombinant, replication-incompetent Ad26
    vector, encoding a stabilized variant of the SARS-CoV-2 Spike (S)
    protein
  - *Inactive ingredients:* Polysorbate-80; 2-hydroxypropyl-ß-cyclo-
    dextrin; Citric acid monohydrate; Trisodium citrate dehydrate;
    Sodium chloride; Ethanol

OTHER COVID-19 VACCINE PROJECTS[12]

Name	What is the vaccine based on?
AstraZeneca / University of Oxford	Chimpanzee adenovirus, which shuttles coronavirus proteins into cells. WHO has approved a EUA to distribute this vaccine worldwide.
Inovio	Potential vaccine is based on the existing work on a DNA vaccine for MERS, which is caused by another coronavirus
Sanofi / Translate Bio	mRNA vaccine Preclinical testing showed that the vaccine could elicit a strong immune response in mice and monkeys
CanSino Biologics	An adenovirus known as Ad5 to carry coronavirus proteins into cells
Gamaleya Research Institute	Includes two adenoviruses, Ad5 and Ad26
Sanofi / GSK / TranslateBio	Two vaccines are being developed: 1. Working with drugmaker GSK on a vaccine based on proteins from the coronavirus. When combined with another compound, called an adjuvant, the proteins elicit an immune response 2. Working with biotech company Translate Bio to develop an mRNA vaccine

(*Continued*)

Name	What is the vaccine based on?
Novavax (Received up to $388 million in funding this spring from the Coalition for Epidemic Preparedness Innovations (CEPI), a group that has funded COVID-19 vaccine development)	Virus proteins attached to microscopic particles
University of Queensland in Australia / CSL	Based on growing viral proteins in cell cultures
Wuhan Institute of Biological Products / Sinopharm	An inactivated virus vaccine developed by Wuhan Institute of Biological Products
Beijing Institute of Biological Products / Sinopharm	An inactivated virus vaccine developed by Beijing Institute of Biological Products
Sinovac Biotech	Inactivated virus vaccine
Bharat Biotech / Indian Council of Medical Research / Indian National Institute of Virology	Inactivated virus vaccine

COVID-19 TREATMENTS[12]

Name of drug/Name of manufacturer	Details
Antivirals (These are preventative drugs that help body fight off certain viruses that can cause disease.)	
Remdesivir (brand name Veklury)	This drug failed in clinical trials against Ebola in 2014, but was found to be generally safe in people. Research with MERS, a disease caused by a different coronavirus, showed that the drug blocked the virus from replicating. A study published in the New England Journal of Medicine showed that this drug shortened the hospital stay of COVID-19 patients by about 5 days. People taking this drug also had a lower risk of dying compared to those who had been given an inactive control substance. A study published in The Lancet reported that participants in a clinical trial who took this drug showed no benefits compared to people who took a placebo.

Name of drug/Name of manufacturer	Details
	The preliminary results from a WHO trial found that this drug had little effect on how long people stayed in the hospital and no effect on their risk of dying.
	This drug is also being tested in many COVID-19 clinical trials around the world, including in combination with other drugs such as interferon beta-1a and a highly concentrated solution of antibodies.
	Eli Lilly announced that in early stage trials their anti-inflammatory drug baricitinib when added to this drug can shorten hospital stays by 1 day for people with COVID-19.
Olumiant (baricitinib)	Used to treat rheumatoid arthritis and other conditions that involve overactive immune systems.
	The drug is also being tested in children with moderate to severe COVID-19.
	FDA issued EUA to use the baricitinib–remdesivir combination therapy for treatment on hospitalized adults and children who need supplemental oxygen.
	Another study concluded that remdesivir provided no clinical benefit to people hospitalized with COVID-19 and may have actually extended their stay in the hospital.
AT-527	Developed by Boston biotech Atea Pharmaceuticals and is being developed in partnership with drugmaker Roche.
	The drug is tested in people hospitalized with moderate COVID-19.
	There are plans to test this drug outside the hospital setting to see if it can work in people recently exposed to the coronavirus.
EIDD-2801	Developed by scientists at a not-for-profit biotech company owned by Emory University.
	Research in mice has shown that it can reduce replication of multiple coronaviruses, including SARS-CoV-2.
	This drug can be taken orally, which would make it available to a larger number of people.
Favipiravir (brand name Avigan)	Manufactured by Japanese company Fujifilm Toyama Chemical Co., Ltd. is approved in some countries outside the United States to treat influenza.
	Testing is underway around the world in people with mild or moderate COVID-19.
	Canadian researchers are testing to see whether the drug can help fight outbreaks in long-term care homes.
	The condition of COVID-19 patients taking the drug improved after 12 days on average versus more than 14 days on average for people taking an inactive placebo.

(Continued)

Name of drug/Name of manufacturer	Details
Fluvoxamine	Drug is used to treat people with obsessive/compulsive disorder. A study with 152 participants reported that the medication was effective in easing symptoms of COVID-19. Another study indicated fluvoxamine could help prevent mild COVID-19 symptoms from becoming worse.
Kaletra	This is a combination of two drugs – lopinavir and ritonavir – that work against HIV. The results of using this combination were found to be mixed. Did not improve outcomes in people with mild or moderate COVID-19 compared to those receiving standard care. The study was not effective for people with severe COVID-19. A study published in Lancet found that people who were given lopinavir/ritonavir along with two other drugs – ribavirin and interferon beta-1b – took less time to clear the virus from their body. Another study found that the drug combo did not reduce the risk of dying, length of hospital stay, or need for mechanical ventilation in COVID-19 patients.
Merimepodib (VX-497)	Developed by ViralClear Pharmaceuticals Inc. has been previously shown to have antiviral and immune-suppressing effects. It was tested against hepatitis C but had only modest effects. People with advanced COVID-19 were randomized to receive either merimepodib with remdesivir, or remdesivir plus a placebo. The phase 2 trial ended after there were concerns about the drug's safety.
Niclosamide	Developed by ANA Therapeutics. The drug has been used for more than 50 years to treat tapeworms. Studies showed the drug had antiviral and immune-modulating activities.
Umifenovir (brand name Arbidol)	This was tested along with the drug lopinavir/ritonavir as a treatment for COVID-19. The three-drug combination didn't improve the clinical outcomes for people hospitalized with mild to moderate cases of COVID-19. A review of 12 studies found that this drug didn't improve outcomes in people with COVID-19.

Name of drug/Name of manufacturer	Details
Monoclonal antibodies (These are laboratory-made proteins that mimic the immune system's ability to fight off harmful pathogens such as viruses.)	
AstraZeneca	A study will be examining whether the drug can provide protection for up to 12 months. The drug is made of two antibodies discovered by Vanderbilt University Medical Center (VUMC), isolated from the blood of a couple from Wuhan, China.
Celltrion (South Korean Company)	Monoclonal antibody treatment - CT-P59. It is being tested in people who have been in close contact with a person with COVID-19 to see whether the drug can prevent infection.
Edesa Biotech Inc.	Monoclonal antibody drug – EB05. Tests will be conducted to see if the drug could reduce the overactive immune responses associated with acute respiratory distress syndrome (ARDS).
Eli Lilly	The treatment was given to people with COVID-19 who hadn't been hospitalized. The results were published in the New England Journal of Medicine (NEJM). People who received the antibodies had significantly reduced virus levels after 11 days. They also had slightly less severe symptoms compared to participants who received an inactive placebo. NIH paused phase-3 trial over potential safety concerns. The drug was being tested in combination with the antiviral remdesivir.
Regeneron Pharmaceuticals Inc.	A two-antibody combination is being tested in four groups: (1) those hospitalized with COVID-19; (2) those with symptoms of the disease but not hospitalized; (3) healthy individuals at high risk for getting sick with COVID-19; and (4) healthy people who have had close contact with someone with COVID-19. A study revealed that the antibody combination reduced the risk of death for people hospitalized with COVID-19 who don't mount an immune defense on their own. The antibody cocktail is being used to help treat people who have been vaccinated but still become ill with COVID-19.
Sorrento Therapeutics	A preprint study found that the antibody protected Syrian golden hamsters that were infected with SARS-CoV-2.
Vir Biotechnology	Has isolated antibodies from people who survived SARS, a disease caused by another coronavirus.

(Continued)

Name of drug/Name of manufacturer	Details
Immune Modulators (These are class of drugs that help to activate, boost, or restore normal immune function after HIV has damaged the immune system.)	
Dexamethasone	This is an inexpensive corticosteroid and approved for other conditions and can be given orally or intravenously. Preliminary results published in NEJM found that a moderate dose of this drug reduced death in people hospitalized with COVID-19 on a ventilator and people receiving supplemental oxygen but not on a ventilator.
Other drugs (Baricitinib, a drug for rheumatoid arthritis, and IL-6 inhibitors.)	Eli Lilly announced that baricitinib in combination with remdesivir reduced recovery time and improved clinical outcomes in people with COVID-19. The largest benefits were seen in those receiving supplemental oxygen or noninvasive ventilation. NIH has started a phase 3 trial of three immune modulators: infliximab, developed by Johnson & Johnson; abatacept, developed by Bristol Myers Squibb; and cenicriviroc, developed by AbbVie. The FDA has also approved a device that filters cytokines out of the blood of people with COVID-19.
Convalescent plasma therapy (Uses blood from people who've recovered from an illness to help others recover.)	
Convalescent plasma therapy	A phase 2 trial published in The BMJ in October found that this treatment didn't prevent people from developing severe COVID-19 or reduce their risk of dying.
Stem cells (These are cells with the potential to develop into many different types of cells in the body.)	
Athersys Inc.	Trials are underway to examine whether the stem cell treatment could potentially benefit individuals with ARDS.
Mesoblast	Trials are underway to examine whether the stem cell treatment could potentially benefit individuals with ARDS.

CONCLUSION

The COVID-19 pandemic has changed the world and put the governments under stress test and challenged the scientific community to race against time to identify treatments to curtail the spiking cases and deaths from the virus. While many of the vaccines and drugs are still a work in progress at least this stressful scenario has highlighted that the vaccinations could be developed at a much faster pace without comprising on the safety standards to save the lives of individuals across the globe.

REFERENCES

1 https://en.wikipedia.org/wiki/COVID-19_pandemic
2 World Bank. 2020a. "Air Transport, Passengers Carried." Accessed August 8, 2021. https://data.worldbank.org/indicator/is.air.psgr
3 https://intermountainhealthcare.org/blogs/topics/live-well/2020/04/whats-the-difference-between-a-pandemic-an-epidemic-endemic-and-an-outbreak/
4 Fleming S.T. Managerial Epidemiology, Cases and Concepts, 3rd Edition. (2015).
5 https://www.redcross.org/about-us/news-and-events/news/2020/coronavirus-what-social-distancing-means.html
6 https://www.hhs.gov/answers/public-health-and-safety/what-is-the-difference-between-isolation-and-quarantine/index.html
7 https://dph.georgia.gov/contact-tracing
8 https://isoponline.org/wp-content/uploads/2015/10/Differences-on-drugs-and-vaccines.pdf
9 https://www.nih.gov/about-nih/what-we-do/science-health-public-trust/perspectives/science-health-public-trust/building-trust-vaccines
10 https://wellcome.org/news/quick-safe-covid-vaccine-development
11 https://www.healthline.com/health-news/heres-exactly-where-were-at-with-vaccines-and-treatments-for-covid-19#Clinical-trial-stages
12 https://www.fda.gov/emergency-preparedness-and-response/mcm-legal-regulatory-and-policy-framework/emergency-use-authorization
13 https://www.cdc.gov/coronavirus/2019-ncov/vaccines/different-vaccines/how-they-work.html

Chapter 17

Value of health information exchanges to support public health reporting

Pradeep S. B. Podila

Methodist Le Bonheur Healthcare

Memphis, TN, USA

CONTENTS

Learning objectives..264
Setting the context..264
Data as the institutional asset..264
Governmental support 265
Healthcare data: Utility and challenges 265
    Gaps in transitions of care 265
Public health is more than about saving money...267
Public health surveillance 267
Health information exchange (HIE) 268
    The focal points of HIE and services offered.....................................268
    Health information exchange models...269
        Federated models 269
        Non-federated models...269
    Common data models (CDMs): Definition, history, utility
        and steps in the process...272
    Key principles related to CDMs 274
    How do the CDMs foster public health surveillance/
        population health efforts? 275
Examples of HIEs work during the COVID-19 pandemic[10, 11] 276
    San Diego Health Connect (SDHC) 276
    Nebraska Health Information Initiative (NEHII) 276
    Indiana Health Information Exchange (IHIE) 276
    Reliance eHealth Collaborative 277
    Arizona's statewide HIE 277
    California's HIE..277
    Other use cases 277
Conclusion..278
References..278

DOI: 10.1201/9781003204138-21

LEARNING OBJECTIVES

1. The necessity of healthcare data for public health efforts.
2. A detailed overview of HIEs.
3. Use-cases of how HIEs have supported ground-level efforts during COVID-19 pandemic.

SETTING THE CONTEXT

The widespread adoption[1] of electronic health records (EHRs), supported by the financial initiatives from the federal government and an exponential increase in the use of consumer electronics like iPhones, and wearable devices has resulted in the continuous generation of electronic health data. EHRs allow for a systematic collection and management of an individual's health information in a form that can be shared across healthcare settings and can help inform public health. About eighty percent of the information collected during healthcare visits is currently documented in electronic format within EHRs. For example, EHRs contain many key variables that can help with public health emergencies. Although EHRs have their own shortcomings they can support with data for studies that inform key public health decisions during the times of emergencies and outbreaks.

For example, a timely availability of information from such data assets for use by hospitals, federal or state entities, and public health agencies (PHAs) is key component for chalking out healthcare/public health strategic visioning and planning preventative and public/population health efforts; and emergency preparedness activities during pandemics such as severe acute respiratory syndrome coronavirus 2 (SARS-CoV-2), i.e., COVID-19. Hence, the utilization of a large number of records from multiple healthcare entities could help provide mission-critical answers to physicians, caregivers, researchers, administrators, public health officials; fill the gaps; and inform the government to better chalk out the strategies.

DATA AS THE INSTITUTIONAL ASSET

Data is considered as a valued asset by many institutions due to its inherent nature to help identify key information and craft strategies for actionable intelligence or insights. Hence, it can also be referred to as the currency of the modern world (or) as the new earth as unless explored valuable resources such as minerals, and fertile lands for crops which are essential for the existence and survival of the humans couldn't be easily found. The ability to tap into the resources to draw insights from data can serve as the ultimate deciding factor as to whether an organization succeeds or fails in meeting the expectations of its customer base.

GOVERNMENTAL SUPPORT

The Health Information Technology for Clinical Health (HITECH) provisions of the bipartisan American Reinvestment and Recovery Act (ARRA) of 2009 provided the largest single national investment and commitment to setting up health information infrastructure. About 38 billion dollars were made available as financial incentives for healthcare systems and physicians to adopt EHRs, and more than 560 million dollars were made available to states to build capacity for health information exchange, within and across state borders, in coordination with state Medicaid and public health programs and health systems.

HEALTHCARE DATA: UTILITY AND CHALLENGES

The data generated by healthcare institutions or hospital systems not only helps the respective institutes where it's been originally collected for carrying out day-to-day business operations as well as supporting health services research and population health efforts but also serves as a great resource for governmental organizations such as the federal or state or local public health agencies in better understanding the needs of the population in those focused regions as well as disease registries in keeping track of the progression of conditions such as cancer, and health vulnerabilities. In other words, the utility of healthcare data goes beyond assisting the parent organization in generating revenue by adding value from a societal aspect.

Gaps in transitions of care

A typical patient is treated by multiple physicians in multiple settings for several comorbid conditions. They are often responsible for coordinating their own care, seeking providers who belong to different delivery systems and are unaware of any given provider's actions thereby receiving needless duplicative clinical workups as a result. According to NEJM about 16 physicians coordinate care for chronic conditions for one patient. Between 42% and 70% of Medicare patients admitted to the hospital received services from a mean of 10 or more physicians during their stay. AHRQ reports that 42% patients routinely fall between the cracks in transfers and have significant problems in information exchange. One in five discharged patients have an adverse event within 3 weeks, missing information necessary for ensuring discharge compliance.

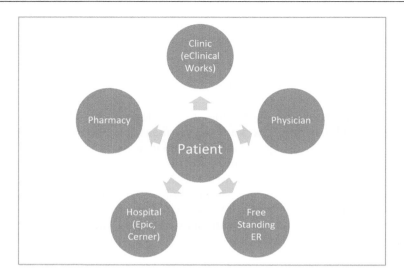

But, the rate at which the data is growing due to the multitude of touch-points and devices that capture the key information during an individual's healthcare encounter is *many fold greater* than the rate at which it could be shared outside of the healthcare entity where it was generated for health services research/population health and/or public health research and surveillance purposes. This is because of the sensitivity that comes with the healthcare data. *Data security* has become the number one priority for healthcare organizations, especially in the wake of an increased number of hacking episodes, ransomware attacks, and high profile data breaches. In addition to this, healthcare also deals with an infinite array of vulnerabilities such as – phishing attacks, malware attacks and thefts of laptops and electronic devices with patient identifiable information (PII) or protected health information (PHI) has not only made healthcare entities as well as federal government bring in more stringent rules to protect the information of an individual.

The Health Insurance Portability and Accountability Act (HIPAA) Security Rule comes with a very long list of necessary technical safeguards for organizations storing PII/PHI in addition to data transmission, security authentication protocols, access controls and audit checks, and integrity checks to ensure information is not tampered with. In spite of all such efforts, the fallibility of humans (staff members) in handling sensitive information and adhering to best practices can complicate matters by resulting in security breaches. Due to this healthcare institutes and hospital systems have been so used to keeping their institutional data close to their chest and always go through serious considerations and essential data governance protocols and procedures such as business associate agreements (BAAs) and data use agreements (DUAs) or data sharing agreements (DSAs) before sharing any sensitive or non-sensitive institutional information outside of their four walls.

PUBLIC HEALTH IS MORE THAN ABOUT SAVING MONEY

Public health is the science of protecting and improving the health of people and their communities. This work is achieved by promoting healthy lifestyles, researching disease and injury prevention, and detecting, preventing, and responding to infectious diseases. Overall, public health is concerned with protecting the health of entire populations. These populations can be as small as a local neighborhood, or as big as an entire country or region of the world. Public health benefits when the health outcomes of the populations increase and costs decrease.

PUBLIC HEALTH SURVEILLANCE

Public health surveillance is considered to be an essential public health function and the best weapon to avert epidemics. It is an ongoing, systematic collection, analysis, interpretation, and dissemination of data regarding a health-related event for use in public health action to reduce morbidity and mortality and to improve health. Data disseminated by a public health surveillance system can be used for immediate public health action, program planning and evaluation, and formulating research hypotheses. For example, data from a public health surveillance system can be used to:

1. guide immediate action for cases of public health importance;
2. guide the planning, implementation, and evaluation of programs to prevent and control disease, injury, or adverse exposure;
3. measure the burden of a disease (or other health-related event), including changes in related factors, the identification of populations at high risk, and the identification of new or emerging health concerns;
4. monitor trends in the burden of a disease (or other health-related event), including the detection of epidemics (outbreaks) and pandemics;
5. evaluate public policy;
6. detect changes in health practices and the effects of these changes;
7. prioritize the allocation of health resources;
8. describe the clinical course of disease; and
9. provide a basis for epidemiologic research.

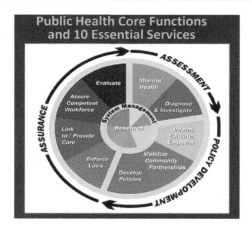

Public health surveillance activities are generally authorized by legislators and carried out by public health officials. Public health surveillance systems have been developed to address a range of public health needs. In addition, public health information systems have been defined to include a variety of data sources essential to public health action and are often used for surveillance. These systems vary from a simple system collecting data from a single source, to electronic systems that receive data from many sources in multiple formats, to complex surveys. The number and variety of systems will likely increase with advances in electronic data interchange and integration of data, which will also heighten the importance of patient privacy, data confidentiality, and system security. Appropriate institutions/agencies/scientific officials should be consulted with any projects regarding public health surveillance.

HEALTH INFORMATION EXCHANGE (HIE)

Health Information Exchange is the process of sharing electronic health-related information which is consistent and interoperable by giving due importance to the aspects of data confidentiality, privacy, and security of the information. It is the electronic mobilization of healthcare information across organizations, communities, or regions. HIEs are often referred by other terms such as Nationwide Health Information Network (NHIN), community health information network (CHIN), etc.

The focal points of HIE and services offered

Uncoordinated care between healthcare providers results in ineffective, inefficient and unsafe care. The fragmented nature of care as well as the lack of a national patient identifier (NPI) makes the records look disjointed as during the care continuum individuals have encounters across various healthcare facilities. The HIE infrastructure helps share the information between two diverse organizations while complying with the standards mandated by the Office of National Coordinator for Health Information Technology (HIT). The services offered by HIE are—(1) integration of clinical services (viewing patient related information and querying and retrieving of information); (2) exchange of medical images and secure messaging services (HIPAA compliant email, and share trusted information via web portals).

Health information exchange models

The HIEs can be separated into two major categories, i.e., federated models, and non-federated models.

Federated models

- Shared databases: A series of databases belong to diverse organizations connected via internet.
- Peer-to-peer network: In this diverse organizations maintain their own health data which is queried by a common querying system based on a common data model (CDM) structure.

Non-federated models

- Cooperation model: In this a small group of community hospitals or systems and exchange information via direct communication.
- Data warehouse: A central database contains the data and this is usually maintained by a HIE site.

HIE Name	Acronym	City	ST
Alabama One Health Record		Montgomery	AL
Arkansas Office of HIT (State Health Alliance Records Exchange)	SHARE	Little Rock	AR
Alaska eHealth Network		Anchorage	AK
Big Sky Care Connect	BSCC	Helena	MT
Bronx RHIO		Bronx	NY
Camden Coalition Health Information Exchange		Camden	NJ
Chesapeake Regional Information System for Patients DC	CRISP DC	Washington	DC
Chesapeake Regional Information System for Patients MD	CRISP MD	Columbia	MD
CIE San Diego		San Diego	CA

HIE Name	Acronym	City	ST
ClinicalConnect Health Information Exchange		Pittsburgh	PA
Coastal Carolina		Wilmington	NC
Colorado Regional Health Information Organization	CORHIO	Denver	CO
ConnectVirginia HIE	ConnectVirginia	Richmond	VA
Connie		Farmington	CT
CyncHealth		Omaha	NE
Delaware HIN	DHIN	Dover	DE
East Tennessee Health Information Network	etHIN	Knoxville	TN
Florida Health Information Exchange		Tallahassee	FL
Georgia Health Information Network	GaHIN	Atlanta	GA
Georgia Regional Academic Community Health Information Exchange	GRAChIE	Sandersville	GA
Greater Dayton Area HIN	GDAHIN	Dayton	OH
Greater Houston Healthconnect	GHH	Houston	TX
Greater New Orleans Health Information Exchange	GNOHIE	New Orleans	LA
Greater Newark Health Care Connect	GNHCC	West Orange County	NJ
Hawaii Health Information Exchange	HHIE	Honolulu	HI
Health Current		Phoenix	AZ
Healthcare Access San Antonio	HASA	San Antonio	TX
healtheConnect Alaska		Anchorage	AK
HealtheConnections		Syracuse	NY
HEALTHeLINK - Western NY		Buffalo	NY
HealtHIE Nevada		Las Vegas	NV
HealthInfoNet		Portland	ME
Healthix		New York	NY
Health Sciences South Carolina	HSSC	Columbia	SC
HealthShare Exchange	HSX	Philadelphia	PA
HIXNY		Albany	NY
Idaho Health Data Exchange	IHDE	Boise	ID
Indiana Health Information Exchange	IHIE	Indianapolis	IN
CyncHealth - Iowa Health Information Network	IHIN	West Des Moines	IA
Integrated Care Collaboration	ICC	Austin	TX

HIE Name	Acronym	City	ST
Kansas Health Information Network	KHIN	Topeka	KS
Kentucky Health Information Exchange	KHIE	Frankfort	KY
Keystone HIE	KeyHIE	Danville	PA
Los Angeles Network for Enhanced Services	LANES	Los Angeles	CA
Louisiana Health Care Quality Forum	LHCQF	Baton Rouge	LA
Manifest MedEx		Riverside	CA
Michigan Health Information Network	MiHIN	East Lansing	MI
Midwest Health Connect	MHC	Columbia	MO
MyHealth Access Network		Tulsa	OK
New Jersey Health Information Network	NJHIN	Newark	NJ
North Carolina HIE Authority	NC HIEA	Raleigh	NC
North Dakota HIN	NDHIN	Bismark	ND
NYU Langone Medical Center		New York	NY
Ohio Health Information Partnership (CliniSync)	OHIP	Hillard	OH
OneHealthPort		Seattle	WA
PHIX		El Paso	TX
Quality Health Network	QHN	Grand Junction	CO
Reliance eHealth Collaborative	Reliance	Medford	OR
Rhode Island Quality Institute	RIQI	Providence	RI
Rio Grande Valley Health Information Exchange	RGVHIE	Harlingen	TX
Rochester RHIO		Rochester	NY
SacValley MedShare		Fairfield	CA
San Diego Health Connect	SDHC	San Diego	CA
Santa Cruz HIO	SCHIO	Scotts Valley	CA
South Dakota Health Link		Madison	SD
St. Joseph Health		Anaheim	CA
Stony Brook University Hospital		Stony Brook	NY
SYNCRONYS		Albuquerque	NM
Texas Health Services Authority	THSA	Austin	TX
The Health Collaborative		Cincinnati	OH
Trenton Health Information Exchange		Trenton	NJ
UHIN		Murray	UT

(Continued)

HIE Name	Acronym	City	ST
Vermont Information Technology Leaders	VITL	Burlington	VT
West Virginia Health Information Network	WVHIN	Charleston	WV
Western Connecticut Health Network	WCHN	Bethel	CT
Wisconsin Statewide Health Information Network	WISHIN	Fitchburg	WI
Wyoming Frontier Information	WYFI	Cheyenne	WY

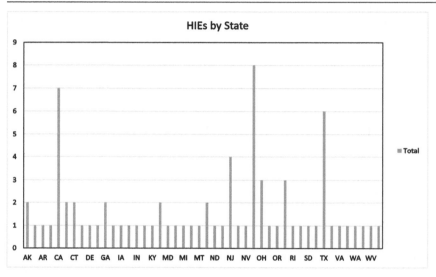

Common data models (CDMs): Definition, history, utility and steps in the process

Definition: A CDM aims to standardize the infrastructure so that many related applications can operate on same shared data in a federated model. So, it can be defined as "*a standard collection of entities, attributes, and relationships that represents business concepts and activities with well-defined semantics, to facilitate data interoperability.*"

History: The popular CDMs in healthcare dates back to 1990 with a collaborative project between the National Immunization Program (NIP) and the U.S. Centers for Disease Control and Prevention (CDC). This effort helped establish a CDM called the Vaccine Safety Datalink (VSD) Shared Data Network (SDN) with several large HMOs to investigate the safety of vaccines.[4]

Utility: A CDM is a way of organizing data into a standard structure and an essential task for multi-organizational collaborative research. The concept behind this approach is to transform data contained within those individual participating institutions databases into a common format (or DM) as well as a common representation (terminologies, vocabularies, coding schemes), and then perform systematic analyses using a library of standard analytic routines (using a platform of choice such as—SAS, R, Python) that have been written based on the common format.

Steps in the Process: Conforming to a CDM ensures that standardized applications and methods can be executed by distributing a query or code using a platform maintained by the hub or linkage unit in order to generate aggregated results from pooled data from participating organizations.

Let's take a look at an example (see Figure 17.1) of a HIE with three diverse organizations (Organization#1: Large Healthcare System with five hospitals, Organization#2: Standalone Hospital, and Organization#3: Psychiatry Clinic) with different EHR systems (Organization#1: Cerner EHR, Organization#2: Epic, and Organization #3: GE Centricity). These organizations have collaborated to support the patient population in the geographic region to address their physical and mental wellbeing. Now, let's take a look at the *administrative, technical*, and *operational* steps in the process.

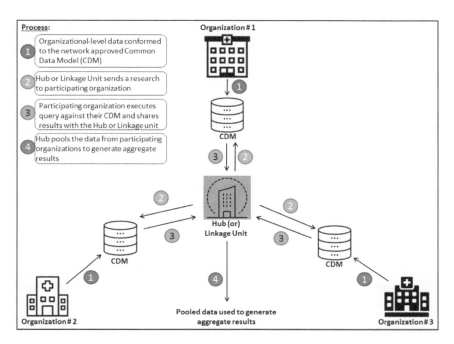

Figure 17.1 A federated model.

Administrative Steps: (a) As a part of the overall HIE governance process, the organizations developed a charter with agreed upon policies, procedures, and guidelines that would need to be followed in order to support the research questions that could be explored as a part of this multi-organizational collaborative. (b) Following the governance process, the collaborative forms a team of researchers to help identify more than a few research questions of interest.

Technical Steps: (a) The Information System (IS) departments at each of these three institutes would then propose the list of data elements that would need to be considered in order to explore the data to find valuable insights. (b) Following this, the IS departments would form a mini-workgroup to help share with each other as to how these elements are documented within each of their systems so that a CDM standard for the collaborative could be proposed to the research team. (c) After going through a rigorous iterative process, the mini-workgroup and the research team would propose their steps to the governance body.

Operational Steps: (a) Organizational data is conformed to the CDM approved by the collaborative. (b) A neutral institute such as a University or a Coordinating Center serves as a Hub or Linkage Unit to facilitate the operations. It sends the query related to the approved research question to the participating organizations using a common tool. (c) Participating organization(s) executes query against their respective institutional CDMs and shares results with the Hub or Linkage Unit. (d) Hub pools the data from participating organizations to generate aggregate results.

Key principles related to CDMs

Usually, the principles that govern the HIEs organically evolve over time and most often by learning from the best practices identified during the development and implementation of other HIEs and technological advancements. Data governance and data provenance are two most important pillars when it comes to the management of HIEs. While the former refers to what kind of data goes into the CDM and how it needs to be handled, the latter refers to the lineage or origin of a data element or a concept from other implemented DDNs. The following are a few principles related to CDMs:

1. **Alleviate privacy and security concerns. The concerns that usually come with privacy and security aspects of health data are alleviated by the *federated nature of the operational mechanism.*** The federated approach is the ability of individual participating institutes to develop the CDM behind the institutes firewall so that no individualized data is exposed to the external organizations. By doing this, more participants would be encouraged to become a part of the collaborative so that the

breadth and depth of the research questions could be expanded. In our earlier example, we have considered three organizations—a large healthcare system, a standalone hospital, and a psychiatric clinic. Now, if a fourth participant such as a pharmacy joins the collaborative then the research questions could be expanded to identify the healthcare utilization in patients with non-adherence to a strict psychiatric medication regimen.

2. **A clear primary purpose.** The primary purpose of the data populated within the CDM should be bound by a clear goal or approach; for example, to(a) foster collaborative research, (b) monitor disease surveillance, and (c) improve patient outcomes by drawing inferences from the knowledge gained from the pooling of the data from multiple participating institutions.

3. **A strict adherence to institutional governance policies.** The CDM and any related tools should strictly adhere to the governance rules set forth by the institution where it has been implemented by following the guidelines set forth by respective organization's Institutional Review Board (IRB) and any other federal/state privacy and data sharing regulations.

4. **Agnostic to source data systems.** The CDM should be agnostic to source data systems as they are defined by data concepts rather than data sources.

5. **Flexible and extensible to accommodate multiple institutes.** The CDM should be flexible and extensible to accommodate the interests and data sources of a wide range of participating institutions.

6. **Ability to easily adapt or clone.** The empty shells of the CDMs can be made available to the public or other institutions so that they could easily adapt or clone to meet their respective organizational needs or while onboarding to an existing collaborative.

How do the CDMs foster public health surveillance/ population health efforts?

In this section, let's take a look at a few scenarios to highlight how the CDMs can help foster both public heath surveillance and population health efforts.

1. **Estimate the burden of disease conditions.** For example, let's say a geographic region contained four diverse healthcare systems, and three of them that have a collective market share area (MSA) of 80 percent in the region have come together as a part of a DDN to collaborate on research efforts. By pooling the data from these three hospitals using their CDMs, a better estimate of the burden or prevalence of chronic disease conditions within the same geographical region could be identified.

2. **Increase the sample size of rare disease conditions.** As CDMs can pool the data from diverse organizations, they can really help researchers by increasing the sample size of individuals with rare disease conditions so that better treatment strategies could be developed.
3. **Assist public health agencies with surveillance efforts.** The prevalence estimates generated using CDMs could help inform the public health agencies in strategizing their localized preventative efforts.
4. **Perform external validation of prior studies.** As CDMs pool the data from multiple organizations, sometimes the research questions that have been solved by organizations in a different region could be tested for external validation purposes to reconfirm the results.

EXAMPLES OF HIES WORK DURING THE COVID-19 PANDEMIC[10, 11]

The following examples highlight how the HIEs have highlighted their importance during the COVID-19 pandemic to the community and both healthcare and public health agencies.

San Diego Health Connect (SDHC)

The San Diego Health Connect (SDHC) helped EMS personnel take appropriate precautions when they are on their way to the residence of a COVID-19 positive patient. This has helped with the safety of the staff when the personal protective equipment (PPE) were in short supply.

Nebraska Health Information Initiative (NEHII)

Nebraska Health Information Initiative (NEHII) launched COVID-19 alerts and reporting system to assist the Nebraska Department of Health and Human Services, healthcare organizations and medical professionals identify and prioritize patients at higher risk of contracting severe forms of the COVID-19 respiratory disease. This also helped in tracking the ICU bed utilization. The program also finds and tracks healthcare facility and ICU bed utilization.

Indiana Health Information Exchange (IHIE)

Indiana's HIE has implemented several critical activities as a part of the COVID-19 resource center. They are:

(1) Sending daily alerts of positive (+) and negative (−) COVID-19 tests from labs to LPHAs, (2) Updating a dashboard that displays counts of patients who are confirmed or suspected positive for COVID-19 and

conditions in that proximity, (3) Generating daily reports for State public health agencies on population who tested positive, and (4) Processing real-time lab results and distributing them to the hospitals that have the original specimen.

Reliance eHealth Collaborative

This HIE in the Pacific Northwest has been effectively agencies the health systems and public health agencies with information related to: (1) Reporting of symptoms and comorbidities, (2) Notification of COVID-19 results by utilizing textual data mining services, (3) aggregating the demographics data using record linkage approaches and filling the gaps in the missing critical information, (4) standardization and normalization of codes, (5) sharing the aggregated patient information with clinical end users across the community for dashboards.

Arizona's statewide HIE

The services offered by this statewide HIE are—(1) receive both positive and negative COVID-19 test results, (2) receive real-time or batch alters at designated times, and (3) push the lab test results into the EHR systems of participating organizations.

California's HIE

While the rest of the world was dealing with the COVID-19 crisis, California was also dealing with the spread of wildfires across the state. The HIEs within California helped connect communities and ensured that the patient medical records are accessible and available at all times so that the first responders, blood banks, and treatment centers can have access to the critical information. The HIEs also leveraged HIE's role as the data steward by seeking their assistance in ensuring that the duplicate medical records are properly sorted out.

Other use cases

In addition to the above examples, HIEs are also playing an important role by directing the encounter related information of individuals across the state lines to appropriate HIEs within the patient's geographical region so that the clinical provider of the patient can have all the relevant information at their disposal. They have also been helping health systems in gathering the data for conducting advanced analytics to monitor any outbreaks or endemic situations, and offering assistance to small healthcare providers who lack the capacity and capability to deal with technological advancements.

CONCLUSION

The primary focus of healthcare is to improve access of quality care at reduced costs while ensuring patient safety. HIEs as data mangers help achieve these goals by making sure that the health information needed by the healthcare facilities or hospitals and their partners are available at the time of need while adhering to appropriate data governance guidelines. Data governance is more than data management and is often referred to as data intelligence as it helps in appropriately handling the data by taken the accountability and role based access into consideration. HIEs as the data stewards play the role of honest broker and ensure that records are appropriate merged and missing demographic information is accurately filled using advanced patient matching methods.

REFERENCES

1 Magnuson JA, and Brian E. Dixon. *Public Health Informatics and Information Systems* (2020).
2 Popovic JR. *Distributed Data Networks: A paradigm shift in data sharing and healthcare analytics* (2015).
3 Weeks J, and Pardee, R. Learning to Share Health Care Data: A Brief Timeline of Influential Common Data Models and Distributed Health Data Networks in U.S. *Health Care Research* (2019).
4 Vaccine Safety Datalink (VSD). (n.d.) Retrieved from: https://www.cdc.gov/vaccinesafety/ensuringsafety/monitoring/vsd/index.html#objectives
5 HCSRN. (n.d.) Retrieved from: https://www.hcsrn.org/en/Tools%20&%20Materials/VDW/
6 OMOP. (n.d.) Retrieved from: https://ohdsi.github.io/CommonDataModel/cdm60.html#Changes_in_v60
7 PCORnet. (n.d.) Retrieved from: https://pcornet.org/wp-content/uploads/2020/12/PCORnet-Common-Data-Model-v60-2020_10_221.pdf
8 CHORDS. (n.d.) Retrieved from: https://www.phidenverhealth.org/health-data-statistics/chords
9 https://www.himss.org/news/times-crisis-hie-front-and-center
10 https://strategichie.com/covid-19/
11 https://ehrintelligence.com/news/how-public-health-crises-enhanced-health-information-exchange

Conclusion

Edward M. Rafalski

University of Illinois School of Public Health
Chicago, IL, USA

University of South Florida College of Public Health
Tampa, FL, USA

Ross M. Mullner

University of Illinois School of Public Health
Chicago, IL, USA

The COVID-19 pandemic, now in its fourth wave, has killed more than twice the number Americans than the 1918 Spanish Flu pandemic. Healthcare analytics have been invaluable in understanding the scope and scale of this public health disaster and much is yet to be learned. There are some known knowns, however (see Figure C.1). The United States knew that there would be another worldwide pandemic, yet, we seemed unprepared. We also knew that the public health system was frayed and lacked the resources to effectively manage a country-wide disaster. There were some known unknowns as well. We were unsure where the next pandemic would originate and we were unsure of the scale and duration. The world has become a much more

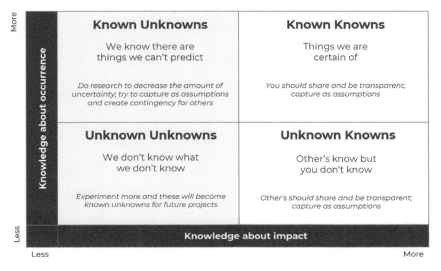

Figure C.1 Knowledge quadrants.

DOI: 10.1201/9781003204138-22

interconnected place with modern travel quickening the pace of transmission of disease yet the pace at which transmission occurs was unknown. There were some things where we did not know what we do not know, and still do not. For example, where did the COVID-19 virus originate and why? It is unclear if there were any unknown knowns, but, at some point those will become available as well.

Regardless of the knowns and unknowns, healthcare analytics have lept forward because of the pandemic. Modeling techniques have evolved and are now arguably much better at incidence and volume prediction. Access to more transparent data will continue to improve the accuracy of predictive modeling and consistent collection of that data will greatly enhance our ability to manage through a disaster. Innovation has occurred and science has lept forward in the understanding of vaccination development techniques. We continue to learn more about behavioral health and the long-term effects of social distancing will need to be understood. Each State in the Union provided its own lessons and those need to be documented and shared for future generations of healthcare professionals and policy makers. That perhaps is the charge going forward – to broaden this body of knowledge so that we may be better prepared for future pandemics and disasters.

Epilogue

Edward M. Rafalski

University of Illinois School of Public Health
Chicago, IL, USA
University of South Florida College of Public Health
Tampa, FL, USA

At the time of writing the pandemic has resulted 44.5 M cases and has claimed 715,000 lives. The United States (US) seems to be on the downward slope of the most recent Delta variant wave which has recently been the dominant strain. There have been multiple strains and waves/peaks since March of 2020. Most would agree that there have been at least three major peaks/waves and perhaps five depending on one's personal opinion (see Figure E.1). From our perspective, the first occurred in the early Spring 2020 when the United States went into shutdown to flatten the curve, the second during the Summer of 2020, the third during the Winter of 2021 and the fourth, most current Delta wave, in the Fall 2021.

There has been seasonality and regional variation to each wave of the pandemic with certain portions of the United States peaking with others

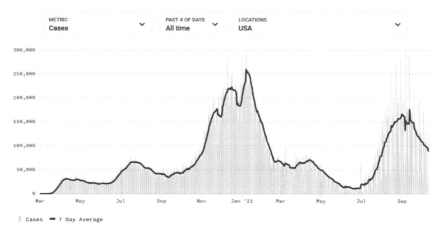

Figure E.1 National COVID-19 waves.

DOI: 10.1201/9781003204138-23

Risk levels

Risk is reduced for those who are vaccinated.

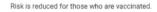

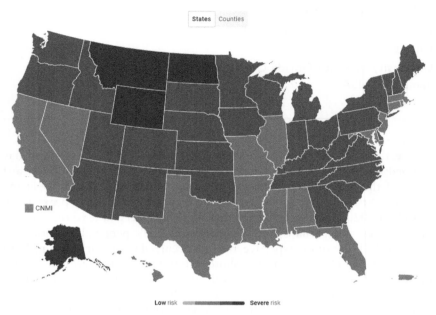

Figure E.2 National risk levels.

trending downward in incidence. Currently, the Upper Midwestern states and Alaska are experiencing higher incidence of the Delta variant. Partly this is due to the onset of colder weather, more people congregating indoors and loosening of restrictions and preventive measures. Further, some states are further along in reaching herd immunity in vaccination rates, such as those in the Northeast and California, where compliance has been greater than the remainder of the country. Last, some states have been more stringent in applying public health measures, such as masking in schools, while others have been more laissez-faire (Figure E.2).

Pfizer has been approved for its Pfizer-BioNTech booster vaccination and Moderna was approved by an FDA advisory panel on October 14, 2021 in a unanimous vote of 19 to 0. At this time the guidance given has been to provide booster vaccinations to those at higher risk such those over the age of 65 and those under the age of 65 with risk factors. The CDC is expected to endorse the additional Moderna dose before it becomes available to the general public. Other variants such as the Lambda and Mu strains are potentially on the horizon but have not taken hold in the United States in any significant way (Figure E.3).

There are six general observations that may be made regarding the pandemic in the United States at this time. First, the pandemic has polarized

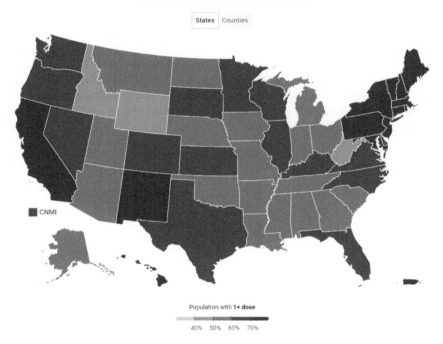

Vaccination progress

65% of the entire U.S. population has received **1+ dose**.

States | Counties

CNMI

Population with **1+ dose**

40%   50%   60%   70%

Figure E.3 National vaccination levels.

the nation. There has been a dynamic tension between public health aware-ness and reactionary policy at the government level. At the personal level, there has been a tension between the worried well abiding by vaccination as a significant tool for preventing disease and fatalists who prefer to take the risk that they will not be infected or that if infected, the body's natural defenses are designed to protect one from disease. Second, the pandemic has changed how people interact. Nowhere has this played out more than in the school setting with some jurisdictions leaving it up to the parent to deter-mine how to protect their child best to others taking more stringent mea-sures such as requiring proof of vaccination to attend school, or testing weekly if there is a religious or clinical reason to abstain from vaccination. Third, the pandemic has accelerated some trends that were in motion prior to the arrival of COVID-19 such as remote working, telehealth and online retail. This has been referred to by some as the "Great Reshuffling" in the case of remote working and the US economy has been transformed into a new normal state affecting how employers will evolve with their respective workforces. Fourth, the pandemic has exposed the weaknesses of the public health system most evidenced by a lack of coordination at all levels of government, from local municipalities, to cities, to states and the federal government. Faults in the public health ecosystem have been exposed, such as the inability to uniformly test and contact trace. Fifth, there has been a failure in the media to distill conflicting information and provide a common source of truth. Perhaps this is a function of the immediate news cycle and the proliferation of subject matter experts on the internet? The opportunity to educate the public on the fundamentals of public health disease prevention was missed. Sixth, the quality of accessible data for analysis has been a challenge; although, it has gotten better as the pandemic has progressed. Having a central source of data truth would be an aspirational goal for future health crisis preparation.

Index

1918 Spanish Flu, 279

A

Accountable Care Organizations, 222
Accountable Care Team, 82
ADC, 49, 54, 187–191
ALOS, 36, 188
Amazon, 67, 229
American College of Healthcare, 79, 80
American Medical Association, 86, 88, 91, 146, 152
American Psychological Association, 199
American Reinvestment and Recovery Act, 265
anthrax, 17
anxiety, 96–98, 196, 199
Arizona's statewide HIE, 277
Arkansas, 167

B

bacterial, 19
behavioral health, 29, 195, 198–199, 203, 214
Big Data, 199, 212–213
BioNTech, 52, 254, 282
bubonic plague, 9, 17, 19
business associate agreements, 267

C

California, 110, 205, 209, 277
California's HIE, 277
CardioSmart, 99
case date, 118, 120, 122–124
case fatality rate, 36

CDC, 10, 14, 37, 90, 93, 108–109, 132–134, 162, 171, 198–199, 213, 227–228, 272, 282
CDPH, 144, 147, 154, 226–229
Center on Budget and Policy Priorities, 198
Centers for Disease Control and Prevention, 10, 37, 108, 272
Centers for Medicare and Medicaid Services, 237
Cerner, 229, 273
CFR, 36
Chartis, 48, 55
Chicago, 47, 54, 144, 146, 148, 150, 152–153, 155–157, 159, 187, 204, 221, 224–225, 228–230
Chicago Cook Workforce Partnership, 155
Chicago Department of Public Health, 152, 155, 159n6, 221, 228
Chicagoland Vaccine Partnership, 155–156
China, 19, 36, 179–180, 182
Cholera, 21, 22, 47
CMIO, 228
CMO, 228
Colorado, 89–102, 270
Columbia, 54
common data model, 269, 272, 276
community health information network, 268
contact tracing, 245–246
continuum, 27–28, 32, 34, 178, 182
Cornell, 54
coronavirus, 9, 25, 35, 49, 90, 108–109, 118–119, 134, 137–138, 167, 199
Coronavirus Aid, Relief, and Economic Security, 63

COVID Act Now, 47, 51
COVID-19, 9–12, 14–15, 18, 26, 28,
        31–32, 36–37, 43–44, 47,
        49–53, 57, 62–68, 94–97,
        99, 101–102, 107–139, 144,
        146, 148, 150, 152–153,
        155–159, 161–172, 177–180,
        182–185, 187–189, 192,
        195–196, 198–199, 201–204,
        206–210, 212–214, 219–230,
        235–238, 241, 243–260, 264,
        276–281, 283
COVID-19 Community Vulnerability
        Index, 154
cumulative case count, 121, *122*
CVS, 67

D

data hub, 226–230
data sharing agreements, 157, 267
data use agreements, 212, 267
Department of Health and Human
        Services, 108
DePaul University, 146, 153, 159, 171
depression, 196, 198–199, 201
DNA sequencing, 10

E

E&Y Parthenon, 55
Ebola, 18, 180, 246
electronic health records, 196, 220–221,
        227, 264
Electronic laboratory reporting, 223
emergency department, 28, 65, 120,
        196, 205, 207, 209
emergency room, 28, 30, 100
EMR, 52, 55, 201, 212–213
Enlace, 152
epidemic curve, *122*
Epic, 221, 229, 273
epidemic, 9–15, 18, 51, 80, 108–109,
        113–114, 118, 121, *122*, 127,
        134–136
epidemiological curve, 38
epidemiologists, 109, 121, 138, 180
ethnicity, 150, 152, 156, 162, 165, 167,
        223, 225
event date, 118, 120–122
exposure, 13, 76, 78, 81, 84, 96, 119,
        170, 201, 244–245, 267

F

FDOH, 108, 110, 119–121, 123,
        132–134, 138
Federal Communications
        Commission, 213
Federal Food, Drug, and Cosmetic
        Act, 252
field hospital, 28, 30, 33
Florida, 38, 107–139
Florida Agency for Health Care
        Administration, 108
Florida Department of Health,
        107–108, 132
Fog of War, 35–40
Food and Drug Administration, 252
Fosun Pharma, 254
FQHCs, 167

G

GDP, 26
GE Centricity, 273
GitHub, 153

H

Health Equity, 157, 159n6, 162, 167
Health Information Exchange, 223,
        263–278
Health Information Technology for
        Clinical Health, 265
Health Insurance Portability and
        Accountability Act, 246, 266
herd immunity, 38, 248, 282
HICS, 56
HIEs, 264, 269–270, 278
HMOs, 272
Home healthcare, 31, 34
Hospital at Home®, 31–33
Household Pulse Survey, 198, 213

I

ICS, 56
ICU, 36–37, 47–50, 53–54, 95, 99,
        178–179, 182, 186, 223,
        225–226, 276
IHME, 37, 47, 54, 110, 185
Illinois, 4, 110, 143–158, 187, 225, 228
Illinois Department of Public Health,
        152, 228

incubation period, 52, 119, 244
Indiana's HIE, 276
influenza, 9–11, 14–15, 19, 21–22, 25,
        38, 180, 186, 247, 257
injustice, 152, 157
isolation, 29, 36, 43, 53, 55, 78–79, 96,
        197–199, 245
Italy, 36, 90, 179–184, 186

J

Janssen Pharmaceuticals, 255
John Snow, 22
Johns Hopkins, 31, 47–49, 54, 153
Johnson & Johnson, 255, 260

K

Kaiser Family Foundation, 162,
        167, 199
Kaufman Hall, 55, 63, 66
Lambda, 282
length of stay, 36, 44, 63, 182, 188

L

Lombardy, 180–181, 184, 186
LOS, 36, 44, 48, 53–54
Loyola University, 152

M

marijuana, 92
McKinsey & Company, 55
measles, 17, 246
Med/Surg, 47–49, 53
Medicaid, 2, 25, 32, 67, 201, 207, 213,
        226, 237, 265
medical countermeasures, 252
Medicare, 2, 25, 32, 67, 100, 201, 207,
        213, 222, 235, 237, 265
Memphis, 162–165, 167, 169–172
miasmas, 19
minorities, 94–96, 213
Mississippi, 20, 164, 167
Moderna, 38, 52, 254, 282
morbidity, 22, 101, 151, 158, 197, 267
mortality, 19, 22, 53, 94–95, 98, 101,
        127, 132, 144–145, 149, 152,
        158, 162–163, 165, 180, 197,
        209, 225–226, 267
mRNA, 253–255

MSA, 38, 164–165, 275
Mu, 282
myocardial infarction, 98

N

N-76, 95
National Health Interview Survey, 198
National Healthcare Safety
        Network, 223
National Immunization Program, 272
national patient identifier, 268
Nationwide Health Information
        Network, 268
Nebraska Health Information
        Initiative, 276
New York, 4, 30, 38, 93, 110, 152, 162,
        178, 184–185, 190, 236, 238,
        270–271
New York City, 184, 236, 238
NIMS, 56
North Lawndale Community
        Coordinating Council, 154
NowPow, 152

O

observation, 49, 52–54, 98, 282
Office of National Coordinator
        for Health Information
        Technology, 269
OHCAs, 96–98
out-of-hospital cardiac arrests, 96–98
overdoses, 99, 196, 207, 209

P

pandemic, 1–6, 9–15, 17–23, 25–33,
        35–38, 43–45, 47, 51–53, 55,
        57, 61–66, 68–69, 74–78,
        80–84, 90–102, 107–109, 113,
        118, 121, 123, 126, 132–134,
        137–138, 146–149, 152–158,
        162–163, 167, 169–171,
        178–180, 182–183, 185–189,
        191, 195–214, 221–227, 230,
        235–238, 244–260
Penn, 48–49, 54, 185
Personal Health Library, 171
Personal Identifiable Information, 246
Pfizer, 38, 52, 254, 282
physical distancing, 5, 28, 51, 245

plague, 9–10, 17–22, 47
Poverty, 18, 22, 92, 163–165, 171
PPE, 15, 37, 45, 49, 54–55, 65, 78–79,
    83–84, 99, 152, 189, 201,
    224, 276
Practice Management Software, 212
predictive analytics, 43, 55, 57, 212
Protect Chicago Plus, 147, 154, 156, 158
psychiatry, 196–197, 199, 201, 203,
    212–213, 273
public health agencies, 2, 11, 26–27,
    107, 138, 171, 228, 245,
    264–265, 276–277
Public Health Emergency of
    International Concern, 244
Python, 273

Q

quarantine, 22, 29, 37, 245–246

R

$R(t)$, 47–48, 50–51
R_0, 51, 182–183, 186
race, 57, 94–96, 118, 147–148, 150–
    156, 162, 165–167, 178, 184,
    186, 201, 207, 223, 225
Racial Equity Rapid Response Team,
    146, 149
randomized trial, 249–251
Reliance eHealth, 271, 277
RERRT, 149–153, 156
r-square, 52
Rush, 55, 152, 220–222, 224–226, 228

S

$S(t)$, 47
San Diego Health Connect, 271, 276
SARS-CoV-2, 1–2, 12–14, 28, 35, 37,
    113, 118–119, 180, 186,
    224–225, 228, 230, 244,
    254–255, 257, 259, 264
SAS, 273
SDoH, 171
SEIR-SD, 52
SG2, 48, 55, 177–179, 182–183,
    185–192
Shared Data Network, 272
Shelby County Health Department,
    162, 167

Sinai Urban Health Institute, 152
SIR, 38, 47–52, 180, 182–184
smallpox, 17, 19–20, 22
SNF, 31–32, 44, 51
social distancing, 38, 48, 52, 146–147,
    180, 182–184, 197, 209,
    245–246, 280
social isolation, 78–79, 197–198
South Shore Works, 152
Spike (S) protein, 254–255
stay at home, 5, 37, 185–191
substance abuse, 196, 198–199
SUHI, 152, 154–155
suicide, 74, 198
Super-SNFs, 30
supply chain, 15, 53–54, 84, 224, 245
supply-chain, 245
surveillance, 37, 44, 107–108, 121,
    138, 170–171, 206, 222–223,
    227–228, 266–268, 275–276
Swiss cheese model of accident
    causation, 28
syphilis, 22

T

Telehealth, 27, 29–31, 33, 99–100,
    196–197, 199, 212–214,
    235–242, 283
tele-mental health, 196–197, 212–213
telepsychiatry, 196–197, 199, 201, 203,
    212–213
tele-psychology, 196
Testing, 27–29, 31, 44, 47–48, 52, 76,
    78–79, 81, 94–96, 100, 107,
    109–118, 120, 123, 125–127,
    153, 156, 167–170, 179, 182,
    184, 186, 189, 191, 225, 249,
    251, 255, 257, 283
Texas, 110, 188, 190–192, 271
The Emergency Use Authorization, 252
trials, 249–253, 256–257, 260
Twitter, 132
typhoid fever, 17, 21
typhus, 17

U

UAB, 74–75, 77, 82–83
Uber, 145
unemployment, 62, 92, 198
United States Census Bureau, 91, 108

United States Preventative Services Task
    Force, 28
University of Chicago, 47, 49, 54, 155
University of South Florida, 54, 108
University of Tennessee Health Science
    Center, 167
Urban Population Health Observatory,
    169–170
Urgent care, 29–30

V

VA, 31, 44
vaccination, 22, 31, 38, 92–93, 107,
    109, 127–132, 147, 153–154,
    156, 162–163, 165, 167, 170,
    244–260, 280, 282–283
Vaccine Safety Datalink, 272
variants, 107, 163, 244, 282
vectors, 12–14, 19

ventilator, 36, 49, 53–54, 99, 178–179,
    260
viral, 13, 19, 113–114, 119, 182,
    253–256, 258–259
Vizient, 55, 187

W

Well-Being Index, 74
WHO, 1, 9–11, 14, 36–37, 244, 255, 257
World Health Organization, 9, 36,
    90, 244
World Medical and Health Policy,
    96–97
Wuhan, 36, 43, 59, 180, 183, 185

Z

Zocdoc, 236, 238–242
Zoom, 100

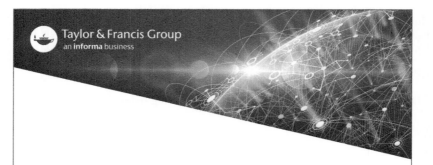